A Practical Guide to Cluster Randomised Trials in Health Services Research

Statistics in Practice

Series Advisors

Human and Biological Sciences
Stephen Senn
CRP-Santé, Luxembourg

Earth and Environmental Sciences
Marian Scott
University of Glasgow, UK

Industry, Commerce and Finance
Wolfgang Jank
University of Maryland, USA

Statistics in Practice is an important international series of texts which provide detailed coverage of statistical concepts, methods and worked case studies in specific fields of investigation and study.

With sound motivation and many worked practical examples, the books show in down-to-earth terms how to select and use an appropriate range of statistical techniques in a particular practical field within each title's special topic area.

The books provide statistical support for professionals and research workers across a range of employment fields and research environments. Subject areas covered include medicine and pharmaceutics; industry, finance and commerce; public services; the earth and environmental sciences, and so on.

The books also provide support to students studying statistical courses applied to the above areas. The demand for graduates to be equipped for the work environment has led to such courses becoming increasingly prevalent at universities and colleges.

It is our aim to present judiciously chosen and well-written workbooks to meet everyday practical needs. Feedback of views from readers will be most valuable to monitor the success of this aim.

A complete list of titles in this series can be found at www.wiley.com/go/statisticsinpractice

A Practical Guide to Cluster Randomised Trials in Health Services Research

Sandra Eldridge • Sally Kerry

*Centre for Primary Care and Public Health, Barts, and The London
School of Medicine and Dentistry, Queen Mary
University of London, UK*

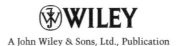

A John Wiley & Sons, Ltd., Publication

Registered office
John Wiley & Sons Ltd, The Atrium, Southern Gate, Chichester, West Sussex, PO19 8SQ, United Kingdom

For details of our global editorial offices, for customer services and for information about how to apply for permission to reuse the copyright material in this book please see our website at www.wiley.com.

Library of Congress Cataloging-in-Publication Data

Eldridge, Sandra.
  A practical guide to cluster randomised trials in health services research / Sandra Eldridge and Sally Kerry.
        p. ; cm. – (Statistics in practice)
  Includes bibliographical references and index.
  Summary: "This book aims to provide that much needed practical guide to the design, execution and analysis of cluster randomized trials in health services research"–Provided by publisher.
  ISBN 978-0-470-51047-6 (hardback) – ISBN 978-1-119-96625-8 (ePDF) – ISBN 978-1-119-96624-1 (oBook) – ISBN 978-1-119-96672-2 (ePub) – ISBN 978-1-119-96673-9 (mobi)
  I. Kerry, Sally M. II. Title. III. Series: Statistics in practice.
  [DNLM: 1. Health Services Research. 2. Randomized Controlled Trials as Topic. 3. Cluster Analysis. W 84.3]
  362.10972–dc23
                                                              2011037453

A catalogue record for this book is available from the British Library.

ISBN: 978-0-470-51047-6

Set in 10/12 pt Times New Roman by Toppan Best-set Premedia Limited

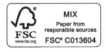

CONTENTS

Preface

Cluster randomised trials differ from the more usual sorts of randomised trials in which individuals are allocated to different trial arms. In cluster randomised trials, it is not individuals, but rather groups (or clusters) of individuals that are randomised. These groups are most usually intact social organisations such as general practices, hospitals, schools or clinics; or geographical areas such as towns or communities. Several books have already been written that bring together some of the methodological literature in this field.

We wrote this book because we felt there was need for one aimed specifically at those working in health services research, not just statisticians, but other trial investigators and those with an interest in the methodological aspects of these trials. Cluster randomised trials have become increasingly common in health services research partly because, when conducted well, they are ideally suited to addressing issues related to policy, practice and organisation of health care. In the past, however, many have failed to produce robust evidence owing to problems with their design, conduct and analysis that could have been avoided with better planning. At a time when the organisation of health care is being re-considered in many countries, high quality research in this area is vital, and our hope is that this book can contribute towards facilitating this research.

In order to make the book accessible to a wide audience, we have introduced and developed the principles underlying good practice in cluster randomised trials through a large number of examples. All of them contain useful features; some, such as COMMIT, are well known as seminal trials which have had considerable influence on the field. Many of the examples are drawn from our own involvement in empirical trials over the past 15 to 20 years, mostly in the UK primary health care setting. We hope that this book will be comprehensible to any researcher with a sound grasp of the basic principles of design and analysis of standard randomised controlled trials. In addition, we have provided an extensive range of references for those who wish to grapple with a more mathematical treatment of some of the book's content.

The book follows, more or less, the order in which investigators might think about the stages of a trial, beginning with recruitment and ethics and ending with reporting. In between we cover the issues that are ubiquitous in books on randomised trials such as design, analysis and sample size calculation. However, we also cover issues which are common in cluster randomised trials in health services research but which have not been covered in detail in other books. These include the potential for bias when recruiting individual participants, problems with estimation of the intra-cluster correlation coefficient and its application in sample size calculations, how to include these trials in systematic reviews, cost effectiveness analysis, and process evaluation. In addition, it is now well recognised that interventions evaluated in health services research need to be thoughtfully and carefully designed and that, because of the organisational complexity of trials evaluating these interventions, a pilot or feasibility study is essential; two chapters provide guidance for those designing interventions and conducting pilot and feasibility studies. Finally, we end the book with a comprehensive elaboration of the use of the CONSORT statement in relation to cluster randomised trials. This statement has become the cornerstone of good reporting of randomised controlled trials. The main statement, updated in 2010, provides the structure for our final chapter, in which we have also incorporated guidance from the extended statements for cluster randomised, pragmatic and non-pharmacological trials.

We are aware of several areas of ongoing research related to cluster randomised trials which would have had a greater influence on the book's contents if we were writing at a later date. For example, a group conducting research on the ethics of cluster randomised trials expect to publish guidelines in 2012. For obvious reasons, we were not able to include these in the book, but refer interested readers to the group's website (http://crtethics.wikispaces.com).

Health economics methods relevant to cluster randomised trials are also currently developing at a rapid pace but neither of us is a health economist. We therefore asked Richard Grieve, from the London School of Hygiene and Tropical Medicine, to write the section in chapter 9 about cost effectiveness. Richard is at the forefront of developments in this area, and we are grateful to him for being willing to contribute and for providing an excellent summary of a fast moving field within the number of pages and in the style that we specified!

Finally, we need to thank other people who have contributed to this book. First and foremost our thanks must go to Lynette Edwards who proof read, not once, but several times, correcting typing and grammatical errors, and inconsistencies; any that remain are entirely our responsibility. We would also like to thank Stephen Bremner, Richard Hooper, Nadine Koehler, Clare Rutterford, Karla Diaz Ordaz, Angela Devine, and Obi Ukoumunne for reading and commenting on draft chapters and for assistance with the index; and our editors at Wiley for efficiency, patience and sound advice. We are indebted to all those who have carried out cluster randomised trials that we were able to use as examples – without them there would be no book; and amongst them we are particularly grateful to Gene Feder, Martin Underwood, Chris Griffiths, Pippa Oakeshott, Tony Kendrick, Franco Cappuccio and Jackie Sturt, whose trials appear in many places in the book, and to Gene and Martin for reading and commenting on various sections. Working with Gene and Chris kindled Sandra's interest in this area and working with Tony and Pippa kindled Sally's. We would not, however, have developed an enduring interest in this field without discussion with and encouragement from Deborah Ashby and Martin Bland. Finally, thanks to Dave and Graham for being longsuffering and supportive over the past year and to Louise for feeding Sandra chocolate while she struggled to meet a publisher's deadline.

Sandra Eldridge
Sally Kerry

Notation

Subscripts

i	Represents clusters
j	Represents individuals
1	Represents intervention arm
2	Represents control arm

Frequently used notation

k	Number of clusters in each arm
N	Sample size (total number of individuals analysed or number of person years) for individually randomised trial
N_c	Sample size (total number of individuals analysed or number of person years) for cluster randomised trial
m	Cluster size (numbers analysed) if cluster sizes are fixed
m_i	Number of individuals in the ith cluster
$\bar{m}$	Mean cluster size
ρ	Intra-cluster correlation coefficient (ICC)
μ	Mean of outcome
σ_b^2	Between-cluster variance (σ_b between-cluster standard deviation)
σ_w^2	Within-cluster variance (σ_w within-cluster standard deviation)
π	Probability of 'success'
λ	Rate

Notation in Chapter 4

p	Proportion of successes in sample
s	Observed total standard deviation of outcome between participants

Notation in Chapter 6

α Constant in generalised estimating equations or mixed effects models

β Effect size

e_{ij} Residual for jth individual in the ith cluster

x_{ij} Dummy variable indicating intervention arm. When there are only two arms, x_{ij} takes the value 1 when the ith cluster is in the intervention arm, and 0 when the ith cluster is in the control arm

Y_{ij} Value of outcome for the jth individual in the ith cluster

Y_i Mean value of outcome in the ith cluster

μ_i Mean effect of being in the ith cluster for cluster-specific models

π_{ij} Probability of 'success' for the ith individual in the jth cluster

Notation in Chapter 7

ρ_m Correlation between matched pairs

cv_c Coefficient of variation of cluster sizes, $cv_c = \dfrac{s_c}{\bar{m}}$

cv_{cs} Coefficient of variation of cluster sizes within strata

s_c Standard deviation of cluster sizes

cv Coefficient of variation for the outcome, $cv = \dfrac{\sigma_{b1}}{\mu_1} = \dfrac{\sigma_{b2}}{\mu_2}$ or $cv = \dfrac{\sigma_{b1}}{\pi_1} = \dfrac{\sigma_{b2}}{\pi_2}$

cv_m Coefficient of variation for the outcome within a matched pair

t Number of person years per cluster

t_h Harmonic mean of the number of person years per cluster

S Number of strata

$Deff$ Design effect

m_a $m_a = \dfrac{\sum m_i^2}{\sum m_i}$

σ_{b1} Between-cluster standard deviation in the intervention arm

σ_{b2} Between-cluster standard deviation in the control arm

σ_{bm} Between-cluster standard deviation for clusters within a matched pair

σ_w Within-cluster standard deviation (consistent with Donner)

μ_1 Mean in the intervention arm (note the subscripts for μ and π have a different meaning in Chapter 7 from their meaning in Chapters 6 and 8, although the usage in each chapter is consistent with the subscripts section at the top of this list)

μ_2 Mean in the control arm (see note above)

π_1 Proportion in the intervention arm (see note above)

π_2 Proportion in the control arm (see note above)

λ_1 Rate in the intervention arm (see note above)

λ_2 Rate in the control arm (see note above)

Notation in Chapter 8

p_s Probability that any two subjects from the same cluster have the same outcome

p_o Probability that any two subjects from different clusters have the same outcome

MSB Mean square between clusters

MSW Mean square within clusters

L Total number of intervention arms

N_s Total number of individuals in a single population

N_l Total number of individuals in arm l of a trial

Y_{li} Mean outcome in cluster i in intervention arm l

Y_l Mean outcome in intervention arm l

Y_{ij} Value of the outcome for the jth individual in the ith cluster

Y_{li} Mean outcome in cluster i in intervention arm l

Y_l Mean outcome in intervention arm l

L Total number of intervention arms

N_s Total number of individuals in a single population

N_l Total number of individuals in arm l of a trial

m_{li} Number of individuals in ith cluster in intervention arm l

σ^2 Total variance

α Constant in generalised estimating equations or mixed effects models

μ_i Mean effect of being in the ith cluster

e_{ij} Residual for jth individual in the ith cluster

Π Pi, mathematical quantity ~3.14159

ρ_1 Proportion of total outcome variance that is due to between-cluster variation on a log scale

σ_S Variance of the ICC as estimated by Swiger's formula

σ_F Variance of the ICC as estimated by Fisher's formula

m_{max} Largest cluster size

Table of cases: Trials used as examples in more than one chapter in the book

Kumasi trial: Health education to prevent stroke
Sections: 1.2, 1.3.3, 1.3.4, 2.2.3, 2.2.5, 2.2.7, 5.1.5, 5.1.8, 5.1.9, 7.5.1
Tables: 1.1, 2.9, 5.4

Guidelines to reduce inappropriate referral for x-ray
Sections: 1.3.1, 2.2.2.2, 7.4.1
Table: 1.2

OPERA: Physical activity in residential homes to prevent depression
Acronym: Older People's Exercise intervention in Residential and nursing Accommodation
Sections: 1.3.1, 1.5.1, 2.2.2.1, 2.2.2.4, 2.2.2.5, 3.7, 5.1.8, 5.1.10, 5.2, 5.6, 6.5, 9.1.1, 9.1.2, 9.1.3, 9.3, 10.2.2, 10.4.3
Tables: 1.3, 2.7, 3.5, 5.9, 6.17, 9.1, 10.8

UK BEAM pilot trial: Active management of back pain
Acronym: United Kingdom Back pain Exercise And Manipulation
Sections: 1.3.1, 1.3.2, 2.3.4, 4.1.1, 4.1.2, 4.2.1, 10.2.1
Table: 1.4

ObaapaVitA: Vitamin A supplementation to reduce maternal and child mortality
(Obaapa means 'good woman')
Sections: 1.5.2, 1.5.6, 2.2.2.1
Tables: 1.5, 2.3

Promoting child safety by reducing baby walker use
Sections: 1.5.3, 1.5.4, 2.3.4, 7.1.2, 7.2.1, 10.4.13
Tables: 1.6, 7.2, 10.11

Trial of home blood pressure monitoring
Sections: 2.1.2, 10.4.10, 10.4.21
Table: 2.1

Diabetes care from diagnosis trial
Sections: 2.2.2.2, 2.2.6, 5.2, 7.1.3, 7.8.4
Tables: 2.4, 5.10, 7.10, 7.11

SHIP: Support following myocardial infarction
Acronym: Southampton Heart Integrated care Project
Sections: 1.5.5, 2.2.2.3, 2.2.6, 3.1, 8.3, 8.3.1
Tables: 2.5, 3.2

Educational intervention to increase depression awareness among students
Sections: 2.2.2.4, 10.4.13
Tables: 2.6, 10.14

Community-based interventions to promote blood pressure control
Sections: 2.2.2, 5.3.3
Table: 2.8

Ekjut project: participatory women's groups to improve birth outcomes and maternal depression
Sections: 2.2.3, 7.3, 7.6
Tables: 2.10, 7.4

Trial of structured diabetes shared care
Sections: 2.3.1, 6.3.1, 10.4.18
Table: 2.11

IRIS: Training to increase identification and referral of victims of domestic violence
Acronym: Identification and Referral to Improve Safety
Sections: 2.3.2, 3.4, 3.7, 4.2.1, 4.2.4, 5.1.6, 6.1, 6.3.3.12, 6.5, 10.4.11
Tables: 2.12, 3.4, 4.1, 5.7, 6.13, 10.12

ELECTRA: Asthma liaison nurses to reduce unscheduled care
Acronym: East London randomised Controlled Trial for high Risk Asthma
Sections: 2.3.3, 5.1.6, 6.3.3.8, 6.3.3.12, 6.3.3.13, 6.6, 7.2.2, 7.4, 7.4.4, 7.6.2, 8.4.4, 10.4.2, 10.4.4, 10.4.8
Tables: 2.13, 5.6, 6.12, 7.3, 10.5

COMMIT: Community-based intervention to increase smoking quit rates
Acronym: COMMunity Intervention Trial
Sections: 3.1, 5.1.9, 6.3.1, 6.4.1, 7.4.2, 7.8.3, 9.3
Tables: 3.1, 5.8

Diabetes Manual trial: Manual and structured care to improve outcomes
Sections: 3.5, 4.1, 4.2.2, 4.3, 5.1.3, 6.3.3.3, 8.4.4, 10.4.2, 10.4.4
Tables: 3.9, 5.3, 6.7, 10.3

Multifaceted intervention to optimise antibiotic use in nursing homes
Sections: 3.4, 3.5, 3.5, 4.2.2
Tables: 3.7, 4.2

1

Introduction

Cluster randomised trials are trials in which *groups (or clusters) of individuals* are randomly allocated to different forms of treatment. In healthcare, the different forms of treatment are sometimes different drugs or, more commonly, different ways of managing a disease or promoting healthy living. These trials are in contrast to conventional randomised trials which randomise *individuals* to different treatments, classically comparing new drugs with a placebo. Cluster randomised trials are common in health services research. This is an area of research concerned with the way healthcare is delivered and with measures taken to prevent ill health and encourage healthy living. It covers a broad range of topics and is an important area in maintaining high standards in a modern health service. New initiatives or interventions in health care may be evaluated by comparing health outcomes in those that are exposed to the new initiative with outcomes in those receiving usual care or an alternative intervention. Since interventions often need to be introduced to a whole organisational unit such as a general practice or geographical area, cluster randomised trials are often the best method of evaluating such interventions.

There are many books written about trials in general, which explain in detail the key features of the design, conduct and analysis of randomised trials; but these are mainly concerned with trials which randomise individual patients to different interventions (Pocock, 1983; Matthews, 2000; Torgerson and Torgerson, 2008). There are now three books that describe the design, analysis and conduct of cluster randomised trials: Murray (1998), Donner and Klar (2000) and Hayes and Moulton (2009). These books have mainly concentrated on large community trials. Hayes and Moulton have a particular emphasis on trials in low-income countries where whole communities have been randomised. Since we have extensive experience in

A Practical Guide to Cluster Randomised Trials in Health Services Research, First Edition.
Sandra Eldridge and Sally Kerry.
© 2012 John Wiley & Sons, Ltd. Published 2012 by John Wiley & Sons, Ltd.

health services research, in this book we have focused on cluster randomised trials in this area, though we have used other examples where useful. This book is intended as a practical guide, written for researchers from the health professions, including doctors, psychologists, and allied health professionals, as well as statisticians, who are involved in the design, execution, analysis and reporting of cluster randomised trials. It is specifically written to address the issues arising from allocating groups of individuals, or clusters, to different interventions, and is primarily concerned with those aspects of cluster randomised trials which differ from randomised trials of individual subjects. Several trials are used as examples throughout the book. These are listed at the front of the book.

1.1   Introduction to randomised trials

A formal definition of a trial is given in Box 1.1. The 'gold standard' for trials is the randomised controlled trial (RCT), originally developed in order to test the efficacy of new drugs. In the earliest example of such a trial (Medical Research Council, 1948), patients were randomly allocated to treatments, each participant having an equal chance of being given the active drug or placebo. As a result any patient characteristics that might have affected the outcome of the treatment would have been randomly distributed between the intervention and control arms, and the observed difference in outcome between the arms could be attributed to the active drug.

Over the years the RCT design has been extended to many other situations: more than two different treatments; crossover trials; non-drug interventions such as surgery, physiotherapy or health education; and in health services research to assess the effectiveness of different models of care.

1.2   Explanatory or pragmatic trials

Randomised trials may be used to test causal research hypotheses. Various epidemiological studies have shown that high salt intake is associated with high blood

---

Any research project that prospectively assigns human subjects to intervention and comparison groups to study the cause-and-effect relationship between a medical intervention and a health outcome. By 'medical intervention' we mean any intervention used to modify a health outcome. This definition includes drugs, surgical procedures, devices, behavioural treatments, process-of-care changes, and the like.

Source: International Committee of Medical Journal Editors, 2009.

Box 1.1   Definition of a trial

Table 1.1   Kumasi trial: health education to prevent stroke.

Aim: To see if a health education programme to reduce salt intake among rural and semi-rural communities in the Ashanti region of Ghana leads to a reduction in blood pressure
Location and type of cluster: Ghana, villages of 500–2000 inhabitants
Number of clusters randomised: 12
Number of villagers randomised: 1013
Interventions: (i) Control: health education not including salt reduction
(ii) Intervention: health education including salt reduction messages
Primary outcome: Reduction in systolic blood pressure after six months

---

Source: Cappuccio *et al.* (2006).

pressure. In order to test whether this relationship was causal, the DASH trial (Moore *et al.*, 2001) recruited a carefully selected group of patients with moderately raised blood pressure and randomised them to take a low salt diet or usual American diet. All the subjects' food was provided by the trial team. Trials such as this, which seek to understand a biological process, are described as explanatory. Explanatory trials may also test the efficacy of treatments under ideal conditions (Roland and Torgerson, 1998). Cluster randomised trials rarely fall into this category.

Pragmatic trials, on the other hand, are designed to help choose between care options applied in routine clinical practice. Providing a low salt diet for people is not a practical option, except perhaps in hospitals and care homes, and a more realistic approach is to reduce dietary salt using health education for the whole community. The Kumasi trial (Table 1.1) took a whole community approach to health promotion: advice on how to reduce dietary salt was dispensed not only to the individuals participating in the trial but also to their families and neighbours, with whom they might share meals. The intervention was therefore not a 'low salt diet' but 'community education to reduce dietary salt'. Many cluster randomised trials are pragmatic trials and share common features with other individually randomised pragmatic trials (Zwarenstein *et al.*, 2008; Eldridge, 2010).

1.3   How does a cluster randomised trial differ from other trials?

A cluster randomised trial is one in which groups or clusters of individuals rather than individuals themselves are randomised to intervention arm. These clusters are often social units. They can range in size from small units such as households, to much larger units such as towns or regions. Often they comprise individuals connected to particular institutions, for example patients attending particular clinics or general practices, or children in particular schools.

While whole clusters form the units of randomisation (or experimental units) in cluster randomised trials, the members of these clusters form the units of observation. These may be all the members of the cluster or a sample from each cluster. It is this distinction between units of randomisation and units of observation which distinguishes cluster randomised trials from the more usual types of randomised trial, with statistical and practical consequences. In this section we briefly describe the consequences of cluster randomisation, covering recruitment, randomisation, consent, analysis, sample size and interventions. All of these issues are dealt with more fully in later chapters.

1.3.1   Recruitment, randomisation and consent

In these key areas, cluster randomised trials exhibit unique features not present in individually randomised trials. Consent to participate may be required from clusters, individuals or both. Even when consent is not required from participants, the methods used to select individuals on whom data will be collected need to be carefully considered in order to avoid bias. This will be discussed in more detail in Chapter 2, but here we describe a few examples to illustrate the wide variability of recruitment, randomisation and consent procedures seen in cluster randomised trials.

A simple trial of radiological guidelines to reduce unnecessary referrals for x-ray by general practitioners is described in Table 1.2. Neither practices nor individuals were asked to consent to participation. Practices regularly referring to one hospital radiology department were identified from the department's records and randomly

Table 1.2   Guidelines to reduce inappropriate referral for x-ray.

Aim: To determine whether postal distribution of radiological guidelines for x-ray referral reduces the number of x-ray referrals from primary care and inappropriate referral for x-ray

Location and type of cluster: UK General practices

Number of clusters analysed: 64

Number of individuals analysed: 2578 (different patients were included at baseline and follow up)

Interventions: (i) Control: no intervention (ii) Intervention: laminated extracts of Royal College of Radiologists' guidelines specifically produced for primary care, posted to general practitioners individually

Primary outcome: Percentage of referrals assessed as conforming to the guidelines using x-ray referral forms collected in the radiology department

Consent required from clusters: No

Consent required from patients: No

Individuals identified prior to randomisation: No, but identified and assessed blind to intervention arm

---

Source: Oakeshott, Kerry and Williams (1994).

Table 1.3 OPERA: physical activity in residential homes to prevent depression.

Aim: To evaluate the impact on depression of a whole-home intervention to increase physical activity among older people

Location and type of cluster: UK residential and nursing homes for older people

Number of clusters randomised: 78

Number of residents recruited: 1060

Interventions: (i) Control: depression awareness programme delivered by research nurses (ii) Intervention: depression awareness programme delivered by physiotherapists plus whole-home package to increase activity among older people, including physiotherapy assessments of individuals and activity sessions for residents

Primary outcome: Prevalence of depression (Geriatric Depression Scale) at 12 months and change in depression score

Consent required from clusters: Yes

Consent required from individuals: Consent was required separately for completion of the Geriatric Depression Scale, access to medical records, and for physiotherapy assessments. All residents were encouraged to take part in activity sessions. Residents of control homes could not access the activity sessions

Individuals consented prior to randomisation: Yes, for individuals resident in the home prior to randomisation but not for individuals moving into the home during the study

Source: Underwood *et al.* (2011).

assigned to an intervention arm or control arm. Individual general practitioners in intervention practices were sent copies of the guidelines through the post, while those in the control arm were sent nothing. Outcomes were assessed through audit of radiology request forms for individual patients held within the radiology department. Identification of the individual patients, who were the units of observation, was carried out after randomisation, but blind to whether or not their practice was in the intervention arm.

A much more complex design is described in Table 1.3. Residential homes for older people were randomised to receive an intervention aimed at reducing depression among the residents. After all residents had been asked for consent to data collection and, if agreeable, had taken part in a baseline assessment, homes were randomised to intervention or control. Part of the intervention was twice-weekly physical activity sessions run in the homes by a physiotherapist. Residents could opt out of attending specific activity sessions but, because they still belonged to a home where the staff had been trained to encourage residents to be more active, they could not opt out of the intervention entirely. Individual residents could refuse to take part in the outcome assessments or refuse to allow researchers access to their medical records. Residential homes were required to give consent and be actively involved in delivering the intervention and assisting the trial team with identification

Table 1.4   UK BEAM pilot trial: active management of back pain.

Aim: To determine whether active management of patients presenting with back
  pain in general practice reduces back pain disability

Location and type of cluster: UK general practices

Number of clusters recruited: 26

Number of patients recruited: 231

Interventions: (i) Control: usual care (ii) Intervention: all clinical and support
  staff were invited to training sessions on the active management of back pain;
  practices were supplied with literature to distribute during consultations and in
  communal areas. Patients were also randomised individually to exercise classes
  or spinal manipulation or neither

Primary outcome: Change in back pain disability

Consent required from clusters: Yes

Consent required from patients: Yes

Individuals consented prior to randomisation: No. Individuals were identified by
  the practice upon presentation to the general practitioner with back pain after
  randomisation. Cluster design abandoned after pilot study due to evidence of
  bias in recruitment

Source: Farrin *et al.* (2005).

of participants and data collection. This trial illustrates the complexities in obtaining
consent that can arise in cluster randomised trials.

In a traditional RCT, consent should always take place before the allocation to
intervention arm is known, thus ensuring that the decision to take part in the study
is not biased by knowledge of the allocation. In cluster randomised trials such an
approach can create major difficulties if the intervention is aimed at managing an
acute condition or the onset of a chronic condition; the patients cannot be identified
and recruited prior to randomisation, but only when they present to the general practitioner. It may therefore be necessary to allocate the clusters to intervention arms
before individual cases are identified. In the UK BEAM trial pilot study (Table 1.4),
26 practices were randomised to offer active management or usual care to patients
presenting with low back pain. Patients within the active management arm were also
individually randomised to receive spinal manipulation, exercise classes or advice
alone. After one year, practices in the control arm (traditional care) had recruited 66
patients, 54% of the number predicted based on practice list size, while those in the
active management arm had recruited 165 patients, 41% more than predicted. In
addition, participants from the active management arm were suffering from milder
back pain than those in control practices. It is likely that the offer of exercise classes
or physiotherapy made participation in the trial an attractive option for the general
practitioners and their patients in the active management arm, whereas there was no
such benefit for patients in the control arm. Following the pilot study, the trial was
redesigned as an individually randomised trial comparing different methods of delivering active management. Here all participants, at the time of consent, would have

an equal chance of receiving an active intervention. This highlights the potential for bias that can arise if individual patients are identified or recruited after randomisation. Chapter 2 discusses identification and recruitment bias in more detail and outlines some approaches which can be used to protect against these biases.

1.3.2   Definition of cluster size

Very often only a subset of individuals in the cluster provides data for the analysis. In this book we will refer to the number of individuals per cluster who contribute data to the analysis as the 'cluster size' and the number of patients in the larger pool from which they come as the 'natural cluster size'. In the UK BEAM trial (Table 1.4), the average cluster size was 5.1 (66 individuals from 13 practices) in the control arm and 12.7 (136 individuals from 13 practices) in the intervention arm, while the average natural cluster size was 7804 in the intervention arm and 8145 in the control arm. These averages are slightly larger than the average for all English practices, which was 6649 in 2009 (Health and Social Care Information Centre, 2011).

1.3.3   Analysis and sample size

The primary aim of a randomised trial is to compare outcome measures in different intervention arms. The simplest analysis is a t-test for comparing two means, or a chi-squared test for comparing two proportions. These tests assume that observations on participants can be regarded as independent of one another. However, in cluster randomised trials, members of the same cluster are more likely to have similar outcomes than a random sample from the same population, and therefore cannot be regarded as independent. Where outcomes relate to participants' own health or behaviour, the effect of clustering is likely to be small. Where outcomes relate directly to the behaviour of the clusters, then the effect of clustering may be much larger. For example, doctor's prescribing behaviour for a particular condition may be more dependent on the doctor's opinions, views and habits than on the patient's condition, while systolic blood pressure may have only a small tendency to be similar among patients attending the same practice. This tendency to have similar outcomes is known as within-cluster homogeneity, and needs to be taken into account in the design and analysis. An alternative expression used to describe this concept is 'between-cluster variability', and this is the term we shall use in this book. The most common measure of between-cluster variability is the intra-cluster correlation coefficient (ICC), which is described in more detail in Chapter 8.

Using analysis methods which fail to take account of clustering may lead to confidence intervals which are too narrow, and increased Type 1 error; that is, results may appear to have a higher level of statistical significance than they actually do. Chapter 6 describes in detail suitable methods to analyse cluster randomised trials.

Since correct methods for analysing cluster randomised trials lead to wider confidence intervals, the sample size also needs to be adjusted for the effect of clustering. In order to detect the same size effect, cluster randomised trials will always require more subjects than individually randomised trials designed to answer identical research questions (assuming it is possible to randomise individuals). Where the number of subjects recruited from each cluster is small and the ICC is small, the increase in the sample size will also be fairly small. However, if the number of participants to be recruited from each cluster is large then even a small ICC may double the sample size required. The Kumasi trial (Table 1.1) used change in systolic blood pressure as an outcome and required 840 participants to be included in the final analysis; if the trial had been individually randomised it would have required less than half that number. Chapter 7 describes how to allow for clustering in sample size calculations.

1.3.4   Interventions used in cluster randomised trials

Cluster randomised trials rarely use interventions which can be delivered blind, except in the case of drugs for the treatment or control of infectious diseases. More commonly, cluster randomised trials are used to assess the effectiveness of educational interventions or management strategies aimed at the whole cluster, and it is not possible to blind the members of the cluster. Ideally the outcome should be assessed blind to the allocation. This situation is not unique to cluster randomised trials, but often presents greater challenges in these trials. If data need to be collected within the cluster it may be difficult to conceal allocation arm from any researcher entering, say, a general practice. Posters or information leaflets may be displayed on the premises, and staff aware of the intervention may inadvertently reveal the allocation. Where patients are interviewed they may be asked not to reveal the allocation of their cluster to the researcher. If an individual patient reveals the arm to which they belong and the trial is individually randomised, only the data from one individual may be compromised, but if it is a cluster randomised trial, assessors are unblinded when assessing all remaining participants from the cluster.

Many interventions used in cluster randomised trials are made up of various connecting parts and can be described as complex interventions. These can be complicated to design, to carry out and to describe. For example the Kumasi trial (Table 1.1) randomly allocated villages to receive a health education package advising villagers to reduce dietary salt in order to reduce their blood pressure. Replication of this trial would require much more detail about what the package entailed, how and when it was delivered, and what both intervention and control arms were told when consenting to take part. Many complex interventions have failed to demonstrate the desired effect of the intervention. In a drug trial, if the trial shows no evidence of benefit and is sufficiently powered, it is usually safe to conclude that the drug does not work, at least at the specified dose. In the case of complex interventions, the interpretation may be more problematic. The intervention *as delivered* has proven to be ineffective, but we need to be sure exactly what the intervention entailed and that the lack of effectiveness is not due to poor implementation, or to changing behaviour in the control arm owing to information provided while obtaining consent. Careful consideration of how different parts of the intervention interact to bring about change in the individual is needed at the design stage. Eldridge *et al.* (2005) modelled the effect of a primary care intervention to screen older people at risk of hip fracture. This showed that the intervention was unlikely to be effective and a large expensive trial was not justified. Complex interventions are described in more detail in Chapter 3.

1.4   Between-cluster variability

In order to understand the effect of clustering on analysis and sample size, it is useful to consider why members of a cluster may be more similar in their outcomes than a random sample of individuals.

1.4.1   Factors that contribute to between-cluster variability

1.4.1.1   Geographical reasons

Most clusters have some kind of geographical basis. Patients registered with a general practice will live near the practice. Social factors such as deprivation are known to affect health outcomes and so will contribute to within-cluster homogeneity. Even stronger effects on between-cluster variance may be observed for lifestyle and behaviours such as smoking and diet.

1.4.1.2   Individuals choose the cluster to belong to

Individuals may be able to choose where they live, which general practice to attend, and which school for their children's education. These choices may be influenced by ethnic, religious or other characteristics, which may in turn influence health outcomes and behaviours, thus contributing to within-cluster homogeneity.

1.4.1.3   Healthcare provided to the cluster

As well as sharing a common environment, members of a cluster will usually be treated by the same healthcare professionals. A general practice which treats hypertension more aggressively is likely to have more patients taking antihypertensive medication, and with consequently lower blood pressure, than one with a more conservative approach.

1.4.2   Measuring between-cluster variability

The variability between clusters in outcomes is often estimated by the intra-cluster correlation coefficient (ICC). This may be thought of as the ratio of the variability between clusters to the total variability in the outcome, although there are alternative ways of defining this quantity (see Chapter 8). Much of the early work on cluster randomised trials by Donner (Donner, Birkett and Buck, 1981) used the ICC, and sample size calculations within health services research also usually use it. The ICC is the measure on which we shall concentrate in this book.

Other methods of estimating the between-cluster variation are the between-cluster variance (Cornfield, 1978), often denoted by σ_b^2, or the between-cluster coefficient of variation of the outcome (σ_b/μ) (Hayes and Bennet, 1999), where μ represents the mean outcome across all clusters. The latter is particularly useful for comparing event rates expressed as number of events per person years (Hayes and Moulton, 2009), and is described in more detail in Chapter 7.

1.5   Why carry out cluster randomised trials?

So far in this chapter we have shown that cluster randomised trials require more subjects than individually randomised trials, are harder to design, are prone to bias in ways that individually randomised trials are not, and give rise to more ethical issues, particularly with regard to informed consent. Consequently they should not be carried out without good justification. We consider seven possible reasons for undertaking cluster randomised trials.

1.5.1   The intervention necessarily acts at the cluster level

Here the intervention is directed towards the whole cluster and could not be implemented for some individuals and not others. Examples include education interventions for healthcare practitioners (Table 1.2), mass education programmes using TV, radio and posters, and changing the environment, for example fluoridation of water. In these examples the whole cluster is subject to the intervention and the intervention could not be implemented in any other way.

In the OPERA trial (Table 1.3), the intervention involved training all staff in the residential home in the importance of remaining active and ways to encourage activity among the residents, provision of activity sessions open to all residents, and assessment of individual mobility needs. The intervention aimed to change the culture within the home and therefore acted at cluster level.

1.5.2   Practical and/or ethical difficulties in randomising at individual level

A trial in Zimbabwe (Murira *et al.*, 1997) of two different antenatal systems, one an existing system in which women had 12 visits and the other a new system in which women had 6 visits during their pregnancy, would have been more difficult to organise on an individual basis. In the ObaapaVitA trial in Ghana (Table 1.5), all

Table 1.5 ObaapaVitA: vitamin A supplementation to reduce maternal and child mortality.

Aim: To see if supplementation with vitamin A would reduce maternal and child mortality in Ghana
Location and type of cluster: Ghana, geographical areas
Number of clusters randomised: 1086
Number of women randomised: 208 145
Interventions: (i) Control: placebo capsules (ii) Intervention: vitamin A capsules
Primary outcome: Pregnancy-related mortality and all-cause female mortality
Length of follow-up: 5–7 years

Source: Kirkwood *et al.* (2010).

Table 1.6 Promoting child safety by reducing baby walker use.

Aim: To evaluate the effectiveness of an educational package provided by midwives and health visitors to reduce baby walker possession and use
Location and type of cluster: UK groups of general practices sharing a health visitor (between 1 and 4 practices)
Number of clusters analysed: 46
Number of individuals analysed: 1008
Interventions: (i) Control: usual care (ii) Intervention: trained midwives and health visitors delivered an educational package to mothers to be, at 10 days postpartum and 3–4 months later, to discourage baby walker use or encourage safe use for those who already had baby walkers
Primary outcome: Possession and use of a baby walker

Source: Kendrick *et al.* (2005).

women in the same cluster, approximately 160 in number, were given identical capsules; for some clusters these contained vitamin A in peanut oil, for others peanut oil only. During monthly visits to the cluster by fieldworkers, the women were given four capsules to be taken once weekly. Fieldworkers were given only one type of capsule at a time. In this way the women could not be given the wrong capsules by mistake in this large trial in a low-income country.

1.5.3 Contamination at health professional level

In a trial of an education package to reduce the use of baby walkers by infants (Table 1.6), the intervention was delivered through midwives and health visitors during routine appointments and visits. In an individually randomised trial it would have been difficult for midwives effectively to discourage the use of baby walkers for some women and not others, and for the researchers to be sure the right women were getting the intervention.

1.5.4   Contamination between members of a cluster

In some trials where randomisation takes place at the individual level, the control arm may be partially exposed to the intervention through interaction with individuals receiving the intervention. In the baby walker trial (Table 1.6), mothers attending the same practice were more likely to use the same baby clinics and support groups, and might have interacted and discussed the use of walkers with one another. The degree of interaction between mothers is likely to be higher than between other adults attending the same general practice. The Family Heart Study (Wood *et al.*, 1994) used two different control arm in a trial of cardiovascular screening among middle-aged adults. Two practices in each town were randomised so that one received cardiovascular risk screening with a risk reduction programme, and the other practice carried on with usual care. Within intervention practices, couples were randomised to the intervention or usual care. The results of the study showed little evidence of contamination between adults attending general practices for this intervention.

Torgerson (2001) has suggested that increasing the sample size of an individually randomised trial to allow for contamination between cluster members may be preferable in some circumstances to randomising clusters with all the attendant difficulties.

1.5.5   Cost or administrative convenience

In health services research, clusters are usually administrative units with participants who are located in a geographical area. Consequently there may be administrative reasons why it is easier to restrict the intervention to fewer clusters. In the SHIP trial (Jolly *et al.*, 1999), specialist nurses worked with the intervention practices to help integrate primary and secondary care of patients suffering from heart attacks. It would have been much more expensive to work with all practices. Trials which involve the use of expensive equipment may also be cluster randomised to avoid having to equip all units.

1.5.6   Ensuring intervention is fully implemented

In the ObaapaVitA trial (Table 1.5), the women might have been tempted to swap capsules with their neighbour in the hope of getting some benefit should they be randomised to placebo. By randomising all women in a village to the same intervention, researchers ensured that this would not matter. In other trials where new technologies are being introduced, they may have greater effect if staff become accustomed to using the new methods by treating everyone in the cluster. In the World Health Organization partograph study (World Health Organization, 1994), centres were randomised to training in the use of the partograph for monitoring progress in labour. Accordingly, midwives could become familiar with the partograph technique and it could become part of routine practice. In other cluster randomised trials, individually administered interventions may be reinforced by publicity at the cluster level.

1.5.7   Access to routine data

In a proposed cluster randomised trial where the intervention was designed to reduce fractures amongst elderly people (Eldridge *et al.*, 2001), the outcome measure chosen was the overall rate of fractured femur in the cluster. These data were easily obtainable from routine sources at the cluster level. Data direct from individuals would have been much more difficult to obtain.

1.6   Quality of evidence from cluster randomised trials

Healthcare professionals, managers and community leaders need to be informed as to which healthcare interventions are effective, and with sufficient information to be able to judge how well the evidence applies to their particular situation. Randomised trials are regarded as the best kind of evidence to inform good practice, but the strength of that evidence can be compromised in two ways. Firstly, to what extent are the results of the trial free from bias, so that the observed effect of the intervention is the result of the intervention itself and not due to characteristics of the subjects recruited to each intervention group or the way the outcome was measured? Secondly, are there key differences between the trial participants and the population to which the results are to be applied, or between the intervention as delivered in the trial and as it might be delivered in a routine setting? These two different aspects of trial quality are known as *internal validity* and *external validity* (Box 1.2). External validity is also referred to as generalisability.

Internal validity   The extent to which differences identified between randomised arms are a result of the intervention being tested.

External validity   The extent to which study results can be applied to other individuals or settings.

Box 1.2   Definition of internal and external validity

1.6.1   External validity

There have been pleas from various researchers to take the issue of external validity more seriously. For example, Glasgow, Vogt and Boles (1999) argue that much research focuses on determining efficacious interventions, thus involving trials with strong internal validity but, partially as a result, weak external validity. Rothwell

(2005) has also argued for greater consideration of external validity in the design and reporting of trials on the grounds that 'Lack of external validity is the most frequent criticism by clinicians of RCTs, systematic reviews, and guidelines, and is one explanation for the widespread underuse in routine practice of many treatments that have been shown to be beneficial in trials and are recommended in guidelines.' Cochrane (1972) and Bradford Hill (Horton, 2000) also recognised the importance of external validity several decades ago.

Table 1.7 describes the different elements of external validity based on Rothwell's paper (Rothwell, 2005) but adapted to include those aspects most relevant to cluster randomised trials; and the selection of clusters as well as participants. With the addition of 'setting', they cover the elements in the PICO (Population, Intervention, Comparator, Outcome) framework often used to define a research question in systematic reviews (Sackett *et al.*, 2000).

Ideally an individually randomised trial would recruit a random sample of individuals from the target population to whom the intervention would be delivered in routine practice if shown to be effective. In practice such a situation rarely arises. Those who take part in randomised trials may be systematically different from the target population. This is known as selection bias. In a cluster randomised trial, selection bias can take place at the individual and the cluster level. This might be due to the setting in which the trial takes place, the inclusion and exclusion criteria for the trial, or the recruitment and consent process (Table 1.7).

1.6.2   Internal validity

A well conducted, double-blind, placebo-controlled trial of sufficient size is likely to have high internal validity. The blinding serves several purposes. Firstly, the subjects are allocated to active or placebo arm without either the investigator or the subject knowing which treatment the patient will receive; knowledge of such allocation may influence the researcher's assessment of the patient's suitability and the patient's decision to participate. Secondly, blinding ensures that knowledge of allocation is unlikely to affect concomitant treatments or lifestyle choices. Finally, outcomes will be assessed blind, thus avoiding any temptation on the part of the patient or the researcher to bias the results in favour of (or against) the new treatment. Blinding of participants to the intervention is uncommon in cluster randomised trials, and selection of individual participants may take place after allocation of clusters to intervention arms. Careful attention to the selection and recruitment of clusters and individual participants, as well as objective assessment of outcomes, can all help protect the trial's internal validity. We consider blinding further in Chapters 9 and 10.

1.6.3   Balancing internal validity, external validity and ethical issues

Godwin *et al.* (2003) discuss the balance between internal and external validity in pragmatic trials in primary care. They make a clear distinction between explanatory

Table 1.7   Elements of external validity.

Element	Application	Example
Setting	Setting	Healthcare system Country Primary, secondary or tertiary
	Selection of clusters	Eligibility criteria Selection process
	Characteristics of clusters	Response rates Reasons for non-response Characteristics of recruited clusters
Population	Selection of participants	Eligibility criteria Selection process
	Characteristics of clusters	Response rates Reasons for non-response Characteristics of recruited participants
Intervention	Differences between protocol and routine practice	Intervention as delivered in the trial compared to the intervention as intended to be delivered in routine care Changes in management/new guidelines/ new policies since the trial began
Control arm	Effect of trial participation	Effect of trial participation on outcomes Effect of informed consent procedures Hawthorne effect
Outcomes	Outcome measures and follow-up	Follow-up rates Relevance of outcomes Relevance of surrogate outcomes and process measures compared with patient-orientated outcomes Appropriateness of timing of follow-up
	Adverse events	Completeness of reporting of adverse events Selection of clusters on basis of skill or experience

Source: adapted from Rothwell (2005).

trials in which the primary aim is to assess efficacy, and pragmatic trials in which the primary aim is to assess effectiveness, or how interventions work in real situations (Section 1.2). For explanatory trials internal validity is paramount, but in pragmatic trials there has to be a 'creative tension' between internal and external validity. This tension exists because promoting internal and external validity requires a certain amount of effort; investigators must judge how much work to put into ensuring each type of validity, depending on their available resources. In addition, issues around participants' consent also need to be considered. In some circumstances ethical issues may compromise either the internal or external validity, or both. In Chapter 2 we will concentrate on ethical issues, selection and recruitment. In Chapter 10 we discuss good practice in reporting internal and external validity.

1.7   Historical perspectives

1.7.1   Early cluster randomised trials

The first cluster randomised trials took place in the field of education, where the clusters were classes, year cohorts or schools. The need to take clustering into account in the analysis was clearly recognised as early as 1940 by Lindquist (1940), who proposed using summary statistics for each cluster as a method of analysis. This was not universally accepted among statisticians at the time, although it is now recognised as a valid method.

1.7.2   Early cluster randomised trials in health up to 2000

Early cluster randomised trials in medical research are difficult to identify as they were not usually described as 'cluster randomised'. Terms such as 'community trials' were used (Isaakidis and Ioannidis, 2003), and the first textbook of cluster randomised trials published by Murray (1998) used the term 'group randomised'. Cluster randomised trials have been used in sub-Saharan Africa since the early 1970s, and have been mainly concerned with reducing rates of infectious diseases such as malaria and sexually transmitted infections (Isaakidis and Ioannidis, 2003). Some of the earliest cluster randomised trials in health services research were in the use of computer-based, clinical decision support systems, beginning in the mid 1970s (Wexler et al., 1975; Chuang, Hripcsak and Jenders, 2000) and extending into screening and treatment of risk factors for coronary heart disease in the late 1970s. Cornfield's landmark paper in 1978 marked the beginning of the extensive development of methods for designing and analysing these trials (Cornfield, 1978). The mid to late 1990s saw the publication of several large cluster randomised trials in UK primary care (Wood et al., 1994; Feder et al., 1995; Kinmonth et al., 1998; Jolly et al., 1999; Feder et al., 1999). A series of statistics notes in the BMJ (Bland and Kerry, 1997; Kerry and Bland, 1998a, 1998b, 1998c) was published in the late 1990s, and a workshop on cluster randomised trials was held in Sheffield, UK in 1999 (Campbell, Donner and Elbourne, 2001). All of these raised the profile of cluster randomised trials and increased the awareness in the research community of the need to allow for clustering in analysis and power calculations. Two key textbooks, Murray (1998) and Donner and Klar (2000), were published at the end of the decade. Medical statistics textbooks also began to highlight the issues surrounding cluster randomised trials and to give some guidance to statisticians who might be involved in these trials (Bland, 2000).

1.7.3   Recent methodological developments

Since then the number of cluster randomised trials published has increased (Bland, 2004), and there has been a growth in awareness of the statistical issues (Eldridge *et al.*, 2008) and a continuing increase in papers describing new methods of analysis and other design issues. Several reviews of methodological developments have been published in the last 10 years (e.g. Murray, Varnell and Blitstein, 2004; Campbell, Donner and Klar, 2007). In this book we describe standard older methods of design and analysis and incorporate new developments in the literature in the last decade, focusing on the following topics.

1.7.3.1   Methods of analysis

Cornfield (1978) and other early methodological papers (Kerry and Bland, 1998a; Donner and Klar, 2000) recommended using summary statistics for each cluster as a valid analysis method, which could be used by researchers with little statistical expertise on readily available software. However, since then there have been considerable advances in available statistical methods such as multilevel modelling, robust standard errors, generalised estimating equations and Bayesian hierarchical models, and their use in cluster randomised trials has been extensively reviewed. These methods are described in Donner and Klar (2000) and in Hayes and Moulton (2009). In Chapter 6 we describe these methods, focusing on the choice of analysis from a practical point of view, with a wide range of examples from the literature where different methods have been used.

1.7.3.2   Sample size

Early methodological papers on sample size assumed that clusters are the same size. This is rarely the case in health services research. In chapter 7 we describe an adaptation of the method proposed by Donner (Donner, Birkett and Buck 1981) to allow for variability in cluster size. Although we concentrate on sample size methods which use the ICC to allow for between-cluster variation but we also discuss the application of other methods to health services research.

1.7.3.3   Estimating the intra-cluster correlation coefficient

One of the key problems for sample size calculations is how to estimate the ICC. There is now much more information available to help the researcher, which will be described in Chapter 8. We describe different methods of calculating the ICC and its precision, and give some guidelines as to the likely value based on published values, type of outcome and other factors.

1.7.3.4   Reporting guidelines

As cluster randomised trials add a level of complexity to design and analysis, they need to be accurately reported. The CONSORT statement was originally developed in 1996 (Begg *et al.*, 1996) to improve the standard of reporting of randomised trials. In Chapter 10 we describe how these guidelines have been extended for cluster randomised trials (Campbell, Elbourne and Altman, 2004), alongside a consideration of the recently updated CONSORT guidelines (Moher *et al.*, 2010) for randomised trials.

1.7.3.5   Recruitment and consent

The recognition of the problems of bias in identification and recruitment of individual participants has been raised in the literature (Puffer, Torgerson and Watson, 2003; Eldridge *et al.*, 2008; Eldridge, 2010) more recently than the need to adjust sample size for clustering. In Chapter 2 we describe the situations which give rise to bias in more detail and suggest some possible solutions.

1.7.3.6   Complex interventions

Many cluster randomised trials have shown no clear evidence to support the intervention being tested. This is partly because the interventions have not been well enough developed and are insufficiently intensive to be able to demonstrate a benefit. The Medical Research Council developed guidance for the development of complex interventions in 2000 (Campbell *et al.*, 2000), which was updated in 2008 (Craig *et al.*, 2008). We shall discuss this in detail in Chapter 3 and consider how to plan appropriate pilot studies in Chapter 4.

1.7.3.7   Other topics

The aim of randomisation is to produce groups of participants that will be similar with respect to characteristics that might affect the outcome. This will work best when a large number of clusters are randomised, but this is not usually the case for cluster randomised trials. Consequently methods such as stratification and matching are used to improve comparability of the intervention arms. Designs which are commonly used in cluster randomised trials are discussed in Chapter 5.

Systematic reviews may include individually randomised trials and cluster randomised trials or be restricted to cluster randomised trials depending on the nature of the intervention. Chapter 9 describes how to apply the principles of systematic reviews to cluster randomised trials, and also includes sections on cost-effectiveness and process evaluation. These topics have not been included in other textbooks of cluster randomised trials.

1.8   Summary

Cluster randomised trials are trials in which groups or clusters of individuals, rather than the individuals themselves, are randomised; this makes their design, analysis and conduct more complicated. Cluster randomised trials are less powerful than individually randomised trials with the same number of individual participants, analysis must take the clustering into account to avoid spurious precision in the confidence intervals, and there is a greater potential for bias when recruiting subjects. Nevertheless, there are several good reasons for adopting this trial design to evaluate a variety of interventions in community healthcare, and these trials are increasingly common. There is also a growing body of methodological literature focusing on these trials. In this book we bring together the literature on these recent developments, with particular emphasis on its implications for those designing and analysing these trials in health services research.

References

Begg, C., Cho, M., Eastwood, S. *et al.* (1996) Improving the quality of reporting of randomized controlled trials. The CONSORT statement. *JAMA*, **276** (8), 637–639.

Bland, J.M. (2000) *An Introduction to Medical Statistics*, 3rd edn, Oxford University Press, Oxford.

Bland, J.M. (2004) Cluster randomised trials in the medical literature: two bibliometric surveys. *BMC Med. Res. Methodol.*, **4**, 21.

Bland, J.M. and Kerry, S.M. (1997) Statistics notes. Trials randomised in clusters. *BMJ*, **315** (7108), 600.

Campbell, M., Fitzpatrick, R., Haines, A. *et al.* (2000) Framework for design and evaluation of complex interventions to improve health. *BMJ*, **321** (7262), 694–696.

Campbell, M.J., Donner A. and Elbourne D.R. (eds) (2001) Special issue: design and analysis of cluster randomized trials. *Stat. Med.*, **20** (3), 329–496.

Campbell, M.J., Donner, A. and Klar, N. (2007) Developments in cluster randomized trials and Statistics in Medicine. *Stat. Med.*, **26**, 2–19.

Campbell, M.K., Elbourne, D.R. and Altman, D.G. (2004) CONSORT statement: extension to cluster randomised trials. *BMJ*, **328** (7441), 702–708.

Cappuccio, F.P., Kerry, S.M., Micah, F.B. *et al.* (2006) A community programme to reduce salt intake and blood pressure in Ghana [ISRCTN88789643]. *BMC Public Health*, **6**, 13.

Chuang, J.H., Hripcsak, G. and Jenders, R.A. (2000) Considering clustering: a methodological review of clinical decision support system studies. *Proc. AMIA Symp.*, **2000**, 146–150.

Cochrane, A.L. (1972) *Effectiveness and Efficiency: Random Reflections on Health Services*, Nuffield Provincial Hospitals Trust, London.

Cornfield, J. (1978) Randomization by group: a formal analysis. *Am. J. Epidemiol.*, **108**, 100–102.

Craig, P., Dieppe, P., Macintyre, S. *et al.* (2008) Developing and evaluating complex interventions: the new Medical Research Council guidance. *BMJ*, **337**, a1655. doi: 10.1136/bmj.a1655

Donner, A. and Klar, N. (2000) *Design and Analysis of Cluster Randomised Trials in Health Research*, Arnold, London.

Donner, A., Birkett, N. and Buck, C. (1981) Randomization by cluster. Sample size requirements and analysis. *Am. J. Epidemiol.*, **114**, 906–914.

Eldridge, S. (2010) Pragmatic trials in primary health care: what, when and how? *Fam. Pract.*, **27**, 591–592.

Eldridge, S., Cryer, C., Feder, G. *et al.* (2001) Sample size calculations for intervention trials in primary care randomizing by primary care group: an empirical illustration from one proposed intervention trial. *Stat. Med.*, **20**, 367–376.

Eldridge, S., Spencer, A., Cryer, C. *et al.* (2005) Why modelling a complex intervention is an important precursor to trial design: lessons from studying an intervention to reduce falls-related injuries in older people. *J. Health Serv. Res. Policy*, **10** (3), 133–142.

Eldridge, S., Ashby, D., Bennett, C. *et al.* (2008) Internal and external validity of cluster randomised trials: systematic review of recent trials. *BMJ*, **336** (7649), 876–880.

Farrin, A., Russell, I., Torgerson, D. *et al.* (2005) Differential recruitment in a cluster randomized trial in primary care: the experience of the UK back pain, exercise, active management and manipulation (UK BEAM) feasibility study. *Clin. Trials*, **2** (2), 119–124.

Feder, G., Griffiths, C., Highton, C. *et al.* (1995) Do clinical guidelines introduced with practice based education improve care of asthmatic and diabetic patients? A randomised controlled trial in general practices in east London. *BMJ*, **311**, 1473–1478.

Feder, G., Griffiths, C., Eldridge, S. *et al.* (1999) Effect of postal prompts to patients and general practitioners on the quality of primary care after a coronary event (POST): randomised controlled trial. *BMJ*, **318**, 1522–1526.

Glasgow, R.E., Vogt, T.M. and Boles, S.M. (1999) Evaluating the public health impact of health promotion interventions: the RE-AIM framework. *Am. J. Public Health*, **89**, 1322–1327.

Godwin, M., Ruhland, L., Casson, I. *et al.* (2003) Pragmatic controlled clinical trials in primary care: the struggle between external and internal validity. *BMC Med. Res. Methodol.*, **3**, 28.

Hayes, J.H. and Moulton, L.H. (2009) *Cluster Randomised Trials*, Chapman & Hall.

Hayes, R.J. and Bennet, S. (1999) Simple sample size calculation for cluster-randomized trials. *Int. J. Epidemiol.*, **28** (2), 319–326.

Health and Social Care Information Centre (2011) General Practice Trends in the UK, http://www.ic.nhs.uk/webfiles/publications/TSC/General_Practice_Trends_in_the_UK.pdf (accessed 20 September 2011).

Horton, R. (2000) Common sense and figures: the rhetoric of validity in medicine (Bradford Hill memorial lecture 1999). *Stat. Med.*, **19**, 3149–3164.

International Committee of Medical Journal Editors (2009) Uniform Requirements for Manuscripts , http://www.icmje.org/publishing_10register.html (accessed 15 May 2011).

Isaakidis, P. and Ioannidis, J.P. (2003) Evaluation of cluster randomized controlled trials in sub-Saharan Africa. *Am. J. Epidemiol.*, **158**, 921–926.

Jolly, K., Bradley, F., Sharp, S. *et al.* (1999) Randomised controlled trial of follow up care in general practice of patients with myocardial infarction and angina: final results of the Southampton heart integrated care project (SHIP). *BMJ*, **318** (7185), 706–711.

Kendrick, D., Illingworth, R., Woods, A. *et al.* (2005) Promoting child safety in primary care: a cluster randomised controlled trial to reduce baby walker use. *Br. J. Gen. Pract.*, **55** (517), 582–588.

Kerry, S.M. and Bland, J.M. (1998a) Analysis of a trial randomised in clusters. *BMJ*, **316** (7124), 54.

Kerry, S.M. and Bland, J.M. (1998b) Sample size in cluster randomisation. *BMJ*, **316** (7130), 549.

Kerry, S.M. and Bland, J.M. (1998c) The intracluster correlation coefficient in cluster randomisation. *BMJ*, **316** (7142), 1455.

Kinmonth, A.L., Woodcock, A., Griffin, S. *et al.* (1998) Randomised controlled trial of patient centred care of diabetes in general practice: impact on current wellbeing and future disease risk. The Diabetes Care From Diagnosis Research Team. *BMJ*, **317** (7167), 1202–1208.

Kirkwood, B.R., Hurt, L., Amenga-Etego, S. *et al.* (2010) Effect of vitamin A supplementation in women of reproductive age on maternal survival in Ghana (ObaapaVitA): a cluster-randomised, placebo-controlled trial. *Lancet*, **375** (9726), 1640–1649.

Lindquist, E.F. (1940) *Statistical Analysis in Educational Research*, Houghton Mifflin, Boston.

Matthews, J.N.S. (2000) *An Introduction to Randomized Controlled Clinical Trials*, Arnold, London.

Medical Research Council (1948) Streptomycin treatment of pulmonary tuberculosis. *BMJ*, **2**, 769–782.

Moher, D., Hopewell, S., Schulz, K.F. *et al.* (2010) CONSORT 2010 Explanation and Elaboration: updated guidelines for reporting parallel group randomised trials. *BMJ*, **340**, c869.

Moore, T.J., Conlin, P.R., Ard, J. *et al.* (2001) DASH (Dietary Approaches to Stop Hypertension) diet is effective treatment for stage 1 isolated systolic hypertension. *Hypertension*, **38**, 155–158.

Murira, N., Munjanja, S.P., Zhanda, I. *et al.* (1997) Effect of a new antenatal care programme on the attitudes of pregnant women and midwives towards antenatal care in Harare. *Cent. Afr. J. Med.*, **43**, 131–135.

Murray, D.M. (1998) *Design and Analysis of Group Randomised Trials*, Oxford University Press, New York.

Murray, D.M., Varnell, S.P. and Blitstein, J.L. (2004) Design and analysis of group-randomized trials: a review of recent methodological developments. *Am. J. Public Health*, **94** (3), 423–432.

Oakeshott, P., Kerry, S.M. and Williams, J.E. (1994) Randomised controlled trial of the effect of the Royal College of Radiologists' guidelines on general practitioners' referral for radiographic examination. *Br. J. Gen. Pract.*, **44**, 197–200.

Pocock, S.J. (1983) *Clinical Trials: A Practical Approach*, John Wiley & Sons, Inc., New York.

Puffer, S., Torgerson, D. and Watson, J. (2003) Evidence for risk of bias in cluster randomised trials: review of recent trials published in three general medical journals. *BMJ*, **327** (7418), 785–789.

Roland, M.O. and Torgerson, D.J. (1998) What are pragmatic trials? *BMJ*, **316**, 285.

Rothwell, P.M. (2005) External validity of randomised controlled trials: 'To whom do the results of this trial apply?' *Lancet*, **365**, 82–93.

Sackett, D.L., Straus, S.E., Richardson, W.S. *et al.* (2000) *Evidence-Based Medicine: How to Practice and Teach*, Churchill Livingstone, London.

Torgerson, D.J. (2001) Contamination in trials: is cluster randomisation the answer? *BMJ*, **322**, 355–357.

Torgerson, D.J. and Torgerson, C.J. (2008) *Designing Randomised Trials in Health, Education and the Social Sciences*, Palgrave Macmillan, Basingstoke.

Underwood, M., Eldridge, S., Lamb, S. *et al.* (2011) The OPERA trial: protocol for a randomised trial of an exercise intervention for older people in residential and nursing accommodation. *Trials*, **12**, 27.

Wexler, J.R., Swender, P.T., Tunnessen, W.W. *et al.* (1975) Impact of a system of computer-assisted diagnosis: initial evaluation of the hospitalized patient. *AJDC*, **129**, 203–205.

Wood, D.A., Kinmonth, A.L., Davies, G.A. *et al.* (1994) Randomised controlled trial evaluating cardiovascular screening and intervention in general practice: principal results of British family heart study. *BMJ*, **308**, 313–320.

World Health Organization (1994) World Health Organization partograph in management of labour. *Lancet*, **343**, 1399–1404.

Zwarenstein, M., Treweek, S., Gagnier, J.J. *et al.* (2008) CONSORT group; Pragmatic Trials in Healthcare (Practihc) group. Improving the reporting of pragmatic trials: an extension of the CONSORT statement. *BMJ*, **337**, a2390.

2

Recruitment and ethics

As we saw in Chapter 1, cluster randomised trials are used in a great variety of settings, and there are a number of ways clusters and individual cluster members are selected and recruited. We showed that cluster randomised trials exhibit unique features not seen in individually randomised trials, and demonstrated the potential for bias. In this chapter we start by considering how clusters and individual participants can be selected in a way that enhances external validity. We then consider how ethical principles apply to cluster randomised trials and consider some of the difficulties around informed consent. Finally we consider how the selection and recruitment of individual cluster members can affect the internal validity of the trial, and some steps that can be taken to reduce the potential for bias.

2.1 Selecting clusters and participants to enhance external validity

2.1.1 Clusters

The first step in any trial is to consider the setting in which the trial will be carried out; this is the first element of external validity listed in Table 1.7. Rothwell (2005) lists a hierarchy of settings from country to healthcare centre to clinician, and includes alongside this a consideration of the healthcare system and the healthcare sector (primary, secondary, tertiary). His framework is clearly designed to apply to individually randomised trials when anything outside the patient can be considered

A Practical Guide to Cluster Randomised Trials in Health Services Research, First Edition.
Sandra Eldridge and Sally Kerry.
© 2012 John Wiley & Sons, Ltd. Published 2012 by John Wiley & Sons, Ltd.

as the 'setting', but within the context of cluster randomised trials it is debateable whether clusters are really 'participants' or 'settings'. From a statistical point of view a good case could be made for adopting the former approach, but we have adopted the latter approach on the basis that viewing a cluster as a setting is the usual view of health professionals who have to treat individual patients.

To enhance external validity in relation to setting, investigators need either to undertake the trial in as wide a range of settings as possible, or to ensure that the settings they use are as representative as possible of those in which the intervention may be used in the future. Cluster randomised trial investigators should consider conducting their trial in as wide a range of clusters as possible and not limiting inclusion unnecessarily. Once approached, clusters may not agree to participate, but this is not within an investigator's control to the same extent as the clusters they approach.

2.1.2   Participants

To enhance external validity, trials should include as wide a range of individuals as possible. One way to do this is to keep exclusion criteria to a minimum; Table 2.1

Table 2.1   Trial of home blood pressure monitoring.

Aim: To assess the effect of home blood pressure monitoring on blood pressure control in hypertensive patients with above-target blood pressure

Location and type of cluster: Canada primary care physicians

Interventions: (i) Control: usual care (ii) Intervention: patient instruction on use of monitor, once weekly measurements of blood pressure at home and reporting of these measurements to family physician at each office visit

Primary outcome: 24-hour ambulatory blood pressure monitoring at 6 and 12 months

Inclusion criteria: Adults, age 18 years and older, who have been diagnosed with essential hypertension and who have not reached their target blood pressure level

Exclusion criteria: Patients with a diagnosis of secondary hypertension; pregnancy; hypertension managed primarily by a consultant; inability to provide informed consent; a physical or mental disability that precludes use of a home blood pressure monitor

Freedom of health professionals in relation to intervention delivery: Physicians may use information provided by patients in whatever way they like; frequency of visits to physician determined by patients and physicians

Freedom of patients in relation to intervention delivery: Patients may use blood pressure monitor as often as they like, but weekly at a minimum; frequency of visits to physician determined by patients and physicians

---

Source: Godwin *et al.* (2003).

describes a cluster randomised trial in which investigators attempted to do this. All adults with uncontrolled essential hypertension who were managed in primary care constituted the target population. No additional tests were required which would not be carried out in routine practice. Most of the exclusion criteria refer to groups who do not form part of the target population or who would not be suitable for the intervention even if applied in routine practice (e.g. inability to use a blood pressure monitor).

Another way to enhance external validity is to encourage a high uptake from eligible patients. Careful consideration should be given to the way individuals are approached, who will be responsible for identifying and consenting eligible patients, whether invitation is through face-to-face encounters or postal invitations, and ensuring that the information about the study provided to participants is accessible. The challenges of recruitment to health research studies, particularly in primary care, should not be underestimated (Bower *et al.*, 2009). Although this applies to both individually randomised and cluster randomised trials, in the latter individuals may be approached after the allocation of the cluster is known. The characteristics of recruited participants may differ if those identifying and/or recruiting individuals are not blinded to allocation. This unblinded allocation should be avoided if at all possible as it has the potential to compromise internal as well as external validity, and we cover this in more detail in Section 2.3.

2.2 Ethics of cluster randomised trials

Over the twentieth century, various codes of research were developed in order to protect the rights, dignity and well-being of subjects taking part in research studies (BMJ, 1996; World Medical Association, 1996). A basic principle is that research should yield some benefit to society by adding to existing knowledge, should minimise harm to individuals, should be fair and should be conducted with integrity. One of the ways of protecting individuals is through voluntary informed consent, where the risks and benefits of taking part in the research are fully explained and the individual is free to decide without coercion. However, it is not possible for individual participants to consent to randomisation in a cluster randomised trial (Section 1.3.1) and, in addition, individual participants may not be able to opt out of the intervention. There are also other situations where consent may be difficult to obtain, such as testing interventions for treating those who are acutely ill or those with severe learning difficulties (Slowther, Boynton and Shaw, 2006). These groups would be disadvantaged if research could not be conducted, and new knowledge thereby obtained, for the want of fully informed consent on the part of individual participants. Therefore while fully informed consent should be obtained wherever possible, not being able to obtain consent is not a reason for not conducting a trial. It is therefore the responsibility of all those involved in the research (researchers, funders, research institutions, ethics review committees, and regulatory bodies) to ensure that research is designed and conducted in such a way as to be ethically sound. For cluster randomised trials this will include community leaders and cluster representatives being involved in decisions about participation and conduct wherever possible.

2.2.1   Components of consent

There are three components of consent which usually occur simultaneously before randomisation in an individually randomised trial. These are consent to (i) randomisation, (ii) participation in the intervention, and (iii) data collection; participants must agree to all three components. In cluster randomised trials individuals cannot usually consent to randomisation, as this takes place at the cluster level. Individuals may or may not have the opportunity to opt out of the intervention and may or may not be required to give consent for data collection, depending on the mode of collection of the outcome data. The ethics of cluster randomised trials were first discussed in detail by Edwards *et al.* (1999), who classified trials into 'cluster-cluster' and 'individual-cluster', and proposed that in 'cluster-cluster' trials individual consent was not possible and therefore not required. The UK Medical Research Council used the same classifications but in relation to *interventions* rather than *trials*; at the same time acknowledging that many interventions in health services research do not fall neatly into these categories (Medical Research Council, 2002. The next section describes an extension of this classification by Eldridge, Ashby and Feder (2005) which is more appropriate for interventions commonly encountered in health services research, while still being applicable to the public health interventions considered by Edwards *et al.*

2.2.2   Classification of interventions and implications for individual participant consent

Table 2.2 lists four categories that classify *interventions* rather than *trials*, based on the reasons for adopting a clustered design. Some trials may have complex interventions where different intervention components will fall into different categories.

2.2.2.1   Individual-cluster interventions

These are interventions directed at the individual. Individual randomisation might be a viable option, but a cluster randomised trial has been chosen to avoid contamination, to increase compliance, or for administrative reasons. Individuals can opt out of these interventions. The ObaapaVitA trial (Table 2.3) randomised women to receive vitamin A capsules or placebo. The intervention was entirely directed at the individual women; in other settings randomisation might have been done at the individual level. The individual women needed to cooperate with the trial team by taking the capsules and so voluntary informed consent was essential.

Table 2.2 Typology of trial interventions based on primary reason for adopting a clustered design.

Intervention classification	Reason for cluster randomisation	Options for opting out of the intervention	Targeting the intervention	Examples
Individual-cluster	To avoid contamination; practical difficulties; ensuring intervention is fully implemented; delivered through a health professional	Individuals can opt out in the same way as in individually randomised trials	Targeted primarily at individuals but may be delivered by a health professional	ObaapaVitA (Table 2.3) Baby walker trial (Table 1.6) Family Heart Study (Wood et al., 1994)
Professional-cluster	Intervention acts at the level of the health professional, not the individual	Individuals can decline to have their data used but the intervention aimed at the professionals is still likely to have an effect on them	Targeted primarily at the health professional with consequences for the individual patient	X-ray guidelines (Table 1.2) Diabetes care from diagnosis trial (Table 2.4) OPERA staff training (Table 2.7)
External-cluster	Cost or administrative convenience	Individuals can opt out by declining to see the additional staff	Targeted at cluster organisation	SHIP (Table 2.5) OPERA physiotherapy assessment (Table 2.7)
Cluster-cluster	The intervention cannot be carried out in any other way	Individuals cannot opt out of the intervention. They may or may not be able to decline to have their data used depending on whether it is collected at an individual level or cluster level (e.g. routinely collected data)	Targeted at cluster organisation, health professional or cluster population	Depression awareness trial (Table 2.6) Kumasi health education (Table 2.9)

The final definitive version of this paper has been published in *Community Dentistry and Oral Epidemiology* (in press) by Sage Publications Ltd. All rights reserved.
© Sage.

Table 2.3   ObaapaVitA: vitamin A supplementation to reduce maternal and child mortality.

Aim: To see if supplementation with vitamin A would reduce maternal and child mortality in Ghana
Location and type of cluster: Ghana, geographical areas
Interventions: (i) Control: placebo capsules (ii) Intervention: vitamin A capsules
Primary outcome: Pregnancy-related mortality and all-cause female mortality
Reasons for cluster randomisation: Administrative convenience; eliminates contamination due to pill swapping within villages
Consent required by individuals: Yes for both intervention and data collection

---

Source: Kirkwood *et al.* (2010).

Table 2.4   Diabetes care from diagnosis trial.

Aim: To assess the effect of additional training of practice staff in patient-centred care on the current well-being and future risk of patients with newly diagnosed type 2 diabetes
Location and type of cluster: UK general practices
Interventions: (i) Control: approach to care developed with practices, based on national guidelines and including patient materials (ii) Intervention: as control plus extra training on patient centred care
Main outcome measures: Quality of life, well-being, haemoglobin A1c and lipid concentrations, blood pressure, body mass index
Reasons for cluster randomisation: Educational intervention aimed at changing consulting style
Consent required from individual participants: For data collection only

---

Source: Kinmonth *et al.* (1998).

2.2.2.2   Professional-cluster interventions

These interventions are directed at the health professional caring for the individual, and include the introduction of guidelines or training. The intervention in the x-ray guidelines trial described in Section 1.3.1 falls into this category. In this trial, consent was not obtained for data collection as the results were obtained from an audit of radiology department records. In the diabetes care from diagnosis trial (Table 2.4), practices were randomised to receive training in a patient-centred approach. To assess the primary outcome, quality of life, patients were required to complete a questionnaire. Patients could not avoid being treated by general practitioners who had received the training, but could opt out of completing questionnaires, or allowing researchers to access their clinical records or blood test results.

2.2.2.3   External-cluster interventions

These interventions involve additional staff from outside the cluster, such as specialist nurses, provided in addition to usual care. In the SHIP trial (Table 2.5), specialist

Table 2.5   SHIP: support following myocardial infarction.

Aim: To assess the effectiveness of a programme to coordinate and support
follow-up care in general practice after a hospital diagnosis of myocardial
infarction or angina

Location and type of cluster: UK general practices

Interventions: (i) Control: usual care (ii) Intervention: programme to coordinate
preventive care led by specialist liaison nurses, which sought to improve
communication between hospital and general practice and to encourage general
practice nurses to provide structured follow-up

Main outcomes: Serum total cholesterol concentration, blood pressure, distance
walked in six minutes, confirmed smoking cessation, and body mass index
measured at one-year follow up

Reasons for cluster randomisation: Cost and administrative convenience

Consent required from individual participants: Yes

Source: Jolly *et al.* (1999).

Table 2.6   Educational intervention to increase depression awareness among
students.

Aim: To assess the effectiveness of an intervention to educate students about
depression

Location and type of cluster: UK colleges of one university

Interventions: (i) Control (ii) Intervention: postcards and posters on depression
and its treatment

Outcomes: Student awareness that depression can be treated effectively

Reasons for cluster randomisation: Intervention implemented at the cluster level
through posters

Consent required from individual participants: No; participants could refuse to
send back questionnaire

Source: Merritt *et al.* (2007).

nurses worked with the intervention practices with the aim of integrating primary
and secondary care more effectively for patients who had been hospitalised for heart
attack or episode of angina. The patients could have declined to see the additional
staff, thus opting out of the intervention, and could also have declined to have their
data used.

2.2.2.4   Cluster-cluster interventions

These interventions operate at the cluster level and cannot be implemented in any
other way. Individuals cannot opt out of the intervention and therefore cannot be
asked to consent to taking part. In a depression awareness trial (Table 2.6), postcards
were sent to students, and posters on depression and its treatment displayed in the

college. The students could not opt out of the intervention, and informing them of the purpose of the study would have compromised the science of the trial (see Section 2.2.5); but they could decline to participate in data collection. Edwards *et al.* (1999) give an example of fluoridation of the water supply. Residents may wish to know that the water supply has been fluoridated or that the area is taking part in an experiment on fluoridation even though they cannot opt out of the intervention except by moving away. Ideally, in such situations some information about the trial should be provided to the individual participants, even though it may increase anxiety. Later discovery that they have been part of an experiment without their knowledge may result in a sense of violation (Hutton, 2001) and mistrust of those agencies and leaders involved, although for some trials in which health services are reorganised any sense of violation is likely to be minimal.

2.2.2.5 Multifaceted interventions

Two-thirds of primary care trials in a review by Eldridge, Ashby and Feder (2005) had multifaceted interventions, in which intervention components fell into more than one of the above categories. In the OPERA trial (Table 2.7), residents were assessed by physiotherapists external to the home (external-cluster); and lived in homes where

Table 2.7 OPERA: physical activity in residential homes to prevent depression.

Aim: To evaluate the impact on depression of a whole-home intervention to increase physical activity among older people

Location and type of cluster: UK residential and nursing homes for older people

Interventions: (i) Control: depression awareness programme delivered by research nurses (ii) Intervention: depression awareness programme delivered by physiotherapists plus whole-home package to increase activity among older people, including physiotherapy assessments of individuals, and activity sessions for residents

Primary outcome: Prevalence of depression (Geriatric Depression Scale) at 12 months and change in depression score

Reasons for cluster randomisation: Whole-home intervention aimed at increasing physical activity

Consent required by individuals: Consent required separately for data collection activities, completion of the Geriatric Depression Scale and access to medical records. Consent required for physiotherapy assessments, but not for whole-home intervention to increase activity through staff education. All residents were encouraged to take part in activity sessions, whether or not they consented to data collection. Residents of control homes could not access the activity sessions

Individuals consented prior to randomisation: Yes, for individuals resident in the home prior to randomisation, but not for individuals moving into the home during the study

Source: Underwood *et al.* (2011).

Table 2.8   Community-based interventions to promote blood pressure control.

Aim: To assess the effectiveness of 2 community-based interventions on blood pressure in hypertensive adults

Location and type of cluster: Communities of approximately 250 households, at least 10 km apart in Karachi, Pakistan

Interventions: (i) Control: no intervention (ii) Individual-level intervention: family-based home health education (HHE) from lay health workers every 3 months (iii) Cluster level intervention: annual training of general practitioners in hypertension management (iv) Both interventions

Primary outcome: Reduction in systolic blood pressure from baseline to end of follow up at 2 years

Reasons for cluster randomisation: Practitioner education intervention and prevention of contamination between households

Consent required by individual: Only for data collection and family-based education. Other patients treated by the same practitioners were unable to consent to the general practitioner education element

---

Source: Jafar *et al.* (2009).

the staff had been trained in promoting physical activity (professional-cluster) and where activity sessions were taking place to which all residents were invited regardless of their participation in the trial data collection (cluster-cluster). In a trial to promote blood pressure control in a low-income country (Table 2.8) communities were randomised. Within the intervention communities, general practitioners were given annual training in hypertension management (professional-cluster), while individual patients with hypertension received home healthcare visits from a trained lay worker (individual-cluster). In trials with multifaceted interventions, the practicalities and scientific implications of obtaining consent can differ for different intervention components. As a general principle, trial investigators should provide an option for individuals to opt out of interventions and data collection if at all possible, as illustrated in Table 2.7. As already discussed, however, the decision to consent to randomisation cannot be made by an individual in a cluster randomised trial, and must be made at the cluster level. We cover this in the next section.

2.2.3   Cluster guardians

Since cluster members cannot act independently in deciding whether or not to be randomised, it is important to consider who should make the decision about randomisation on behalf of the cluster members. Many clusters are formed from existing administrative units, for which there is a clear authority figure or committee who normally makes decisions that affect the whole cluster. This role is referred to by Edwards *et al.* (1999) as the 'guardian' of the cluster; examples of these are the chief executive of a hospital, head teacher of a school, or community leaders in a village.

Identifying the guardian in trials which randomise healthcare organisations is often straightforward. For example, if randomising general practices in the UK, it

Table 2.9   Kumasi trial: health education to prevent stroke.

Aim: To see if a health education programme to reduce salt intake among rural
and semi-rural communities in the Ashanti region of Ghana leads to a reduction
in blood pressure

Location and type of cluster: Ghana, villages of 500-2000 inhabitants

Interventions: (i) Control: health education not including salt reduction (ii)
Intervention: health education including salt reduction messages

Primary outcome: Reduction in systolic blood pressure after six months

Reason for cluster randomisation: Health education delivered to all members of
the village, through presentations in the village, usually in the open

Consent from clusters: Chiefs and elders of each village gave consent after
meeting with the trial team

Consent required from participants: Yes, for data collection, and they were
informed the trial was about 'changing diet', not specifically about salt.
Individuals could opt out of attending the education sessions but might receive
some of the messages through family or neighbours. Those who did not
consent could still attend

Source: Cappuccio *et al.* (2006).

will usually be the senior partner in the practice. However, in other situations it may
not be so simple. Firstly, there may be political instability at either local or national
level, with different parties claiming authority for the cluster. In the Kumasi trial
(Table 2.9), one potential cluster was not invited to take part because of a local
dispute over who should be the next village chief. Osrin *et al.* (2009) gives an
example from Nepal of running a trial in an area with two governments, each considered illegitimate by the other, after the country's Maoist insurrection. Secondly,
the cluster may be geographically defined but unrelated to existing political or
administrative demarcations. A smoke alarm give-away trial in London (DiGuiseppi
et al., 2002) randomised electoral wards, which are much smaller than local authori-
ties, the smallest administrative geographical unit. The trial was developed by a
working group representing local government, health agencies and community
groups. In this trial, clusters were not asked to consent to the intervention, although
individual households receiving a smoke alarm were asked to sign a consent/
indemnity form. Finally, several clusters may share the same administrative authority. For example, the chief executive or medical director of a hospital may be the
guardian while wards are the clusters. A similar situation arises where units of time
are chosen as the cluster. Here the guardian may still act to protect members of the
cluster from harm but will not represent the particular interests of a cluster.

In acting in the best interests of the cluster, guardians should consider the potential benefits of the research; that is, it would be useful to know whether a new
intervention actually works before investing time and money in it. This needs to be
weighed against possible harm to individuals as a result of taking part. However,
those who have responsibility for a community cannot always be relied upon

Table 2.10   Ekjut project: participatory women's groups to improve birth outcomes and maternal depression.

Aim: To see whether a community mobilisation through participatory women's groups might improve birth outcomes and maternal depression

Location and type of cluster: India rural communities, with a mean population of 6338 per cluster (range 3605–7467)

Interventions: (i) Control: no intervention (ii)Intervention: a facilitator convened 13 groups every month to support participatory action and learning for women, and facilitated the development and implementation of strategies to address maternal and newborn health problems

Primary outcome: Neonatal mortality rate and maternal depression scores

Reason for cluster randomisation: Participatory women's groups in the community

Consent from clusters: Open community meetings with village elders, opinion leaders and headmen. And written consent obtained from village elders

Consent required from participants: Yes, verbal consent for data collection. The agenda of the first women's group meeting was to seek consent for future meetings

---

Source: Tripathy *et al.* (2010).

accurately to reflect its views (Onwujekwe, Shu and Okonkwo, 1999). The Ekjut project (Table 2.10) was designed to ascertain whether a community mobilisation through participatory women's groups might improve birth outcomes and maternal depression in Jharkhand and Orissa, India. The cluster guardians were predominantly men, who may have seen the intervention as challenging the status quo, and therefore socio-politically destabilising (Osrin *et al.*, 2009). Although this decision-making process is sometimes necessary in individually randomised trials, the role of the cluster guardian is more important in cluster randomised trials. In individually randomised trials, while cluster guardians can decide whether an individual can be approached to take part in the trial, once approached individuals are free to choose for themselves. In cluster randomised trials, guardians of the cluster are asked to consent to randomisation on behalf of the cluster, and the individual cluster members may not be able to opt out. The Medical Research Council (2002) recommends establishing a 'cluster representation mechanism', independent from the research team, to safeguard the interests of cluster members, with details of how the mechanism has been selected given in the trial protocol. Lay participation in the cluster representation mechanism could contribute to judging the benefits and risks of intervention.

2.2.4   Timing of cluster consent

In most cluster randomised trials, clusters are informed of the study and give consent prior to randomisation. Even where cluster representatives are unfamiliar with research ideas, randomisation can be regarded as similar to a lottery; many will be familiar with this. However, some trials have informed the intervention arm only after randomisation; Osrin gives four examples from developing countries (Osrin *et al.*, 2009). In one of these, a trial of women's groups to improve birth outcomes in Bangladesh (Azad *et al.*, 2010), community leaders were approached for permission to establish women's groups within the intervention arm. Although consent for data collection was sought from all women, those in the control clusters may not have been aware of the existence of the intervention. In this large trial, no clusters dropped out of the trial post-randomisation, but this will not always be the case, and post-allocation consent from clusters is best avoided. If clusters decline to participate after randomisation, there is a potential for bias unless outcome data can be collected through routine sources on all clusters, including those declining to participate. Finally, post-randomisation consent of the clusters may also increase the possibility of bias in the selection of the individual participants (Section 2.3), as identification and recruitment of individuals cannot usually take place until clusters have consented. We recommend that representatives of all clusters give consent to randomisation prior to allocation. It may be appropriate to give additional information describing the intervention, such as how it will be carried out, to the intervention clusters after consent, but this should be considered as part of the intervention and not part of the consent process.

2.2.5   Fully informed consent for educational and awareness campaigns

Intervention and control clusters, and individuals within these clusters, should be given similar information about the trial before consent. However, fully informing the control participants of the intervention could dilute the intervention effect, causing bias. In the Kumasi trial (Table 2.9), the information sheet did not mention salt but referred to 'changing diet', and all participants were asked to attend health education sessions on a variety of subjects, with the addition of salt reduction in the intervention clusters. How much information control participants should receive in these circumstances has been the subject of debate (Little and Williamson, 1997). This problem is not restricted to cluster randomised trials (Little *et al.*, 1997), but in a cluster randomised trial there may be a temptation to have very different information sheets for the intervention and control arms. This should be avoided. If fully informed consent cannot be obtained then the scientific merit of the trial should be weighed against the potential harms to the individual. In practice the harm of withholding information will be negligible in many cluster randomised trials, because of the nature of the interventions involved.

2.2.6   Protecting the privacy of individuals

Before individuals can give consent to participate in a trial they need to be selected and approached, and their right to privacy and confidentiality must be respected.

This may be an issue for trials which identify patients, for example as the result of their consulting for a specific condition, or by using information contained in their medical records, even if this is only their contact details. The SHIP trial (Table 2.5) and the diabetes care from diagnosis trial (Table 2.4) are both examples from primary care. Patients often need to be recruited through an approach from a healthcare professional. Researchers may not be able to access identifiable information prior to consent. This affects the validity of trials, including cluster randomised trials in two ways. Firstly, it is difficult to get busy practice staff, for whom research is not their main priority, to offer patients invitations face to face, and letters often lead to poor response rates. Secondly, the amount of information that can be collected on those who do not consent to take part may be restricted. This can make it difficult to assess whether or not trial participants are representative of those eligible to take part. However, some anonymised summary data may be available for each cluster.

2.2.7 Duty of care to control participants

Generally in cluster randomised trials the control arm is allocated to usual care, to measure what would happen in the absence of the intervention. The control arm should experience the existing healthcare norms as far as possible (Osrin *et al.*, 2009), but in some cases this may be less than optimal care. This may be seen as unethical, as control patients would not necessarily receive best care. However, many primary care and public heath trials aim to test ways of improving the delivery of care in a real-life setting. For example, optimal care for patients with hypertension would normally include treatment with antihypertensive medication, increasing the dose or number of drugs until blood pressure is controlled. However, in developing countries individuals may have poor access to medical facilities and may be unable to afford the most effective drugs. It was in this context that the Kumasi stroke prevention trial (Table 2.9) was carried out, to see if reducing salt in the diet would reduce blood pressure in the population as a whole and so reduce the need for medication. Thus, if recruitment to the study involved identification and treatment of all individuals with hypertension, the control arm would not reflect usual care in this population. This is most likely to occur in pragmatic trials, where interventions are being tested in the 'real world' rather than under ideal conditions. Intervention strategies for improving the management of patients in primary care, and public health interventions, are almost always cluster randomised. The PINCER trial (Avery *et al.*, 2009) aimed to determine the effectiveness of a pharmacist-led, information-technology-based complex intervention to reduce the proportion of patients at risk from potentially hazardous prescribing and medicines management in general practice. Practices were randomised to either computer-generated feedback, or a pharmacist-led intervention comprising computer-generated feedback, educational outreach and dedicated support. There was no control arm that did not receive any intervention at all, as it was considered unethical not to give any feedback on individuals at risk of prescribing errors. The control arm received a minimal intervention compared to the intervention arm.

In other trials, medical problems may come to light during baseline data collection, showing a participant to be at significant risk. From a scientific viewpoint intervening in the control arm should be avoided, but it may be considered negligent to ignore the problem entirely. In the Kumasi trial (Table 2.9), many villagers had never had their blood pressure measured. Even when they knew they had hypertension, very few villagers were taking adequate medication owing to the cost of drugs and the poor access to medical facilities in the rural and semi-urban villages recruited. One rationale for the study was to try a simple, cheap, population approach to reducing blood pressure that would reduce the need for antihypertensive treatment. In these circumstances it was considered acceptable not to actively intervene for the majority of patients found to have undiagnosed hypertension. However those with very high blood pressure were referred to the teaching hospital in the city for treatment. A protocol should be agreed in advance, after carefully considering the risks and benefits, so that individuals are treated consistently and without unnecessary risk.

2.2.8 Summary of consent issues

Given the variety of interventions employed in cluster randomised trials, the conduct and ethics of each trial should be considered carefully. Box 2.1 gives some recommendations for trial investigators designing cluster randomised trials.

2.3 Selection and recruitment of participants to enhance internal validity

Allocation concealment is seen as the cornerstone for avoiding bias in randomised trials. It means making sure that the individuals are enrolled into a trial without either the recruiter or the participants knowing which intervention the participants will receive prior to the point of allocation, even if it is impossible to blind the

---

1. Be aware of the different types of intervention and different elements that need consent within a cluster randomized trial.

2. Consider practical reasons and scientific arguments for not obtaining consent to various elements of an intervention.

3. Consider lay involvement in cluster representation mechanisms or as part of trial planning specifically to consider ethical issues.

4. Consider whether opportunities for patient opt out can be incorporated into trial design.

Source: Eldridge, Ashby and Feder (2005).

Box 2.1   Recommendations for trial investigators

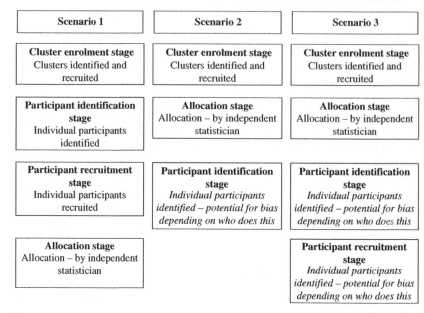

Figure 2.1   Ordering stages of allocation and recruitment. Text in italics indicates potential for bias.

participants to the intervention once allocated. This is usually straightforward in an individually randomised design and for clusters in a cluster randomised design. However, in a cluster randomised design it is important that those selecting and enrolling individuals are also blind to allocation status up to the point of allocation. This important issue has been raised in the literature in recent years (Puffer, Torgerson and Watson, 2003; Farrin *et al.*, 2005; Eldridge *et al.*, 2008). The potential for bias and what can be done about it depends to a large extent on the nature of the randomisation and recruitment process, as described in Eldridge, Kerry and Torgerson (2009).

In general there are four stages to the randomisation and recruitment in a cluster randomised trial, and a variety of ways in which the stages can be ordered, although cluster enrolment always comes first. This is illustrated in Figure 2.1, where potential for bias is indicated by italics. There is a fourth possible scenario, discussed in Section 2.2.4, where clusters are consented after randomisation. We have not considered this separately, as we are not aware of any health services research trials which have done this, and the implications for recruitment of individual participants will be the same as scenarios 2 and 3.

2.3.1   Trials which identify and recruit individual participants before randomisation (scenario 1)

In scenario 1, identification and recruitment are carried out before allocation is known, and there is no potential for bias as a result. In a trial of structured diabetes

Table 2.11   Trial of structured diabetes shared care.

Aim: To assess the feasibility and effectiveness of a structured diabetes shared
    care service in a mixed healthcare system and to analyse the impact on total
    patient care

Location and type of cluster: General practices, north Dublin, Ireland

Interventions: (i) Control: usual care (ii) Intervention: education to practice nurses
    to support target-setting and achievement amongst patients (a diabetes
    specialist nurse was available for support and to administer the intervention to
    patients when practice nurses were not available). Annual review in specialist
    outpatient clinic and 3 monthly in practice reviews

Primary outcome: HbA1c level

Consent required by clusters: Yes

Consent required by participants: Yes; only patients willing to attend general
    practice for diabetes care were recruited

Consent from participants before randomisation: Yes

Source: Smith *et al.* (2004).

care (Table 2.11), patients were selected from practice diabetes registers that were
compiled *de novo* in the three-month period prior to the start of the trial. Consent
was obtained from all participants in each cluster prior to randomisation.

2.3.2   Trials where individual participants are not recruited (scenario 2)

Even in today's increasingly restrictive research environment it may sometimes be
ethically acceptable not to recruit individual participants. Table 2.12 describes the
IRIS trial, which aimed to increase the identification and referral of women who
are victims of domestic violence. The intervention is a combination of cluster-
professional and cluster-cluster components (see Section 2.2.2), and outcomes are
collected from routine data. However, bias can still occur in trials without individual
patient recruitment if individual participants are identified by people who know the
allocation status. The potential for bias will be greater if the inclusion or exclusion
criteria are more subjective. A trial to improve secondary prevention of ischaemic
heart disease in primary care (Sondergaard *et al.*, 2006) used general practitioners
to identify patients with ischaemic heart disease after the allocation to intervention
arms was known. Fewer patients with recent myocardial infarction were identified
in the intervention practices compared to the control practices, indicating that there
may have been a bias in the application of the inclusion criteria between the
two arms. Common ways of identifying individuals which avoid bias are: all cluster
members are included; a random sample of individuals individuals are included;
only certain cluster members are included but they are identified in a way that
is not open to interpretation (i.e. those for whom a prescription/test has been
ordered or who are identified electronically in some other way). In the IRIS trial

Table 2.12   IRIS: training to increase identification and referral of victims of domestic violence.

Aim: To test the effectiveness of a training and support programme for general practice teams targeting identification of women experiencing domestic violence, and referral to specialist domestic violence advocates

Location and type of cluster: UK general practices

Intervention: (i) Control: usual care (ii) Intervention: multidisciplinary training sessions held in each practice (professional-cluster intervention), electronic prompts in the patient records and referral pathway to a named domestic violence advocate as well as feedback on referrals and reinforcement over the course of a year. Posters were displayed in the practice and leaflets were available (cluster-cluster intervention)

Primary outcome: Number of referrals of women aged over 16 years to advocacy services based in specialist domestic violence agencies recorded in the general practice records

Consent required by clusters: Yes

Consent required by participants: No

Comment: Outcome data were obtained from practice notes by researchers, and no patient identifiable data were taken outside practices.

Source: Gregory *et al.* (2010).

(Table 2.12), the only inclusion criteria were age (over 16) and sex (female), which are clearly defined, and information was obtained for all women in the practice.

2.3.3   Trials where participants are recruited after randomisation but blind to allocation status (scenario 3)

When the intervention aims to improve care of an acute condition or the onset or exacerbation of a chronic condition it will be difficult to identify participants prior to randomisation. However it may still be possible for individuals to be recruited by someone outside the cluster masked to the cluster allocation. In the ELECTRA trial (Table 2.13) patients were identified from the Accident and Emergency department or general practitioner out-of-hours service, and invited to take part by a researcher unaware of the allocation status of the practice with which the patient was registered. After consent was obtained, the patient was handed over to a different research nurse who then informed the patient which arm his/her practice was in. In this way selection and recruitment of patients was masked to allocation status even though the clusters had already been randomised and clusters knew their allocation status.

It is sometimes possible to recruit participants on cluster premises using someone blind to allocation status. In a trial of the impact of counselling on the care-seeking behaviour of families with sick children, project staff enrolled mothers bringing children for curative care at each health centre involved; the precise objectives of the study were not disclosed to these fieldworkers (Table 2.14).

Table 2.13   ELECTRA: asthma liaison nurses to reduce unscheduled care.

Aim: To determine whether asthma specialist nurses, using a liaison model of
    care, reduce unscheduled care in a deprived multiethnic setting
Location and type of cluster: UK general practices
Interventions: (i) Control: a visit promoting standard asthma guidelines; patients
    were checked for inhaler technique (ii) Intervention: patient review in a
    nurse-led clinic, and liaison with general practitioners and practice nurses
    comprising educational outreach, promotion of guidelines for high risk asthma
    and ongoing clinical support
Primary outcome: Unscheduled care for acute asthma over one year, and time to
    first unscheduled attendance
Consent required by cluster: Yes
Consent required by patient: Yes. Consent was taken when patients attended for
    unscheduled care by a researcher unaware of the allocation of the practice

Source: Griffiths *et al.* (2004).

Table 2.14   Counselling training to improve help-seeking behaviour of families
with sick children.

Aim: To assess whether training doctors in counselling improves care-seeking
    behaviour in families with sick children
Location and type of cluster: Primary healthcare centres in rural India
Interventions: (i) Control: doctors received one to three days of training in
    clinical skills only (ii) Intervention: five-day training of doctors in counselling,
    communication and clinical skills; card to give to mothers
Primary outcome: Occasions when mothers sought appropriate care for children
    with danger signs

Source: Mohan *et al.* (2004).

2.3.4   Trials where recruitment is carried out after randomisation and where the recruiter knows the allocation (also scenario 3)

In some trials, the only option is for an individual who knows the allocation of a
patient's cluster to identify and recruit the participants. However, it needs to be
recognised that there is a potential for bias, because knowledge of the allocation
may influence the likelihood of the individual being recruited. Farrin *et al.* (2005)
were the first explicitly to describe an example of bias resulting from this type of
patient identification and recruitment, in the UK BEAM trial, in which clinicians in
the intervention arm were more attuned to identifying relevant participants and
recruited more patients. The intervention also offered the patients treatment options
which would not have been so readily available outside the trial. In contrast the
Change of Heart trial (Steptoe *et al.*, 1999a) had lower recruitment rates in the

intervention arm. Practice nurses in the intervention practices were trained to offer brief behavioural counselling to reduce smoking and dietary fat intake and to increase regular physical activity among those at increased risk of coronary heart disease. Lack of confidence in their ability to influence patients (Steptoe *et al.*, 1999b), as well as increasing workload, probably contributed to the low recruitment rate in the intervention practices. More recently, Kendrick *et al.* (2005) recruited pregnant women to a trial of education by midwives and health visitors to reduce baby walker use. In this trial midwives recruiting the women knew the allocation of the practice. In the trial report, similar percentages of women from each intervention arm agreed to take part. The possibility of bias was recognised in the discussion, but thought to be unimportant to the interpretation of the results. It is, however, unwise to conclude that no bias has occurred if the numbers in the two arms are balanced, since balance in numbers does not necessarily imply balance in characteristics.

2.3.5   Identification and recruitment bias: Summary

In the previous sections we have presented a variety of scenarios and discussed ways of reducing the possibility of bias for each. Figure 2.2 gives a flowchart to assess the potential for bias for various different ways of identifying and recruiting participants.

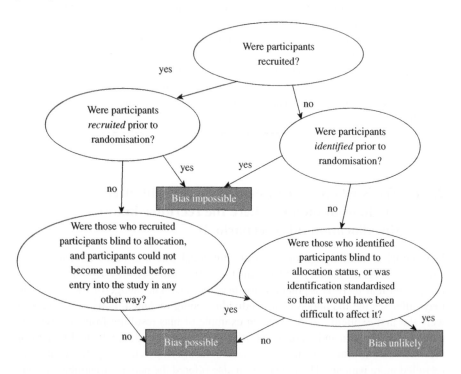

Figure 2.2   Flow chart to estimate the potential for identification and recruitment bias.

2.4   Retention of participants in the trial

In all randomised trials, high numbers of participants dropping out of the trial after randomisation will increase the possibility of bias, particularly if the characteristics of participants dropping out are different in the two intervention arms. At the recruitment stage there can be a tension between selecting only those participants who are most likely to continue in the study, and being more inclusive and therefore more generalisable. At the follow-up stage, having to complete long questionnaires or attend a facility for physical examination or undergo blood tests can all reduce follow-up rates. Comprehensive information at the outset may help to ensure that those who consent are fully aware of how burdensome the follow-up will be, but may deter others from participating. This will reduce the external validity of the trial, particularly if it is the data collection rather than the intervention that is the reason for poor follow-up rates. In cluster randomised trials these factors can be applied to both the clusters and the individual members of the cluster, but when the cluster withdraws then all the members withdraw as well. However, in practice the risk of clusters dropping out of a trial is in general small. Drop outs are discussed in more detail in Section 7.5.

2.5   Summary

The choice of control and intervention, methods of patient and practice recruitment, ways in which consent is obtained, loss to follow-up and adherence of professionals to trial protocol can all affect the validity and hence usefulness of the results of a cluster randomised trial. It is important to consider all of these aspects of a trial carefully at the design stage. They cannot be considered in isolation from the design of the intervention itself, however; the next chapter deals with this.

References

Avery, A.J., Rodgers, S., Cantrill, J.A. *et al.* (2009) Protocol for the PINCER trial: a cluster randomised trial comparing the effectiveness of a pharmacist-led IT-based intervention with simple feedback in reducing rates of clinically important errors in medicines management in general practices. *Trials*, **10**, 28.

Azad, K., Barnett, S., Banerjee, B. *et al.* (2010) Effect of scaling up women's groups on birth outcomes in three rural districts in Bangladesh: a cluster-randomised controlled trial. *Lancet*, **375**, 1193–1202.

BMJ (1996) The Nuremberg Code (1947). *BMJ*, **313**, 1448.

Bower, P., Wallace, P., Ward, E. *et al.* (2009) Improving recruitment to health research in primary care. *Fam. Pract.*, **26**, 391–397.

Cappuccio, F.P., Kerry, S.M., Micah, F.B. *et al.* (2006) A community programme to reduce salt intake and blood pressure in Ghana [ISRCTN88789643]. *BMC Public Health*, **6**, 13.

DiGuiseppi, C., Roberts, I., Wade, A. *et al.* (2002) Incidence of fires and related injuries after giving out free smoke alarms: cluster randomised controlled trial. *BMJ*, **325** (7371), 995.

Edwards, S.J., Braunholtz, D.A., Lilford, R.J. *et al.* (1999) Ethical issues in the design and conduct of cluster randomised controlled trials. *BMJ*, **318**, 1407–1409.

Eldridge, S., Ashby, D. and Feder, G.S. (2005) Informed patient consent to participation in cluster randomized trials: an empirical exploration of trials in primary care. *Clin. Trials*, **2**, 91–98.

Eldridge, S., Ashby, D., Bennett, C. *et al.* (2008) Internal and external validity of cluster randomised trials: systematic review of recent trials. *BMJ*, **336** (7649), 876–880.

Eldridge, S., Kerry, S. and Torgerson, D.J. (2009) Bias in identifying and recruiting participants in cluster randomised trials: what can be done? *BMJ*, **339**, b4006.

Farrin, A., Russell, I., Torgerson, D. *et al.* (2005) Differential recruitment in a cluster randomized trial in primary care: the experience of the UK back pain, exercise, active management and manipulation (UK BEAM) feasibility study. *Clin. Trials*, **2** (2), 119–124.

Godwin, M., Ruhland, L., Casson, I. *et al.* (2003) Pragmatic controlled clinical trials in primary care: the struggle between external and internal validity. *BMC Med. Res. Methodol.*, **3**, 28.

Gregory, A., Ramsay, J., Agnew-Davies, R. *et al.* (2010) Primary care Identification and Referral to Improve Safety of women experiencing domestic violence (IRIS): protocol for a pragmatic cluster randomised controlled trial. *BMC Public Health*, **10**, 54.

Griffiths, C., Foster, G., Barnes, N. *et al.* (2004) Specialist nurse intervention to reduce unscheduled asthma care in a deprived multiethnic area: the east London randomised controlled trial for high risk asthma (ELECTRA). *BMJ*, **328** (7432), 144.

Hutton, J.L. (2001) Are distinctive ethical principles required for cluster randomized controlled trials? *Stat. Med.*, **20**, 473–488.

Jafar, T.H., Hatcher, J., Poulter, N. *et al.* (2009) Community-based interventions to promote blood pressure control in a developing country. A cluster randomized trial. *Ann. Intern. Med.*, **151**, 593–601.

Jolly, K., Bradley, F., Sharp, S. *et al.* (1999) Randomised controlled trial of follow up care in general practice of patients with myocardial infarction and angina: final results of the Southampton heart integrated care project (SHIP). *BMJ*, **318**, 706–711.

Kendrick, D., Illingworth, R., Woods, A. *et al.* (2005) Promoting child safety in primary care: a cluster randomised controlled trial to reduce baby walker use. *Br. J. Gen. Pract.*, **55** (517), 582–588.

Kinmonth, A.L., Woodcock, A., Griffin, S. *et al.* (1998) The Diabetes Care from Diagnosis Research Team. Randomised controlled trial of patient centred care of diabetes in general practice: impact on current wellbeing and future disease risk. *BMJ*, **317** (7167), 1202–1208.

Kirkwood, B.R., Hurt, L., Amenga-Etego, S. *et al.* (2010) Effect of vitamin A supplementation in women of reproductive age on maternal survival in Ghana (ObaapaVitA): a cluster-randomised, placebo-controlled trial. *Lancet*, **375** (9726), 1640–1649.

Little, P. and Williamson, I. (1997) Informed consent in medical research. *BMJ*, **314**, 1478.

Little, P., Williamson, I., Warner, G. *et al.* (1997) Open randomised trial of prescribing strategies for sore throat. *BMJ*, **314**, 722–727.

Medical Research Council (2002) *Cluster Randomised Trials: Methodological and Ethical Considerations*. MRC Clinical Trials Series, Medical Research Council, London.

Merritt, R.A., Price, J.A., Mollison, J. *et al.* (2007) A cluster randomized controlled trial to assess the effectiveness of an intervention to educate students about depression. *Psychol. Med.*, **37**, 363–372.

Mohan, P., Iyengar, S.D., Martines, J. *et al.* (2004) Impact of counselling on careseeking behaviour in families with sick children: cluster randomised trial in rural India. *BMJ*, **329**, 266.

Onwujekwe, O., Shu, E. and Okonkwo, P. (1999) Can community leaders' preferences be used to proxy those of the community as a whole? *J. Health Serv. Res. Policy*, **4**, 133–138.

Osrin, D., Azad, K., Fernandez, A. *et al.* (2009) Ethical challenges in cluster randomized controlled trials: experiences from public health interventions in Africa and Asia. *Bull. World Health Organ.*, **87**, 772–779.

Puffer, S., Torgerson, D. and Watson, J. (2003) Evidence for risk of bias in cluster randomised trials: review of recent trials published in three general medical journals. *BMJ*, **327** (7418), 785–789.

Rothwell, P.M. (2005) External validity of randomised controlled trials: 'To whom do the results of this trial apply?'. *Lancet*, **365**, 82–93.

Slowther, A., Boynton, P. and Shaw, S. (2006) Research governance: ethical issues. *J. R. Soc. Med.*, **99**, 65–72.

Smith, S., Bury, G., O'Leary, M. *et al.* (2004) The North Dublin randomized controlled trial of structured diabetes shared care. *Fam. Pract.*, **21**, 39–45.

Sondergaard, J., Hansen, D.G., Aarslev, P. *et al.* (2006) A multifaceted intervention according to the Audit Project Odense method improved secondary prevention of ischemic heart disease: a randomised controlled trial. *Fam. Pract.*, **23**, 198–202.

Steptoe, A., Doherty, S., Rink, E. *et al.* (1999a) Behavioural counselling in general practice for the promotion of healthy behaviour among adults at increased risk of coronary heart disease: randomised trial. *BMJ*, **319**, 943–948.

Steptoe, A., Doherty, S., Kendrick, T. *et al.* (1999b) Attitudes to cardiovascular health promotion among GPs and practice nurses. *Fam. Pract.*, **16**, 158–163.

PG(36; Tripathy, Nair, Barnett et al; 2010)Tripathy, P., Nair, N., Barnett, S. *et al.* (2010) Effect of a participatory intervention with women's groups on birth outcomes and maternal depression in Jharkhand and Orissa, India: a cluster-randomised controlled trial. *Lancet*, **375**, 1182–1192.

Underwood, M., Eldridge, S., Lamb, S. *et al.* (2011) The OPERA trial: protocol for a randomised trial of an exercise intervention for older people in residential and nursing accommodation. *Trials*, **12**, 27.

Wood, D.A., Kinmonth, A.L., Davies, G.A. *et al.* (1994) Randomised controlled trial evaluating cardiovascular screening and intervention in general practice: principal results of British family heart study. *BMJ*, **308**, 313–320.

World Medical Association (1996) Declaration of Helsinki. *BMJ*, **313**, 1449–1450.

3

Designing interventions

In this chapter we consider the design of interventions in cluster randomised trials. Results from previous cluster randomised trials suggest that the interventions they evaluated were often ineffective or only minimally effective; it is possible that better designed interventions might have been more effective. We begin this chapter by discussing evidence for lack of effectiveness of interventions. Most of the interventions in these trials can be classed as complex, where 'complex' has a particular interpretation, as we describe in Section 3.2. The key guidance on how to improve the design of complex interventions comes from the UK Medical Research Council (MRC) (Campbell *et al.*, 2000; Craig *et al.*, 2008). In Section 3.3 we outline this guidance. The original guidance (Campbell *et al.*, 2000) identifies three separate phases in the development of complex interventions, although it is generally accepted now that these 'phases' are not necessarily distinct or sequential, but rather represent three elements that should be considered in the design of a complex intervention. We describe these three elements in Sections 3.4 (Identifying evidence for potential intervention effect), 3.5 (Understanding more about intervention components) and 3.6 (Developing the optimum intervention and study design).

In developing any intervention it is important to be able to define exactly what the intervention is, because this ensures correct interpretation of the results. For drug trials definition of the intervention is usually straightforward, but for the types of intervention evaluated in cluster randomised trials it often requires more thought. In Section 3.7 we draw on some examples presented in earlier sections of this chapter to illustrate this.

A Practical Guide to Cluster Randomised Trials in Health Services Research, First Edition.
Sandra Eldridge and Sally Kerry.
© 2012 John Wiley & Sons, Ltd. Published 2012 by John Wiley & Sons, Ltd.

3.1   Lack of effectiveness of interventions evaluated in cluster randomised trials

An example of lack of effectiveness of interventions evaluated in cluster randomised trials comes from the COMMIT trial (Table 3.1), one of the earliest community intervention trials, in which an intervention to increase smoking cessation rates was introduced through multiple community sectors and organisations in 11 communities. Although primarily aimed at heavy smokers, there was no statistically significant effect on their quit rate at the end of the four-year intervention; there was a small effect on the quit rates of moderate-to-light smokers. The authors of the trial report concluded that new policies and programmes might be required to reach heavy smokers. Later trials embedded in the health service, such as the SHIP trial (Table 3.2), have drawn similar conclusions. In this trial, the intervention appeared

Table 3.1   COMMIT: community-based intervention to increase smoking quit rates.

Aim: To assess whether a community-level, multi-channel, 4-year intervention would increase quit rates among cigarette smokers, with heavy smokers (≥ 25 cigarettes per day) a priority
Location and type of cluster: Communities (20 in United States, 2 in Canada)
Number of participants: 20 347
Interventions: (i) Control: no intervention (ii) Intervention: each community formed a community board. The intervention focused on public education, healthcare providers, worksite and other organisations, and cessation resources
Primary outcome: Smoking quit rates

Source: COMMIT Research Group (1995).

Table 3.2   SHIP: support following myocardial infarction.

Aim: To assess the effectiveness of a programme to coordinate and support follow-up care in general practice after a hospital diagnosis of myocardial infarction or angina
Location and type of cluster: UK general practices
Interventions: (i) Control: usual care (ii) Intervention: programme to coordinate preventive care led by specialist liaison nurses, which sought to improve communication between hospital and general practice and to encourage general practice nurses to provide structured follow-up
Main outcomes: Serum total cholesterol concentration, blood pressure, distance walked in six minutes, confirmed smoking cessation, and body mass index measured at one-year follow-up

Source: Jolly *et al.* (1999).

effective in promoting follow-up in general practice, but did not improve health outcomes, and the authors concluded that simply coordinating and supporting existing National Health Service care was insufficient to change health; greater efforts to institute a systematic approach to caring for these patients were needed.

There may be many reasons why interventions are not successful. Indeed it is the task of a randomised controlled trial to identify whether interventions are successful or not; so lack of success should not surprise us. Not only are interventions often unsuccessful, however, but investigators frequently identify problems with their interventions after the event, or state that their interventions were not 'strong enough'. The two trials mentioned above are examples of this. A similar result in a drug trial might suggest that a different formulation or a stronger dose is needed. The equivalent for most of the interventions used in cluster randomised trials is better, stronger, interventions or, as suggested in Section 1.3.4, more effective implementation of interventions. In recent years this area has attracted a great deal of attention. The key guidance on developing and evaluating complex interventions comes from the UK MRC's framework for developing complex interventions (Campbell *et al.*, 2000), and updated guidance based on this framework (Craig *et al.*, 2008).

3.2   What is a complex intervention?

In the original UK MRC framework (Campbell *et al.*, 2000), complex interventions are defined as being 'built up from a number of components, which may act both independently and interdependently.' The authors based this on a dictionary definition of the word 'complex'. However, once you start to unpick this definition it becomes difficult to interpret because of the difficulty of precisely defining components. It has also been suggested that any intervention mediated by the action of human beings is a complex intervention, or that any non-drug intervention is a complex intervention. None of these three definitions is wholly satisfactory. Nevertheless, in spite of the difficulty of defining complex interventions, it is relatively easy to recognise those interventions generally denoted as complex; usually they have some element of each of these three definitions, as we discuss below. There is now a growing science around complex interventions.

Our contention is that almost all interventions evaluated in cluster randomised trials in health services research are complex, having components that could be administered separately, and/or effects mediated by human action to a larger extent than some other interventions, and/or being non-pharmacological. In Tables 3.3–3.5 we describe several interventions evaluated in cluster randomised trials. Not only do all three interventions exhibit all three of these qualities, but they all aim in some way or another to change professional and patient behaviour and/or to change the organisation of healthcare; a common aim of complex interventions. The descriptions of these interventions in the tables are adapted from the protocols or funding applications for the trials, which usually contain more detail than a trial report published in a journal.

Table 3.3   FIAT: financial incentives for patients with psychotic disorders to take medication.

Aim: To test the use of financial incentives to achieve medication adherence for patients with psychotic disorders living in the community

Location and type of cluster: UK assertive outreach teams (AOTs)

Number of clusters: 67 randomised

Interventions: (i) Control: usual care (ii) Intervention: see below

Primary outcomes: Adherence to antipsychotic maintenance medication

Detailed description of intervention:

(i)   *Financial incentives:* Patients in the AOTs allocated to the intervention were offered a financial incentive for each injection of antipsychotic medication for a 12-month period. Patients received £15 for one injection, with the total sum not exceeding £60 for a 4-week period (the maximum number of injections is 4 per month). The administering clinician gave money in cash directly after the injection. Patients signed a receipt

(ii)   *Training programme:* Members of the research team attended meetings of each AOT in the intervention group, and discussed the practice of offering financial incentives and the nature of the study. Following that there was a brief training programme on the exact procedure

(iii)   *Written manual:* The procedure of the intervention was outlined in a written manual. All teams were regularly visited by the research assistants and, if required, also by members of the team of applicants. The procedure was discussed at a team meeting after 6 months of the intervention period

---

Source: Priebe *et al.* (2009).

Table 3.4   IRIS: training to increase identification and referral of victims of domestic violence.

Aim: To test the effectiveness of a training and support programme for general practice teams, targeting identification of women experiencing domestic violence and referral to specialist domestic violence advocates

Location and type of cluster: UK general practices

Number of clusters: 51 randomised, 48 analysed

Interventions: (i) Control: usual care (ii) Intervention: see below

Primary outcome: Number of recorded referrals of women aged over 16 years to domestic violence agencies recorded in general practice records

Detailed description of intervention:

(Continued)

Table 3.4   (*Continued*)

(i) *Training:* Two 2-hour multidisciplinary training sessions, scheduled at lunchtime on practice premises, targeted at the clinical team: general practitioners, directly employed practice staff (practice nurses and counsellors), and those employed by Primary Care Trusts (midwives, health visitors, district nurses) who have contact with patients registered in the practice. The training sessions were designed to address the expressed and tacit barriers to improving the response of clinicians to women experiencing abuse, through improved identification, support and referral to specialist agencies. They incorporated case studies and role-play in relation to asking about violence and responding appropriately. They were delivered by an advocate educator based in one of the two collaborating specialists' agencies, a clinical psychologist specializing in domestic violence and an academic general practitioner

(ii) *Advocate educator:* A single advocate educator in each of two non-statutory domestic violence agencies, Nia Project (East London) and Next Link (Bristol), combined a training and support role to the practices with provision of advocacy to women referred from the practices. The training sessions were followed by periodic contact with the practice in clinical meetings, feeding back anonymised practice data on disclosure and referral to the advocacy service, and reinforcing guidance on good practice with regard to domestic violence, as well as ad hoc telephone conversations with clinicians about referrals or advice. One-hour meetings with administrative staff highlighted issues of confidentiality and safety for patients experiencing abuse, and introduced the IRIS information materials signposting domestic violence agencies. Ongoing support to clinicians in the practices was provided by the named advocate educator, with the aim of consolidating the initial training

(iii) *Practice champion:* Intervention practices were asked to identify a 'champion' for the project; with the agreement of the practice, a member of staff from any of the clinical disciplines was invited to attend additional training about domestic violence and to integrate this into the work of the practice

(iv) *Pop-up template:* Linked to diagnoses (such as depression, anxiety, irritable bowel syndrome, pelvic pain and assault), this acted as a prompt to remind clinicians to ask questions about domestic violence and to record this in the electronic medical record

(v) *Referral pathway:* An explicit referral pathway to the named advocate in the Nia Project or Next Link

(vi) *Publicity materials in practices:* Materials about domestic violence were visible in the practices (waiting rooms and women's toilets)

Source: Gregory *et al.* (2010).

Table 3.5   OPERA: physical activity in residential homes to prevent depression.

Aim: To evaluate the impact on depression of a whole-home intervention to increase physical activity among older people

Location and type of cluster: UK residential homes for older people

Number of clusters and individual participants: 78 randomised and analysed; 1060 participants recruited

Interventions: (i) Control: depression awareness programme delivered by research nurses (ii) Intervention: depression awareness programme delivered by physiotherapists, plus physical activation programme (see below)

Primary outcomes: Prevalence of depression (Geriatric Depression Scale) at 12 months, and change in depression score

Detailed description of intervention:

(i) *Depression awareness programme:* Staff education package on identifying and managing depression in older people

(ii) *Physical activation programme: (a) For staff:* Physiotherapists promoted safe physical activity by improving knowledge and awareness of the benefits of physical activity in the staff, residents and relatives; the main activity targeted in the physical activation programme was safe walking. They also provided an individualised review of mobility safety; ensured that appropriate and safe walking aids (including grab rails where needed) and footwear were available to each individual, and reinforced the need for use; and provided advice on activation strategies for individual clients, including the level of supervision needed, and support for the staff and residents in their implementation. With the Director of Nursing/Home Manager, they reviewed the policies and strategies in place to promote physical activity; where appropriate, they involved volunteers and families in the supervision and promotion of physical activity. *(b) For residents:* All residents were encouraged to attend twice-weekly group exercise sessions in the communal space of the homes. The groups were led by a physiotherapist experienced in managing frail older people. Scheduling was undertaken carefully to facilitate maximal likelihood of attendance. The physiotherapists used mixed training stimuli, combining aerobic conditioning, progressive strength and balance training and utilising music and rhythmic, simple movement patterns. The groups lasted 40 minutes to an hour depending on the tolerance and ability of the group. Prior to the groups, the physiotherapists obtained agreement to participate, gave each participant a brief risk assessment; determined any absolute contraindications to exercise, and the optimal exercise intensity for each participant. In larger homes, where there was a need for several groups, physiotherapists grouped together participants with similar levels of ability, and set the intensity of exercise accordingly.

Source: Underwood *et al.* (2011).

3.3   Phases in the development of a complex intervention

The MRC framework for complex interventions sets out a process of designing interventions to be evaluated, similar to the process for developing and testing drugs via phase I, phase II and phase III trials. The original MRC framework paper lists five phases of the development of a complex intervention: pre-clinical phase (using theory), phase I (modelling), phase II (exploratory trial), phase III (definitive randomised controlled trial) and phase IV (long term implementation) (Campbell *et al.*, 2000). Table 3.6 shows the tasks that a researcher is expected to carry out at each phase, but a more flexible approach is advocated in Campbell *et al.*, (2007). The authors state that they found it helpful to consider the first three phases as 'all part of one larger activity' geared towards designing an intervention for evaluation in a randomised controlled trial. A subsequent update to the framework takes the same view that the phases are not necessarily sequential, and identifies a number of other issues which the original framework did not address, amongst them a lack of evidence for its recommendations and limited guidance on how to approach developmental and implementation phases (Craig *et al.*, 2008).

While the MRC framework has now become the definitive guide for those wishing to develop complex interventions in a structured way, it would be incorrect to assume that no complex interventions prior to the framework were developed rigorously. For example, the REACT trial (Luepker *et al.*, 2000) used similar principles to those set out in the framework prior to the framework's publication. The investigators used social cognition theory and self-regulatory theory to underpin their intervention. They also used focus groups and community profiling to develop their intervention and an iterative process of intervention development. Those who follow the MRC framework undertake similar activities in their development work, as outlined in the following sections.

While there is general agreement that developing a complex intervention may not follow a straightforward linear process, here we discuss the three phases relevant to developing a complex intervention – pre-clinical, modelling and exploratory – in separate sections because these phases have distinct purposes. It is not necessary to identify three separate sequential activities in any intervention development, but it is important to make sure that the aims of each phase have been addressed in any pre-trial work.

3.4   Identifying evidence for potential intervention effect (pre-clinical phase)

The purpose of the pre-clinical phase is to 'identify evidence that the intervention might have the desired effect' (Campbell *et al.*, 2000). Most investigators look for evidence for the potential effect of an intervention in empirical literature. This is often via one or more focused systematic literature reviews. For example, in

Table 3.6 Phases of the MRC framework for complex interventions.

Pre-clinical	Phase I	Phase II	Phase III	Phase IV
Theory	Modelling	Exploratory trial	Definitive randomised controlled trial	Long term implementation
Explore relevant theory to ensure best choice of intervention and hypothesis and to predict major confounders and strategic design issues	Identify the components of the intervention and the underlying mechanisms by which they will influence outcomes to provide evidence that you can predict how they relate to and interact with each other	Describe the constant and variable components of a replicable intervention and a feasible protocol for comparing the intervention with an appropriate alternative	Compare a fully defined intervention with an appropriate alternative using a protocol that is theoretically defensible, reproducible, and adequately controlled, in a study with appropriate statistical power	Determine whether others can reliably replicate your intervention and results in uncontrolled settings over the long term

Source: Campbell *et al.* (2000).

Table 3.7   Multifaceted intervention to optimise antibiotic use in nursing homes.

Aim: To assess whether a multifaceted intervention can reduce the number of prescriptions for antimicrobials for suspected urinary tract infections in residents of nursing homes

Location and type of cluster: Nursing homes in Canada and the United States

Number of clusters: 24 (4217 residents)

Interventions: (i) Control: no intervention (ii) Intervention: presentation of diagnostic and therapeutic algorithms to nurses and physicians in homes and relevant general practitioners; nursing home member of staff acted as champion; regular visits to nursing homes by research teams

Primary outcome: Number of prescriptions for antimicrobials

Pre-clinical phase: From the systematic review there were no data to support reducing antibiotics for lower respiratory or skin infections, but there were data to support reducing antibiotic use for urinary indications

Sources: Loeb *et al.* (2005), Loeb (2002).

Table 3.8   Within-practice meetings to alter general practitioner referral behaviour.

Aim: To assess the effectiveness of in-practice educational meetings in reducing general practice referral rates

Location and type of cluster: UK general practices

Number of clusters: 26

Interventions: (i) Control: usual care (ii) Intervention: in-practice meetings

Primary outcome: Referral rate change

Pre-clinical phase: Literature review showed that peer discussion, rehearsal of communication skills, patient-centred activities, feedback and educational meetings can be effective in changing doctors' behaviour

Source: Rowlands, Sims and Kerry (2005).

preparation for a trial evaluating an intervention to optimise antibiotic use in nursing homes (Table 3.7), Loeb (2002) carried out a systematic literature review for data on strategies to reduce antibiotic use. Similarly, in preparation for a trial examining the effectiveness of in-practice meetings for reducing referral rates, investigators reviewed literature on factors that can change clinical practice (Table 3.8). Prior to the IRIS trial (Table 3.4), investigators conducted systematic reviews of (i) interventions to improve response of healthcare providers to abused women, (ii) interventions to improve outcomes for abused women by providing advocacy, and (iii) studies of what abused women want from health providers. Whether investigators choose to conduct one systematic review or several will depend on the evidence they require to identify the potential effect of an intervention.

It is also recommended, and now common, to adopt a specific theoretical framework in this phase; for example, in the trial of in-practice meetings to alter general practitioner referral behaviour (Table 3.8), investigators adopted androgogic education principles as a basis for alteration of referral behaviour. The principles are that learning is learner centred; educational needs and approaches are identified by the learner; and educational needs are usually best met using small-group work and role-play rather than more traditional approaches. Combining this theoretical perspective with evidence from literature, they developed a hypothesis that in-practice educational meetings would alter general practitioner referral behaviour as evidenced by reduction in referral rates.

Many theories are available on which to base a non-pharmacological intervention. For interventions that attempt to change behaviour, there is a growing body of literature regarding theory. Some of it is useful in facilitating the design of interventions. In particular, Michie *et al.* (2008) explored how behaviour change techniques relate to desired changes in behaviour, mapping specific techniques to specific behaviour changes. For example, appropriate techniques to change skills include goal setting, monitoring, rewards, and modelling of skills by others. If investigators can identify a behaviour that they wish to change, this mapping work can be used to identify appropriate behaviour change techniques.

In general it is good practice to use both theory and empirical evidence to develop ideas about possible interventions, because they can provide complementary insights. In addition, where these two approaches concur there is stronger evidence for a potential positive effect. Where they conflict, this may indicate that further investigation of existing literature is necessary before a possible intervention can be suggested.

3.5   Understanding more about intervention components (modelling phase)

The purpose of the modelling phase is to 'improve the understanding of the components of an intervention and their interrelationships' to identify 'the components of the intervention and the underlying mechanisms by which they will influence outcomes to provide evidence that you can predict how they relate to and interact with each other' (Campbell *et al.*, 2000). This is open to a wide range of interpretations, perhaps not surprisingly, because the aim is to understand more about components, and understanding can be facilitated in a number of ways.

Many investigators use qualitative methods to understand more about the components of an intervention, the mechanisms by which they will influence outcomes, and their interactions. In the development of the intervention to reduce antibiotic prescribing in nursing homes (Table 3.7), the investigators gathered opinions from focus groups of physicians and nurses involved in the process of prescribing antibiotics. In the Diabetes Manual trial (Table 3.9), diabetes professionals were interviewed to gather their views on self-management (Sturt *et al.*, 2006). We describe this and other development work carried out for this trial in more detail in Section 4.1.

Questionnaires can also be used in this phase. In developing the Diabetes Manual (Table 3.9), investigators used questionnaires to elicit the views of

Table 3.9 Diabetes Manual trial: manual and structured care to improve outcomes.

Aim: To determine the effects of the Diabetes Manual on glycaemic control, diabetes-related distress and confidence to self-care of patients with type 2 diabetes

Location and type of cluster: UK general practices

Interventions: (i) Control: usual care (ii) Intervention: education of nurses, followed by one-to-one structured education of patients via a self-completed manual and nurse support, and audiotapes

Primary outcome: HbA1c level

Modelling work: Interviews with professionals and questionnaires with patients eliciting views about self-management contributed to the development of the Diabetes Manual

---

Sources: Sturt *et al.* (2008), Sturt *et al.* (2006).

healthcare professionals and people with type 2 diabetes on self-management interventions (Sturt *et al.*, 2006).

Alongside eliciting views on the intervention, the modelling phase may also involve considerable thought and discussion by the team developing the intervention and/or the construction of a 'causal' or 'logic' model. Hardeman, Sutton and Griffin (2005) describe 'the development of a specific causal model to guide the design of a programme to support behaviour change.' The causal modelling described covers both the pre-clinical and modelling phases of the MRC framework. Although the intervention described was not evaluated in a cluster randomised trial, the principles illustrated are applicable to the pre-trial work for most complex interventions. Causal modelling involves the mapping of mechanisms and pathways expected to lead from the intervention to the outcome. This can often be depicted by a flow chart.

For an intervention designed to reduce falls and fractures in older people, Eldridge *et al.* (2005) used a flow chart to represent the flow of older people through stages of the intervention leading to treatment which could potentially reduce falls and fractures. They attached quantitative data from routine sources and from a pilot study to the transitions in the flow chart and, using these data, showed that there was little chance of this intervention being successful. Partly as a result of this finding, the intervention was never evaluated in a full trial. Because much of the data used in the modelling exercise was obtained from a pilot study, this work encompassed both the modelling and exploratory stages outlined by the MRC framework. This pilot study was mentioned in Section 1.3.4 and we discuss it further in Section 4.2.2.

A salutary lesson about the importance of modelling in developing an intervention is provided by Rowlands, Sims and Kerry (2005). The investigators proceeded to a full trial of an intervention to alter general practitioner referral behaviour on the basis of a preliminary hypothesis and a pilot study in one general practice which indicated a 25% reduction in practice referral rates. The full trial did not show any evidence of an effect, however. The authors conducted a qualitative study alongside their full trial which highlighted the complexity of the settings in which the trial took place. They suggest that if they had modelled the intervention before proceeding to a full trial they might have found out some of this information sooner, which would have enabled them to alter both the design and implementation of the intervention. They describe how they might have modelled the intervention starting with an explicit articulation of the assumptions inherent in the intervention design. Articulation and checking of assumptions is an important part of modelling an intervention.

3.6   Developing the optimum intervention and study design (exploratory trial phase)

The exploratory trial phase is designed to 'develop the optimum intervention and study design' (Campbell *et al.*, 2000). The goal of most trial investigators is to develop an intervention that is both effective and easily implemented in routine practice. Designing an optimum intervention should therefore consider both of these aspects. Most studies used to develop the optimum intervention and study design are pilot trials in which investigators implement an intervention they have developed to assess its feasibility, whether it needs refining, and whether it is worth proceeding to a full trial. Other features of the pilot trial such as the design, outcomes, population and setting are usually as close as possible to what is expected to occur in the main trial, so that the feasibility of all aspects can be assessed. Thus, such pilot trials are generally used for more than optimising the intervention. We describe some examples of refining and optimising interventions via pilot studies more fully in the next chapter (Section 4.2.2), which focuses on pilot studies. Here we focus on other designs for exploratory trials and a framework for understanding issues of implementation.

Intervention modelling experiments are an alternative to a standard pilot study for developing optimum interventions. These experiments mimic many aspects of a planned trial but involve measuring an intermediate outcome regarding health professional behaviour rather than the eventual planned outcome measured on an individual trial participant. For example, Bonetti *et al.* (2005) conducted an intervention modelling experiment to see whether audit and feedback and/or educational reminder messages influenced behavioural intentions or simulated behaviour of general practitioners in England and Scotland in relation to lumbar x-rays. Individual patients were not involved, which made the experiment considerably cheaper than a full trial. The assumption was that the general practitioner outcomes might be (at least partially) predictive of patient outcomes. In fact in this example that was not true; the experiment provided evidence for effectiveness of the interventions on practitioner behaviour, but neither intervention was effective in changing patient outcomes in a full trial involving patients. To illustrate the method, Bonetti *et al.* conducted this particular experiment *after* conducting a full trial involving patients.

Nevertheless, they present intervention modelling experiments as a means of selecting interventions more likely to be successful prior to a full trial.

Fractional factorial trials are another type of exploratory trial that can be used prior to a full trial to optimise interventions. Each randomised unit receives a combination of various potential intervention components. In a full factorial design (Section 5.3.3), all possible combinations are represented, but in a fractional factorial design only some are represented. The combinations are chosen to maximise statistical efficiency bearing in mind the most important questions the investigators wish to answer. The results enable investigators to screen out the least effective from amongst a pool of potential intervention components (Collins *et al.*, 2005; Chakraborty *et al.*, 2009), and can therefore be particularly useful if there is considerable uncertainty about which components might be most effective in combination. To date, intervention modelling and fractional factorial experiments have been little used in the context of optimising interventions.

Normalisation process theory, developed by Carl May, considers the issues that need to be addressed to enable successful implementation and integration of interventions into routine practice (May *et al.*, 2009; Murray *et al.*, 2010). This theory can be useful in helping researchers to think through issues regarding implementation at the design stage of their trial. The theory is based on three propositions shown in Box 3.1. One example of an application of this theory to the development of an intervention to be evaluated in a cluster randomised trial is illustrated by Kennedy *et al.* (2010). In an exploratory study involving two general practices in the UK, investigators developed the WISE (Whole system Informing Self-management Engagement) approach to implement appropriate self-care support for those with long term conditions. Normalisation process theory was used to focus on the ease

---

1. Material practices become routinely embedded in social contexts as the result of people working, individually and collectively, to implement them. From this follows specific propositions [that define] a mechanism (i.e. embedding is dependent on socially patterned implementation work).

2. The work of implementation is operationalized through four generative mechanisms (coherence, cognitive participation, collective action and reflexive monitoring). From this follows specific propositions that define components of a mechanism (i.e. those factors that shape socially patterned implementation work).

3. The production and reproduction of a material practice requires continuous investment by agents in ensembles of action that carry forward in time and space. From this follow specific propositions that define actors' investments in a mechanism (i.e. how the mechanism is energized).

Source: May *et al.* (2009).

Box 3.1   General propositions of normalisation process theory of implementing and embedding the intervention in practice, specifically on the work that staff involved were doing and how they were doing it. The development of the intervention drew on qualitative work carried out in the exploratory study, with normalisation process theory as the underlying framework.

3.7   What is the intervention?

One key question to be addressed in designing any intervention is 'Exactly what is the intervention?' In a cluster randomised trial this is not always straightforward to answer, because the intervention being evaluated very often aims to change behaviour and is multi-component and multi-layered (aimed partly at clusters and partly at individuals). In Section 2.2.2 we classified interventions into four categories: individual-cluster, professional-cluster, external-cluster and cluster-cluster. For the purposes of the discussion in this section, we treat the last three of these categories as one group of interventions all aimed at the cluster. We distinguish intervention components in this group from components aimed at individual participants.

The multi-layered nature of many interventions evaluated in cluster randomised trials is illustrated in the trials described in Section 3.2. In the FIAT trial (Table 3.3), *patients* were offered financial incentives by assertive outreach teams (AOTs), and *clusters* were given training. Similarly in the OPERA trial (Table 3.5), the depression awareness and staff-orientated physical activation programmes were aimed at the *clusters*, while the exercise classes delivered by physiotherapists were aimed at *individual participants*. It is important that in any description of an intervention all components aimed at clusters and individuals are included.

In some cases the intervention will be entirely or largely aimed at the clusters. For example, in the IRIS trial (Table 3.4), training, provision of advocate educator, identification of practice champion, pop-up template, and introduction of new referral pathways were all aimed at the clusters; only the publicity materials in the waiting rooms and toilets were aimed at individual women. In this trial it was expected that professionals in the clusters would change their behaviour towards women, for example screening for domestic violence more often, in response to the training and other intervention components aimed at them. However, this behaviour change, although induced by the intervention, cannot be seen as part of the intervention. A useful distinction here is between change in professional behaviour that is *prescribed* by the intervention (for example, the offer of incentives by the intervention arm AOTs in FIAT), and behaviour change that is *induced* by the intervention but not prescribed, as just described for IRIS. The former can be seen as part of the intervention, but the latter cannot.

Any intervention components that prescribe change impacting directly on participants need to be defined carefully because of the ethical imperative to allow participants choice at the point of treatment. Thus, in FIAT, the financial incentives component prescribed by the intervention is strictly defined as the *offer* of financial incentives, not the financial incentives themselves. Similarly, the intervention component aimed at individual participants in OPERA is the *offer* of exercise classes; residents within the nursing homes retained the option to attend the classes or not.

Finally, if investigators wish to consider the fidelity of the intervention by, for example, monitoring the way the intervention is implemented, this monitoring may induce behaviour change. Two questions then arise. (i) Is this something the investigators wish to pursue? (ii) Are there circumstances in which monitoring should then be seen as part of the intervention? When the purpose of the monitoring is purely to provide evidence of fidelity for reporting purposes, then as long as this can be done in a way which induces as little change in behaviour as possible, it does not need to be seen as part of the intervention. If, however, the purpose of the monitoring is to feed back to professionals in the clusters during the trial in order to maintain fidelity, then this should be seen as part of the intervention. We cover monitoring in more detail in Section 9.4.

3.8   Summary

In this chapter we have described the lack of effectiveness of interventions evaluated in cluster randomised trials, and explained why we think most of these interventions are complex interventions. There is now a growing science around the development and evaluation of complex interventions which we have summarised in relation to developing interventions for cluster randomised trials. Some of the development work can be conducted within pilot or feasibility studies and we describe these in the next chapter.

References

Bonetti, D., Eccles, M., Johnston, M. *et al.* (2005) Guiding the design and selection of interventions to influence the implementation of evidence-based practice: an experimental simulation of a complex intervention trial. *Soc. Sci. Med.*, **60** (9), 2135–2147.

Campbell, M., Fitzpatrick, R., Haines, A. *et al.* (2000) Framework for design and evaluation of complex interventions to improve health. *BMJ*, **321** (7262), 694–696.

Campbell, N.C., Murray, E., Darbyshire, J. *et al.* (2007) Designing and evaluating complex interventions to improve health care. *BMJ*, **334** (7591), 455–459.

Chakraborty, B., Collins, L.M., Strecher, V.J. *et al.* (2009) Developing multicomponent interventions using fractional factorial designs. *Stat. Med.*, **28** (21), 2687–2708.

Collins, L.M., Murphy, S.A., Nair, V.N. *et al.* (2005) A strategy for optimizing and evaluating behavioral interventions. *Ann. Behav. Med.*, **30** (1), 65–73.

COMMIT Research Group (1995) Community Intervention Trial for Smoking Cessation (COMMIT): I. cohort results from a four-year community intervention. *Am. J. Public Health*, **85** (2), 183–192.

Craig, P., Dieppe, P., Macintyre, S. *et al.* (2008) Developing and evaluating complex interventions: the new Medical Research Council guidance. *BMJ*, **337**.

Eldridge, S., Spencer, A., Cryer, C. *et al.* (2005) Modelling a complex intervention is an important precursor to trial design: lessons from studying an intervention to reduce falls-related injuries in older people. *J. Health Serv. Res. Policy*, **10**, 133–142.

Gregory, A., Ramsay, J., Agnew-Davies, R. *et al.* (2010) Primary care Identification and Referral to Improve Safety of women experiencing domestic violence (IRIS): protocol for a pragmatic cluster randomised controlled trial. *BMC Public Health*, **10**, 54.

Hardeman, W., Sutton, S. and Griffin, S. (2005) A causal modelling approach to the development of theory-based behaviour change programmes for trial evaluation. *Health Educ. Res.*, **20** (6), 676–687.

Jolly, K., Bradley, F., Sharp, S. *et al.* (1999) Randomised controlled trial of follow up care in general practice of patients with myocardial infarction and angina: final results of the Southampton heart integrated care project (SHIP). *BMJ*, **318** (7185), 706–711.

Kennedy, A., Chew-Graham, C., Blakeman, T. *et al.* (2010) Delivering the WISE (Whole Systems Informing Self-Management Engagement) training package in primary care: learning from formative evaluation. *Implement. Sci.*, **5**, 7.

Loeb, M., Brazil, K., Lohfeld, L. *et al.* (2005) Effect of a multifaceted intervention on number of antimicrobial prescriptions for suspected urinary tract infections in residents of nursing homes: cluster randomised controlled trial. *BMJ*, **331** (7518), 669.

Loeb, M.B. (2002) Application of the development stages of a cluster randomized trial to a framework for evaluating complex health interventions. *BMC Health Serv. Res.*, **2** (1), 13.

Luepker, R.V., Raczynski, J.M., Osganian, S. *et al.* (2000) Effect of a community intervention on patient delay and emergency medical service use in acute coronary heart disease: The Rapid Early Action for Coronary Treatment (REACT) Trial. *JAMA*, **284** (1), 60–67.

May, C.R., Mair, F., Finch, T. *et al.* (2009) Development of a theory of implementation and integration: normalization process theory. *Implement. Sci.*, **4**, 29.

Michie, S., Johnston, M., Francis, J. *et al.* (2008) From theory to intervention: mapping theoretically derived behavioural determinants to behaviour change techniques. *Appl. Psychol.*, **57** (4), 660–680.

Murray, E., Treweek, S., Pope, C. *et al.* (2010) Normalisation process theory: a framework for developing, evaluating and implementing complex interventions. *BMC Med.*, **8**, 63.

Priebe, S., Burton, A., Ashby, D. *et al.* (2009) Financial incentives to improve adherence to anti-psychotic maintenance medication in non-adherent patients – a cluster randomised controlled trial (FIAT). *BMC Psychiatry*, **9**, 61.

Rowlands, G., Sims, J. and Kerry, S. (2005) A lesson learnt: the importance of modelling in randomized controlled trials for complex interventions in primary care. *Fam. Pract.*, **22** (1), 132–139.

Sturt, J., Taylor, H., Docherty, A. *et al.* (2006) A psychological approach to providing self-management education for people with type 2 diabetes: the Diabetes Manual. *BMC Fam Pract.*, **27** (7), 70.

Sturt, J.A., Whitlock, S., Fox, C. *et al.* (2008) Effects of the Diabetes Manual 1:1 structured education in primary care. *Diabet. Med.*, **25** (6), 722–731.

Underwood, M., Eldridge, S., Lamb, S. *et al.* (2011) The OPERA trial: protocol for a randomised trial of an exercise intervention for older people in residential and nursing accommodation. *Trials*, **12**, 27.

4

Pilot and feasibility studies

So far in this book we have considered the selection and recruitment of individuals (Chapter 2) and the development of the intervention (Chapter 3). These aspects of trial design require good quality information at the planning stage in order to ensure that a trial has a good chance of answering the research question successfully, and that it is internally and externally valid. Information will also be required on the outcomes, and estimates of their variability, both within and between clusters, for the sample size calculations. Many trial designs are based on a number of assumptions which may turn out to be over optimistic when the trial is carried out. Cluster randomised trials tend to be large and expensive, with more assumptions and decisions to be made at the design stage than individually randomised trials, making preliminary work all the more important. We have already touched on this in Chapter 3. In this chapter we will first describe some of the principles of pilot and feasibility studies and then discuss different situations where they may be useful, concentrating on those aspects of particular relevance to cluster randomised trials or complex interventions, and using pilot or feasibility studies from cluster randomised trials as examples.

4.1 What is a pilot study?

At the planning stage, information may be obtained from previous similar trials, systematic reviews, routine data, local sources of information and so on. However, it is likely that there will be some aspects of a trial that would benefit from empirical testing prior to the full trial. A pilot study can be defined as a small scale study conducted in advance of a main research study with the aim of refining or improving the

A Practical Guide to Cluster Randomised Trials in Health Services Research, First Edition.
Sandra Eldridge and Sally Kerry.
© 2012 John Wiley & Sons, Ltd. Published 2012 by John Wiley & Sons, Ltd.

design of the main study or assessing its feasibility. There has been a tendency to describe small trials with limited resources and/or time scales or even small student research projects as 'pilot' studies in order to justify the small sample size or lack of formal power calculations. This is not an appropriate use of the term (Thabane *et al.*, 2010); investigators should always embark on a pilot study with an expectation that a main trial will follow. Nevertheless, because one of the aims of a pilot study is to assess feasibility of a main trial, not all pilot studies result in a main trial. An example of pilot work which resulted in the full trial being abandoned is that reported by Eldridge *et al.* (2005); this pilot study is described in more detail in Section 4.2.2. The publication of the pilot study results allowed the information to be accessible to other researchers who might wish to carry out similar interventions.

A general introduction to good practice in pilot studies is provided by Lancaster, Dodd and Williamson (2004) and Thabane *et al.* (2010). Sometimes there may be a series of feasibility studies testing different aspects of a main trial.

In developing the intervention for the Diabetes Manual trial (Sturt *et al.*, 2005), the researchers carried out a series of small feasibility studies. Firstly, they conducted a needs assessment, using focus groups to find out what diabetic patients would want from an educational intervention package. This was followed by semi-structured interviews with eight healthcare professionals to ascertain their views on self-management interventions, followed by a questionnaire to 300 patients. The Diabetes Manual was then developed, guided by both lay and professional expert panels. Finally, two focus groups of people with type 2 diabetes confirmed that the penultimate draft of the Diabetes Manual had face validity (Sturt *et al.*, 2006). In contrast, investigators may assess different aspects of the trial in a single pilot study, which may be very similar to a small scale version of the main study but with different aims. Pilot studies are particularly important for cluster randomised trials owing to the greater complexity of these trials. They are usually larger and more expensive than pilot studies for individually randomised trials, particularly if they involve more than one cluster.

4.1.1 Is there a difference between pilot studies and feasibility studies?

So far we have used the term 'pilot' study to mean any preliminary study in advance of the main trial; others have used the terms 'pilot' and 'feasibility' interchangeably. Farrin *et al.* (2005) described the UK BEAM pilot as a 'feasibility' study in the title of their publication; while in the abstract they also used the term 'pilot'. However, a useful distinction can be made between the two (Arain *et al.*, 2010). The most helpful definitions are given by The National Institute for Health Services Research Evaluation, Trials and Studies Coordinating Centre (NETSCC, 2011) in the UK, and are shown in Box 4.1. Using these definitions, a feasibility study addresses the question 'Can this study be done?' by looking at the individual components, whereas a pilot study tests whether the components can all work together. A pilot study will usually take place further on in the development process.

Feasibility studies

Feasibility studies are pieces of research done before a main study in order to answer the question 'Can this study be done?' They are used to estimate important parameters that are needed to design the main study.

Pilot studies

Pilot studies are a version of the main study that is run in miniature to test whether the components of the main study can all work together. It is focused on the processes of the main study, for example to ensure recruitment, randomisation, treatment, and follow-up assessments all run smoothly.

Source: NETSCC (2011).

Box 4.1   Definitions of pilot and feasibility studies from NETSCC (2011)

Feasibility studies for randomised controlled trials need not themselves be randomised, unless assessing the randomisation process. When a pilot or feasibility study is randomised, it may be advantageous to set the allocation ratio so that more clusters are randomised to the intervention arm to obtain more information about the intervention.

4.1.2   Internal and external pilot studies

A pilot study may be the first phase of a main trial, and data from the pilot phase may contribute to the final analysis; this is usually referred to as an *internal* pilot. The advantage is that all the data collected can contribute to answering the main research question, and therefore an internal pilot may be seen as an efficient use of resources. However, it also limits the changes which can be made to the protocol at the end of the internal pilot without compromising the trial's validity. One exception is checking the sample size assumptions. Internal pilot studies could be considered to be an adaptive design (Arnold *et al.*, 2009; Thabane *et al.*, 2010; Chow and Chang, 2008). Researchers need to consider what information will be collected and analysed at the end of the pilot phase and how this information will be used to make decisions about the trial design after the pilot phase. It may be useful to set some stopping rules at the outset of the study; these may be based on satisfactory recruitment rate or satisfactory retention rate. Criteria for feasibility are discussed in more detail in Section 4.3. Internal pilots may also be used for sample size re-estimation. Lancaster, Dodd and Williamson (2004) and Wittes and Brittain (1990) argue that sample sizes should only be increased, and not decreased, as a result of internal pilot study data, in order to preserve the type 1 error rate (the chance of rejecting the null hypothesis), but Lake *et al.* (2002) show that this restriction may not be necessary for cluster trials with large numbers of small clusters.

An internal pilot should always be described in the protocol, with clear aims, objectives and mechanisms for decision making. An external data monitoring or trial steering committee may be useful to advise on the decisions, including whether any information collected during the pilot phase should lead to termination of the trial. In some circumstances it may be better to stop after the pilot than to carry on with a trial that is unlikely to be able to provide a satisfactory answer to the research question.

External pilot studies are small scale versions of the main study which are not intended to be part of the main study. There is therefore greater freedom to change the trial design for the main study once the results of the pilot are available. This may be one reason why external pilots are much more common than internal pilots. The UK BEAM pilot (Farrin *et al.*, 2005) is an example of an external pilot. The results of this pilot led to a change from a cluster randomised trial to an individually randomised trial: a complete change of design (see Section 1.3.1). If a substantial change of design is not required, it may be tempting to include participants from an external pilot in the main study analysis. This should be avoided as the decision to proceed with the main study will not have been made independently of the results of the pilot study (Lancaster, Dodd and Williamson, 2004).

4.2   Reasons for conducting pilot and feasibility studies

Box 4.2 lists a number of reasons for conducting a pilot study, using the same headings as Thabane *et al.* (2010), who give more detail for process measures. We have listed items of most relevance for cluster randomised trials. In the following sections we describe the key components for cluster randomised trials in more detail.

4.2.1   Piloting randomisation and recruitment

Key aspects of recruitment to be tested in a pilot study will be acceptability, recruitment rates and potential for recruitment bias (Section 2.3.5). In these three respects, cluster randomised trials often differ from other trials. In individually randomised trials, consent to be randomised to different interventions may be a considerable barrier to recruitment. Potential participants may be willing to provide data and attend for follow-up appointments, but may have strong preferences for one of the treatments being tested and be unwilling to agree to random allocation. In cluster randomised trials, individual participants cannot opt out of randomisation and will not always be able to opt out of the intervention. If this is the case, then their consent is for data collection only and it may be less important to pilot individual recruitment in a randomised pilot study. On the other hand, recruitment bias is unlikely to occur in an individually randomised trial but may be a real threat to the validity of a cluster randomised trial. Figure 2.2 (Section 2.3.5) shows how to identify whether such bias is likely to occur.

The pilot trial for UK BEAM is probably one of the best known pilots of a cluster randomised trial. We have already discussed this in Section 1.3.1. UK BEAM

Process:

Acceptability of trial to clusters and participants

Feasibility of recruitment process, including assessing recruitment bias

Number of eligible clusters and participants, and participation rates

retention rates.

Resources:

Research staff time involved in recruitment and follow-up of clusters and participants

Research investigator time required to implement the intervention

Costs of implementing the intervention and whether they relate to the number of clusters or number of participants.

Outcomes:

Designing a new outcome measure or checking the performance of an existing one

Standard deviation of a continuous outcome for sample size calculations

Baseline proportion for binary outcomes

Estimation of mean or proportion in the control arm to ensure change is feasible

Acceptability of outcome measures to health professionals and participants

Intra-cluster correlation coefficient (ICC) of outcome.

Intervention:

Testing the components of the intervention

Measuring adherence to intervention

Estimate of likely intervention effect.

Box 4.2   Reasons for conducting pilot and feasibility studies

Table 4.1 IRIS: training to increase identification and referral of victims of domestic violence.

Aim of main trial: To test the effectiveness of a training and support programme for general practice teams targeting identification of women experiencing domestic violence, and referral to specialist domestic violence advocates

Location and type of cluster: UK general practices

Interventions: (i) Control: usual care (ii) Intervention: multidisciplinary training sessions held in each practice, electronic prompts in the patient records and referral pathway to a named domestic violence advocate as well as feedback on referrals and reinforcement over the course of a year

Aim of pilot: (i) To test recruitment strategies (ii) To test data collection (iii) To determine most appropriate outcome (iv) To test feasibility of the intervention

Proposed outcome measure for main trial: Depression and anxiety in women suffering domestic violence

Design of pilot: Three clusters randomized to intervention and one to control; testing all components simultaneously

---

Source: Feder *et al.* (2011).

was originally designed with practices randomised to active management or usual care, and then within the active management practices individual patients were randomised to exercise classes, spinal manipulation or neither. The pilot study showed that more patients than predicted were recruited to the intervention arm, while fewer than predicted were recruited to the control arm, and in addition the patients in the intervention arm had less severe back pain. Following the pilot study, randomisation of practices was abandoned; all practices were trained in active management and only the individual randomisation was retained. Thus the randomisation strategy was changed in this trial as a result of piloting.

In a pilot study for the IRIS trial (Table 4.1), four general practices were allocated to intervention (three practices) or control (one practice). The outcomes were depression, and anxiety. In order to detect any changes in these outcomes as a result of the intervention, investigators had to recruit women and measure these outcomes on them. The planned recruitment strategy involved researchers in practice waiting rooms identifying women who had experienced abuse in the past year. The women then attended their appointment with a health professional as planned. While the researchers were present in the waiting rooms, 2213 women attended the practices; but researchers found it was feasible to approach only a quarter of these, and only half consented to be screened. Of these, about 20% were identified as experiencing abuse, and only 28 of these women agreed to be followed up and have their data collected at the end of the study. Additionally it was difficult to follow the women up because of issues of safety and confidentiality; in the end investigators were able to follow-up only a handful of women. Because of the large amount of effort expended in recruitment in relation to numbers actually providing outcome data, the investigators decided not to recruit in this way in the main trial. The main trial did not recruit individual women at all; the outcomes were changed to the intermediate outcomes of identification of abuse and referral to specialist agency that could be measured from practice records. A further reason for changing these outcomes was that very few of the *recruited* women were actually exposed to the intervention by being asked about abuse and referred to advocates, even though the intervention did substantially increase the number of women who were asked and referred on. Thus an assessment of recruitment strategies within this pilot resulted in a change in the recruitment, data collection and choice of outcome in the main trial.

4.2.2   Piloting the intervention

In assessing an intervention in a pilot study, investigators may wish to consider its delivery, its form, its content and its intensity. For example, training for health professionals could be delivered by a similar health professional or a researcher (delivery), face to face or via the internet (form), over two days or two hours (intensity), using structured guidance or a series of scenarios and reflection/discussion pointers (content). Ideally these elements should already have been considered in developing an intervention (Chapter 3), possibly using one or more feasibility studies in the process, as in the development of the Diabetes Manual (Sections 3.5 and 4.1). A pilot study can then be used to test how the different components fit together, and to make small refinements. These small refinements can sometimes be extremely important in optimising the effectiveness of an intervention. If part of the intervention is delivered to health professionals who then have to deliver a specific part to individual participants, it may be important to consider the delivery, form, content and intensity at both levels.

Loeb (2002) conducted a three-month pilot study which resulted in a change to the design of an intervention (Table 4.2). Originally, the investigators planned to

Table 4.2   Optimising antibiotic use in nursing homes.

Aim of main trial: To assess whether a multifaceted intervention can reduce the number of prescriptions for antimicrobials for suspected urinary tract infections in residents of nursing homes

Location and type of cluster: Nursing homes in Canada and the United States

Interventions: (i) Control: no intervention (ii) Intervention: presentation of diagnostic and therapeutic algorithms to nurses and physicians in homes, and relevant general practitioners; nursing home member of staff acted as champion; regular visits to nursing homes by research teams

Primary outcome: Number of prescriptions for antimicrobials

Design of the pilot: Implementation of the intervention in four nursing homes over 3 months, without a control arm

Change to intervention as result of pilot: Research team trained all staff in homes directly rather than training the home's infection control practitioner to train the home staff

Source: Loeb (2002).

use the research team to train infection control practitioners who were part of the nursing home staff, and then the trainers would train the other staff. This strategy was based on the opinion of staff in nursing homes that this process would be the best to use. However, it did not prove successful, and the design of the intervention delivery was altered so that in the main trial the research team trained the staff directly. This highlights the importance of conducting a pilot of the intervention process alongside gathering opinion about the best options for the intervention; if the investigators had proceeded to a main trial without the pilot they would have used their original training strategy based on nursing staff opinion, and this would probably have been less effective. In addition to removing the trainers from the delivery of the intervention, the investigators also introduced regular on-site visits to the homes to give feedback on adherence to the protocol and discuss barriers to implementation with the nursing staff.

Sometimes, however, a pilot study can have more serious implications for the intervention design. Eldridge *et al.* (2005) describe modelling conducted after a pilot study designed to assess the feasibility of a trial evaluating an intervention to reduce falls and fractures in older people (Table 4.3). UK Primary Care Trusts (PCTs) were to be the clusters. (PCTs were introduced in the UK in 1999 to be responsible for the healthcare needs of the local population. Each PCT comprised a group of general practices covering a population of approximately 100 000 patients.) These are relatively large units to randomise, and partly because of that, and the complexity of the intervention, the pilot was conducted in only one PCT. A facilitator was employed within the trust to coordinate the intervention, and there was a programme of falls risk assessments via a short questionnaire that could be used by all health and social care professionals who might see older people. Those at risk of falling could be referred to a falls clinic. The investigators collected data within the pilot on the use of the falls risk assessment tool, and within a separate questionnaire study on the

Table 4.3   Pilot study for a falls prevention programme.

Aim of the intended trial: To assess whether a falls prevention programme would reduce the rate of hip fractures in older people

Location and type of cluster: UK Primary Care Trusts (approximately 100 000 patients in each)

Intervention: A facilitator was assigned to the Primary Care Trust to introduce a programme of falls risk assessment and referral. The intervention included enhancement of existing referral systems, the establishment of a falls clinic if none existed, and the introduction of a specially designed two-part tool for assessment of falls risk in older people (falls risk assessment tool or FRAT)

Primary outcome: Fractured neck of femur

Design of feasibility study: Intervention was implemented in one cluster with community survey of patients' experiences of falls and additional data on service use. This was combined in a model to assess potential impact of the intervention

---

Source: Eldridge *et al.* (2005).

outcomes from the tool. These data and other routine data were combined into a model (Section 3.5). The model indicated that it was very unlikely that this intervention would show the sort of effect the investigators were hoping for, and that the effect could be increased only if more older people were exposed to the falls risk assessment tool. This might be achieved through a public awareness campaign via leaflets and posters so that older people themselves would become aware and initiate assessment. In fact, a full trial was never conducted. Nevertheless, the finding from the pilot study was, in itself, important, and influenced the UK's National Institute for Health and Clinical Excellence (NICE) guidelines on falls prevention (NICE, 2004).

4.2.3   Acquiring information to help with sample size

Very often investigators use information from pilot studies to estimate the variability in their primary outcome, in order to estimate sample size. In cluster randomised trials there are two elements of variability to be estimated: within and between cluster. Alternatively, the total variability and the ICC can be calculated; these measures provide essentially the same information in a different format (Section 7.1.1).

One problem with estimating total variation and ICC from pilot studies is that the ICC tends to have extremely wide confidence intervals, and so the value found in a pilot study is likely to be imprecise. A further problem is that statistical inference from a pilot to a main study may be problematic. These issues are discussed further in Chapter 8 (Section 8.3.2).

4.2.4   Refining outcome measures

The success of a randomised trial depends on choosing an appropriate outcome measure, and there may be many potential outcome measures. A trial of an intervention to improve care of asthmatic patients could consider mortality, lung function, exacerbations, use of health service, or quality of life, each of which could be measured in a number of ways. Some outcomes, such as mortality, may be very important but extremely rare; this would lead to a trial of unmanageable size. Other outcomes may not be very sensitive to the intervention or be difficult to measure.

Waters *et al.* (2011) used a pilot study to see how the use of evidence in decision making could be measured, for a trial to assess an intervention to increase the use of evidence in developing local government policies. This was a new area where little background information was available. The pilot study was designed as an exploratory trial, randomising clusters, but with the aim of testing the feasibility and acceptability of the intervention and trial outcome measures. Specific aims are shown in Table 4.4.

Pilot work may indicate that the preferred outcome is not reliably measured by the method intended. Ka'opua *et al.* (2011) used questionnaires to measure uptake

Table 4.4   Knowledge translation to increase use of evidence in local government decision making.

Aim of full trial: To assess whether a knowledge translation strategy to support evidence-informed decision making in local government increases use of evidence

Location and type of cluster: Local government councils in Victoria, Australia

Interventions: (i) Control: improved access to research evidence via provision of summaries of intervention research on topics of relevance in childhood obesity prevention for local government (ii) Intervention: improved access to research evidence as for control arm, and building capacity of local government to use research evidence to inform public health decision making by providing facilitated support

Primary outcome: Use of evidence in decision making

Aims and objectives of pilot:

1. What knowledge transfer strategies show promise to increase the use of research evidence in policy and programme decision making in local government?

2. How can we measure evidence use and the key sub-components of evidence use that are to be targeted by the intervention, at decision maker and council level?

3. What are the estimates of ICC by council of outcomes and of the change in such outcomes that a larger trial would need to be powered to detect?

Source: Waters *et al.* (2011).

of breast cancer screening by native Hawaiian women. They used self-completed questionnaires asking whether the women had had a mammogram in the past year. Inconsistencies in the questionnaire responses, such as reporting a mammogram in the past year but providing a date two years in the past led researchers to investigate other ways to collect the data. Sometimes pilot data can lead to a complete change of outcome, as described for the IRIS trial pilot in Section 4.2.1.

4.3   Designing a pilot or feasibility study

Pilot or feasibility studies should have specific objectives and these should relate to, but be distinct from, the aim of the intended main trial. Thabane *et al.* (2010) stress the importance of clear aims in their useful tutorial on how to design pilot studies and how to present these in patient information sheets. Feasibility studies may be more suitable where key components need to be tested, for which a control arm may not be necessary. A full pilot study, which will often be larger and more expensive, and take longer to conduct, may be carried out later. Qualitative studies may be useful to gain insight into participants' views of the intervention, recruitment

Table 4.5   Pilot trial of intervention to reduce inappropriate antibiotic prescribing.

Aim: To assess the feasibility and acceptability of the study design, procedures, and intervention

Location and type of cluster: Canadian general practices

Interventions: (i) Control: usual care (ii) Intervention: DECISION+ programme, which included 3 three-hour workshops over a four to six month period

Primary outcome: Number of prescriptions for antimicrobials

Feasibility criteria: (i) The proportion of contacted family medicine groups participating in the pilot study would be 50% or greater (ii) The proportion of recruited family physicians participating in all three workshops would be 70% or greater (iii) The mean level of satisfaction from family physicians regarding the workshops would be 65% or greater (iv) The proportion of missing data in each completed questionnaire would be less than 10%

Source: Leblanc *et al.* (2011).

or study materials, and to understand why elements of the study design are not working well. These may be independent or integrated into a larger study. The choice of study design will depend on the objectives of the pilot or feasibility study. For example in the Diabetes Manual trial (Sturt *et al.*, 2006), the intervention was developed through a series of studies which did not have a control arm, as described in Section 4.1, while Leblanc *et al.* (2011) designed a pilot study to assess the feasibility and acceptability of the study design, procedures, and intervention in a trial to reduce inappropriate prescribing of antibiotics for acute respiratory tract infections in primary care (Table 4.5). Here the pilot study involved recruitment of clusters and participants and implementation of the intervention in those clusters randomised to the intervention. Although the trial looked like the main study, it was much smaller and, importantly, it had different aims: to establish whether the trial was feasible and acceptable. The investigators had established an a priori threshold for specific feasibility and acceptability criteria as listed in Table 4.5.

4.3.1   Size of pilot study

The size of a pilot study will depend on study aims. It should not be powered to detect a difference on the primary outcome, as this should not be a pilot study aim. Many aspects of feasibility will result in the calculation of proportions; for example recruitment rates, drop-out rates or proportion of successfully completed questionnaires. The size of the sample will depend on how precisely the researchers wish to estimate these proportions. Precision can be usefully expressed as a 95% confidence interval. The following formula gives a value for the width of the 95% confidence interval for a single proportion, p, where n is the number of individuals required.

$$p - 1.96\sqrt{\frac{p(1-p)}{n}} \quad \text{to} \quad p + 1.96\sqrt{\frac{p(1-p)}{n}}$$

This formula assumes that the data are not clustered, however, and will be too narrow if clustering is present. If there is considerable variability between clusters in the pilot it may be more useful to consider the reasons for this rather than to adjust the confidence interval for variability between clusters.

If the aim of the study is to calculate the standard deviation between individual participants, s, then the following formula gives the 95% confidence interval, assuming no clustering.

$$\sqrt{\frac{(n-1)s^2}{\chi^2_{0.025,n-1}}} \quad \text{to} \quad \sqrt{\frac{(n-1)s^2}{\chi^2_{0.975,n-1}}}$$

where $\chi^2_{0.025,n-1}$ and $\chi^2_{0.975,n-1}$ are the values corresponding to the upper and lower tails of the χ^2_{n-1} distribution. Lancaster, Dodd and Williamson (2004) recommend choosing 30 subjects as a ballpark figure in order to estimate the standard deviation. The value of $\chi^2_{0.025,29}$ is 45.7 and $\chi^2_{0.975,29}$ is 16.0. The resulting 95% confidence interval is $0.79s$ to $1.34s$. Thus we can expect the true value to be not greater than a third more than the estimated value. The sample size of the pilot study can be increased for greater accuracy. This guidance was given for individually randomised trials but for cluster randomised trials, most pilots should ideally be larger. It is difficult to power a pilot study to estimate the ICC with any degree of precision, as discussed in Section 8.3.2.

4.3.2 Protocols for pilot studies

A methodologically rigorous pilot study with clear aims will also have a clear protocol. Arnold *et al.* (2009) recommend that pilot studies should be subject to the same scrutiny as full trials in order to ensure their scientific rigour, and should be registered in the same way as full trials (see Section 10.2.1). Protocols for pilot studies can also be published. For example, Waters *et al.* (2011) is a protocol publication of a pilot study which is a version of the intended main study in miniature and is registered in the Australia and New Zealand Clinical Trials Register (ANZCTR). Another registered study is, Brach and Hontikainen (2011). This study focuses on an intervention in one nursing home. The intervention aims to increase nurses' movement support skills relating to residents' daily activities. Data are obtained from nurses themselves, from observing them supporting residents and from the residents. Any future trial would clearly be cluster randomised. but it is not clear whether nurses or residential homes would be randomised. The publication contains a clear list of criteria on which the feasibility of the main trial will be judged.

4.4   Reporting and interpreting pilot studies

External pilot studies and feasibility studies should always be reported where possible. Internal pilot studies inform the main study directly, and data is included in the main analysis, so the contribution of participants and the effort expended is not wasted, but insights may have been gained which would be useful to other researchers, and there may be insufficient space in the main paper to report these in detail. If studies are not reported then information gained will not be accessible to the research community, and other trialists cannot benefit. Pilot studies, owing to the nature of their aims, are less likely to be considered by many traditional (paper) journals as interesting to their target audience, who are mainly clinicians and policy makers, and these journals may be more reluctant to publish pilot studies. Online, open access journals such as the BMC group of journals have published many of the examples in this chapter. These journals have a policy to publish based primarily on validity and coherence rather than interest to their readership.

Pilot studies should not be reported as main trials, as they have different aims. Thabane *et al.* (2010) gives a detailed guide based on the CONSORT statement. The key areas of difference between pilot studies and full trials are given in Box 4.3. It is inappropriate to place undue emphasis on hypothesis testing, as no formal power calculations will have been carried out.

Nevertheless, pilot studies are sometimes used to estimate the likely effect of the intervention. It is important in this case to use the limits of confidence intervals in making any judgements about likely effect, not the effect estimate itself or the *p*-value from a significance test. The limits of the confidence interval for effect estimate will show the likely extreme boundaries of effect in a main trial, and these can be used to identify whether a specific effect is potentially possible or not. The confidence intervals are likely to be wide and a full trial will still be justified to give greater certainty to the estimate of effect, even when they do not contain the null value.

4.5 Summary

Cluster randomised trials are often large and expensive to carry out. Carefully designed pilot studies can help avoid inconclusive results, which often arise because of over-optimistic assumptions at the planning stage. Pilot studies help to ensure

---

The title should indicate that this is a pilot study.

The aims of the main trial should be described.

The specific aims of the pilot study should be clearly stated.

Statistical analysis should relate to the aims of the pilot study.

Analysis should be mainly descriptive, and significance tests should be avoided.

Formal sample size calculations are not always appropriate.

Box 4.3 Guidelines for reporting pilot studies

assumptions are reasonable and that the components of the intervention and trial work together. In this chapter we have described the ways in which pilot studies can be and have been used in preparation for cluster randomised trials.

References

Arain, M., Campbell, M.J., Cooper, C.L. *et al.* (2010) What is a pilot or feasibility study? A review of current practice and editorial policy. *BMC Med. Res. Methodol.*, **10**, 67.

Arnold, D.M., Burns, K.E.A., Adhikari, N.K.J. *et al.* (2009) The design and interpretation of pilot trials in clinical research in critical care. *Crit. Care Med.*, **37** (Suppl.), S69–S74.

Betschon, E., Brach, M. and Hantikainen, V. (2011) Studying feasibility and effects of a two-stage nursing staff training in residential geriatric care using a 30 month mixed-methods design [ISRCTN24344776]. *BMC Nurs.*, **10**, 10.

Chow, S. and Chang, M. (2008) Adaptive design methods in clinical trials – a review. *Orphanet. J. Rare Dis.*, **3**, 11. doi: 10.1186/1750-1172-3-11

Eldridge, S., Spencer, A., Cryer, C. *et al.* (2005) Why modelling a complex intervention is an important precursor to trial design: lessons from studying an intervention to reduce falls-related injuries in older people. *J. Health Serv. Res. Policy*, **10** (3), 133–142.

Farrin, A., Russell, I., Torgerson, D. *et al.* (2005) Differential recruitment in a cluster randomized trial in primary care: the experience of the UK back pain, exercise, active management and manipulation (UK BEAM) feasibility study. *Clin. Trials*, **2** (2), 119–124.

Feder, G., Agnew Davies, R., Baird, K. *et al.* (2011) Identification and Referral to Improve Safety (IRIS) of women experiencing domestic violence: a cluster randomised controlled trial of a primary care training and support programme. *Lancet*, 2011 Oct 12 [Epub ahead of print].

Ka'opua, L.S.I., Ward M. E., Park, S.H. *et al.* (2011) Testing the feasibility of a culturally tailored breast cancer screening intervention with Native Hawaiian women in Rural Churches. *Health Soc, Work* **36** (1), 55–65.

Lake, S., Kamman, E., Klar, N. and Betensky, R. (2002) Sample size re-estimation in cluster randomization trials. *Stat. Med.*, **21**, 1337–1350.

Lancaster, G.A., Dodd, S. and Williamson, P.R. (2004) Design and analysis of pilot studies: recommendations for good practice. *J. Eval. Clin. Pract.*, **10**, 307–312.

Leblanc, A., Légaré, F., Labrecque, M. *et al.* (2011) Feasibility of a randomised trial of a continuing medical education program in shared decision-making on the use of antibiotics for acute respiratory infections in primary care: the DECISION+ pilot trial. *Implement. Sci.*, **6**, 5.

Loeb, M.B. (2002) Application of the development stages of a cluster randomized trial to a framework for valuating complex health interventions. *BMC Health Serv. Res.*, **2** (1), 13.

NETSCC (2011) NIHR Evaluation, Trials and Studies Coordinating Centre. Glossary, http://www.netscc.ac.uk/glossary/ (accessed 17 July 2011).

NICE (2004) *CG21 Falls: The Assessment and Prevention of Falls in Older People.* Clinical Guideline, National Institute for Clinical Excellence, London, http://www.nice.org.uk/CG021NICEguideline (accessed 22 July 2011).

Sturt, J., Hearnshaw, H., Barlow, J. *et al.* (2005) Supporting a curriculum for delivering type 2 diabetes patient self-management education: a patient needs assessment. *Prim. Care Res. Deve.*, **6**, 291–299.

Sturt, J., Taylor, H., Docherty, A., *et al.* (2006) A psychological approach to providing self-management education for people with type 2 diabetes: the diabetes manual. *BMC Fam. Pract.*, **7**, 70.

Thabane, L., Ma, J., Chu, R. *et al.* (2010) A tutorial on pilot studies: the what, why and how. *BMC Med. Res. Methodol.*, **10**, 1.

Waters, E., Armstrong, R., Swinburn, B. *et al.* (2011) An exploratory cluster randomised controlled trial of knowledge translation strategies to support evidence-informed decision-making in local governments (the KT4LG study). *BMC Public Health*, **11**, 34.

Wittes, J. and Brittain, E. (1990) The role of internal pilot studies in increasing the efficiency of clinical trials. *Stat. Med.*, **9**, 65–72.

5

Design

Once investigators have decided to carry out a cluster randomised trial, some of the basic principles of recruitment and ethics have been understood (Chapter 2) and an intervention has been developed (Chapter 3), and any piloting or feasibility work undertaken (Chapter 4), the next step is to consider in more detail how the trial should be designed. The majority of cluster randomised trials involve the comparison of outcomes in two arms of a trial concurrently; one arm which receives an intervention and the other which receives treatment as usual. In a review of cluster randomised trials in primary care, 123 out of 152 trials had this two-arm parallel design (Eldridge *et al.*, 2004). These trials can be completely randomised, or employ a method of allocation to intervention arms in which investigators try to ensure balance between arms in terms of prognostic factors (stratified, minimised or matched designs) or to fix more precisely the number of clusters in each arm for some other reason (using blocking). In Section 5.1 we cover the different methods of allocation in two-arm trials, including whether to use an equal or unequal number of clusters in each arm. If investigators wish to collect information at more points than just the primary endpoint, for example at baseline, this information can be collected from the same participants or different participants, an option unique to those conducting cluster randomised trials; we cover this in Section 5.2. For most readers of this book, these two sections contain what they need to make decisions about the design of their trial. However, in some cases, investigators may wish to have more than two arms in their trial. These types of trial are covered in Section 5.3. Further sections cover less common designs such as crossover (Section 5.4) and stepped wedge and pseudo cluster designs (Section 5.5).

A Practical Guide to Cluster Randomised Trials in Health Services Research, First Edition.
Sandra Eldridge and Sally Kerry.
© 2012 John Wiley & Sons, Ltd. Published 2012 by John Wiley & Sons, Ltd.

5.1   Parallel designs with only two arms

5.1.1   Introduction

Many of the trials we have encountered so far in this book are parallel trials with only two arms; for example, Oakeshott, Kerry and Williams, 1994 (Section 1.3.1), Cappuccio *et al.*, 2006 (Section 1.2). In the review by Eldridge *et al.* (2004), approximately half of the trials with parallel designs were completely randomised, a third were stratified or minimised, and a sixth were pair matched. The following sections cover these three types of randomisation. For those unfamiliar with the general principles of these designs, a straightforward introduction is provided in Roberts and Torgerson (1998) or can be found in most standard textbooks on trials, such as those referenced at the start of Chapter 1.

5.1.2   Completely randomised designs

The principle of complete randomisation is that each cluster has a pre-specified (usually equal) chance of being included in each of the trial arms. In theory this could be achieved by tossing a coin, but this method is not recommended because of the potential for bias, for example if a coin is not perfectly balanced or some tosses of the coin are, for whatever reason, ignored. In practice, randomisation is generally carried out using computers. While many cluster randomised trials have used completely randomised designs in the past, these may become less common as the advantages of stratification (see Section 5.1.4) are being increasingly recognised. The main advantage of the completely randomised design is its simplicity. One example of such a design is a trial of an intervention designed to improve intercultural communication (Table 5.1).

Table 5.1   Educational intervention to improve intercultural communication.

Aim: To assess the effectiveness of an educational intervention on intercultural communication aimed to decrease inequalities in care provided between western and non-western patients

Location and type of cluster: Dutch general practitioners

Number of clusters and individual participants: 38 clusters recruited, and 35 analysed; 986 individual participants analysed

Interventions: (i) Control: (details not specified) (ii) Intervention: educational intervention to patients (12-minute videotape in waiting rooms) and for general practitioners (2.5 days of training spread over 2 weeks)

Primary outcome: Mutual understanding between patients and general practitioners (on a validated scale)

Randomisation: GPs randomly allocated to an intervention or a control arm

---

Source: Harmsen *et al.* (2005).

One disadvantage of a completely randomised design is that imbalances in certain prognostic factors may arise between the trial arms by chance. Although this does not in itself lead to bias, trial results often appear more plausible if the arms look balanced. Peto *et al.* (1977) argues that, in most individually randomised trials of a reasonable size, factors are very unlikely to be imbalanced between intervention arms and a completely randomised design will suffice; while Lasagna (1976) argues that it is worth protecting against extreme imbalance, even if this is very rare. In cluster randomised trials, the argument in favour of using a method more likely to achieve balance between arms is stronger, because there are often relatively few clusters. Imbalance in factors is then more likely by chance; results appear less plausible, and analyses which take account of baseline factors (Sections 6.3.2 and 6.3.3) are statistically less efficient if applied to imbalanced rather than balanced designs. Several methods of allocation are available to try to balance arms with respect to prognostic or other factors. These are often referred to as restricted designs. We describe these designs in Sections 5.1.4–5.1.9. In the next section we focus on how to choose which particular factors to attempt to balance.

5.1.3   Choosing factors to balance in designs that are not completely randomised

The most common factors that investigators try to balance between intervention and control arms are: (i) a feature of the cluster, for example the make-up of staff in a cluster; (ii) cluster size, although often this is not known in advance and a proxy for cluster size must be used; (iii) geographic location, for example region; (iv) a feature of the cluster population, for example a measure of socio-demographic characteristics; and (v) baseline characteristics of trial participants.

Choice of which factors to try and balance depends on which factors investigators think may be most important in influencing outcome or in influencing the effectiveness of the intervention. For an outcome measuring the process of care such as whether patients are referred from primary to secondary healthcare, features of the cluster may be most likely to affect that process.

For a clinical outcome or an outcome measuring other individual patient characteristics or behaviour, for example blood pressure or quality of life, it may be more important to balance by characteristics of patients. It is not possible to balance individual participant factors directly using usual methods of stratification, minimisation or matching within a cluster randomised trial, because in these trials any balancing factors have to be specified at the cluster level. Instead, individual-level data, either routine or collected directly from patients, are summarised at the cluster level and used as the balancing factor. When using routine data, a summary is often obtained from the cluster population or from a population located in the same geographical area as the cluster, even though not all the individuals in the cluster population or area will eventually form part of the actual cluster. For example, in Hampshire *et al.* (1999) socio-demographic characteristics of the practice area were used (Table 5.2).

Table 5.2   Action research to promote child surveillance reviews.

Aim: To assess the benefits of using action research in primary care to increase child surveillance reviews

Location and type of cluster: UK general practices

Number of clusters and individual participants: 28 clusters recruited and analysed; 2015 records of individuals analysed

Interventions: (i) Control: anonymised feedback reports on child health surveillance (ii) Intervention: anonymised reports plus visits by researchers who facilitated practice team meetings

Primary outcome: Return rate of child surveillance reviews

Randomisation: Practices were randomly allocated to the action research arm or a control arm. Stratification factors: (i) single-handed practice versus larger practices (ii) socio-demographic characteristics of the practice area

Note: action research is a process of reflection and progressive problem solving by individuals working in a particular environment to improve their working practices, often facilitated by researchers from outside that environment.

Source: Hampshire *et al.* (1999).

Table 5.3   Diabetes Manual trial: manual and structured care to improve outcomes.

Aim: To determine the effects of the Diabetes Manual on glycaemic control, diabetes-related distress and confidence to self-care of patients with type 2 diabetes

Location and type of cluster: UK general practices

Number of clusters and individual participants: 48 practices were randomised and analysed; 245 individual participants were recruited, and 202 analysed

Interventions: (i) Control: delayed intervention (ii) Intervention: education of nurses, followed by one-to-one structured education of patients via a self-completed manual and nurse support, and audiotapes

Primary outcome: HbA1c level

Randomisation: Practices were allocated in blocks to intervention or delayed intervention arms by a statistician blind to practice identity using computer-aided minimisation

Minimisation factors: (i) Mean HbA1c of consented patients (ii) Number of patients recruited per practice (iii) Practice-level Quality and Outcomes Framework aspirational points score

Source: Sturt *et al.* (2008).

However, to achieve balance in participant characteristics it may be most effective to use a factor which is a cluster-level summary measure of baseline data from actual trial participants. This may be important for the face validity of the trial, but is only possible if patients are recruited prior to allocation. An example of this occurs in the Diabetes Manual trial (Table 5.3). Baseline values of HbA1c were obtained from trial participants at recruitment; the mean HbA1c level was calculated for each cluster and then clusters were allocated to intervention or control arms using mini-misation, with mean HbA1c at the cluster level as one of the minimisation factors. When there is a large pool of potential participants in each cluster, known in advance, from whom a small sample must be drawn to participate in the trial, an alternative method of balancing arms using patient characteristics is stratified random sampling of participants within clusters (Section 5.1.5).

If cluster sizes vary considerably it may be advisable to balance by cluster size, in order to prevent all large clusters being randomised into one intervention arm. Even if cluster size does not influence the outcome or intervention effectiveness, very uneven-sized intervention arms will reduce the power of the study to show an effect. If the main reason for balancing by cluster size is to ensure reasonably bal-anced arms in terms of numbers, the most effective way of doing this is to balance by the number of participants in each cluster, as in the Diabetes Manual trial (Table 5.3). Nevertheless, as for individual participant characteristics, unless participants are recruited before allocation to intervention arms (or there is no recruitment), the number of individual participants in each cluster may be unknown at the point of allocation. In trials where recruitment has to take place after allocation, investigators can use the number of professionals in a healthcare organisation as a proxy for cluster size, or the natural cluster size (see Section 1.3.2) if this is available.

5.1.4   Stratified designs

In stratified designs investigators choose the factors that they want to balance between the different arms of the trial and the number of levels of each factor. For example, in the trial in Table 5.2, one stratification factor was size of practice: single-handed versus larger practices. This factor had two levels. If investigators wish to balance on the basis of a continuous factor this must be categorised into a number of discrete categories first. Each of these categories then becomes a separate level. Caria *et al.* (2011) describe this process for a trial in which schools in a number of different countries were randomised. The investigators stratified by a social-status index, which they created using different social-status indicators in each country. In each country the index was divided into tertiles, so the overall index of social status was a stratification factor with three levels.

Following identification of factors and levels, clusters are then divided into strata, each containing only clusters with identical levels of each factor, and within each stratum blocking (Section 5.1.8) is used to ensure equal (or as near equal as possible) numbers of clusters from each stratum in each arm of the trial. For example, with 2 factors each with 2 levels, the number of strata needed is 4 (2×2). If one factor has 2 levels and one has 3, then 6 (2×3) strata are needed. Thus, as the number of factors or the number of levels within each factor increases, the number of strata increases. If the number of strata is large compared with the number of clusters this can result in some very small, or even empty, strata. In these cir-cumstances, it is often difficult to achieve balance within strata and the whole point of stratification is lost. There is, however, an alternative to stratification which is better able to cope with several stratification factors: minimisation, which we describe in Section 5.1.6.

5.1.5   Stratified random sampling within clusters

This technique is unique to cluster randomised trials in which participants are sampled from a larger pool of participants in each cluster (the natural cluster –Section 1.3.2), and baseline characteristics of participants that investigators wish to balance can be easily identified in advance of recruiting participants. Such characteristics might be, for example, age, sex, or routinely recorded clinical information. The technique was used in the Kumasi trial in rural Ghana; data were available on age and sex of residents in each village prior to recruitment of residents and randomisation of clusters (Table 5.4). The investigators purposely selected, as far as possible, the same proportions of residents in particular age and sex bands from each village, in order to achieve balance on these characteristics between intervention and control arms. An additional design feature of this trial was blocked randomisation. This was used to ensure that the time between participant and village recruitment and the start of the intervention was as short as possible, and is described in more detail in Section 5.1.8.

5.1.6   Minimisation

Minimisation does something slightly different from stratification (Taves, 1974; Pocock and Simon, 1975). Important prognostic factors are identified at the start of

Table 5.4   Kumasi trial: health education to prevent stroke.

Aim: To see if a health education programme to reduce salt intake among rural and semi-rural communities in the Ashanti region of Ghana leads to a reduction in blood pressure

Location and type of cluster: Ghana, villages of 500–2000 inhabitants

Number of clusters and individual participants: 12 clusters were recruited and analysed; 1031 individual participants were analysed

Interventions: (i) Control: health education not including salt reduction
(ii) Intervention: health education including salt reduction messages

Primary outcome: Reduction in systolic blood pressure after six months

Randomisation: (i) Blocks of 2 villages were formed (ii) Individuals within each village in the block were stratified by age (four levels) and sex so that as far as possible participants with the same age and sex structure were selected from each village (iii) Villages were randomly allocated to intervention or control arms in blocks of size 2, and allocation was conducted only when subject recruitment was complete in the whole block

---

Source: Cappuccio *et al.* (2006); Kerry *et al.* (2005).

Table 5.5   Characteristics of first 15 clusters minimised in a cluster randomised trial.

Factor	Level	Intervention arm	Control arm
Natural cluster size	Large	5*	4*
(dichotomised)	Small	3	3
Deprivation score of area in	Deprived	4*	2*
which cluster is located	Less deprived	4	5
System of referral	A	5*	3*
	B	3	4

the trial, and experimental units (in our case, clusters) are assigned sequentially. Each unit's assignment depends on the assignment of previous units and is made so that the imbalance between arms in terms of the prognostic factors is minimised. There are different methods of calculating the imbalance between the arms (Taves, 2010); here we illustrate one method.

Suppose clusters are to be minimized using three factors, each of which has two levels. Table 5.5 shows the numbers allocated to each arm by subgroup after 15 clusters have been randomised. Suppose the next cluster is large, deprived, with referral system A. We have shown the numbers already in these categories with asterisks in the table. These numbers sum to 14 in the intervention group and 9 in the control group. Placing the new cluster in the arm in which the sum is lower (control arm) will result in better balance (the new sums will be 14 and 12 respectively).

Minimisation has advantages over stratification when the number of units to be allocated is small – as in the case of a relatively small number of clusters – but the number of stratification factors is large (Pocock and Simon, 1975; Altman, 1991). Minimisation performs better than some other methods of balancing arms in these circumstances (Scott *et al.*, 2002).

Disadvantages of minimisation are that it is essentially a deterministic method, but statistical analyses of trials assume random allocation; that the allocation of an experimental unit depends on the characteristics of units already allocated and as a result the next assignment can sometimes be predicted; that it may be complex to use; and that it ensures only that *overall* the intervention arms will be balanced for each factor, not that factors in combination will be balanced (as in stratification). An adaptation of the simple deterministic approach assigns a new experimental unit to the arm which would achieve the better balance with a probability of, say, 0.75. Using this method on the example in Table 5.5, the new cluster would have a 75% chance of being allocated to the control arm and a 25% chance of being allocated to the intervention arm. This introduces an element of randomness and avoids the certain prediction of intervention allocation. Minimisation with a random element does not, however, resolve the issues of how to carry out appropriate inference, or what to do about interaction between factors. These disadvantages of minimisation

Table 5.6   ELECTRA: asthma liaison nurses to reduce unscheduled care.

Aim: To determine whether asthma specialist nurses, using a liaison model of
   care, reduce unscheduled care in a deprived multiethnic setting

Location and type of cluster: UK general practices

Number of clusters and individual participants: 44 clusters were randomised and
   analysed; 324 participants were recruited, and 319 analysed

Interventions: (i) Control: a visit promoting standard asthma guidelines; patients
   were checked for inhaler technique (ii) Intervention: patient review in a
   nurse-led clinic, and liaison with general practitioners and practice nurses
   comprising educational outreach, promotion of guidelines for high risk asthma,
   sand ongoing clinical support

Primary outcomes: Unscheduled care for acute asthma over one year, and time to
   first unscheduled attendance

Randomisation: General practices were allocated to intervention and control arms
   using minimisation

Minimisation factors: (i) Partnership size (ii) Training practice status (iii) Hospital
   admission rates for asthma (iv) Employment of practice nurse (v) Whether the
   practice nurse was trained in asthma care

Source: Griffiths *et al.* (2004).

are partially a consequence of its development for trials in which allocation is necessarily sequential (Senn, 1997). In cluster randomised trials, the characteristics of all
clusters are often known at the start of a trial and other methods of achieving balance
could be used instead, although this is an area which is, as yet, relatively under-
explored. Currently, it is not uncommon for minimisation to be used even when all
clusters and their characteristics are known prior to randomisation. In this case the
clusters should be minimised in a random order, as for example in a trial of teaching
general practitioners to carry out structured assessments of their long term mentally
ill patients (Kendrick, Burns and Freeling, 1995).

Minimisation was used in the ELECTRA trial (Table 5.6). Sometimes both
minimisation and stratification are used in the same trial. This was the case in the
IRIS trial (Table 5.7). Clusters were stratified by region and then minimised on other
factors. Twenty-four clusters were recruited in each of two regions. In both trials,
the MINIM program was used to perform the minimisation. This program is currently freely available over the web (Evans, Royston and Day, 2004).

A recent review has indicated that minimisation is not always used correctly and
in many trials is poorly described (Taves, 2010). For example, in the ELECTRA
trial (Table 5.6), a random element was used in the minimisation, but this is not
reported, and the factors should have been described as 'minimisation' rather than
'stratification' factors. If using minimisation, investigators should make clear that
minimisation was used and describe whether or not a random element was included,
and if possible give more detail of the precise method used.

Table 5.7   IRIS: training to increase identification and referral of victims of domestic violence.

Aim: To test the effectiveness of a training and support programme for general practice teams targeting identification of women experiencing domestic violence and referral to specialist domestic violence advocates

Location and type of cluster: UK general practices

Number of clusters: 51 clusters were randomised, and 48 analysed

Interventions: (i) Control: usual care (ii) Intervention: multidisciplinary training sessions in each practice, electronic prompts in the patient record and a referral pathway to a named domestic violence advocate, as well as feedback on referrals and reinforcement over the course of a year. Posters were displayed in the practice and leaflets were available

Primary outcome: Number of recorded referrals of women aged over 16 years to advocacy services based in specialist domestic violence agencies recorded in the general practice records

Randomisation: (i) General practices were stratified by area (ii) Allocated to intervention or control arm using minimisation

Minimisation factors: (i) Proportion of whole-time-equivalent female doctors in the practice (ii) Postgraduate training status (iii) Number of patients registered with the practice (iv) Percentage of the practice population on low incomes

Source: Feder *et al.* (2011).

5.1.7   Other techniques for balancing factors between trial arms

There are other ways of trying to achieve balance in prognostic factors between intervention groups. Raab and Butcher (2001), for example, calculate an index of balance for every possible allocation of clusters to treatment groups. An allocation can then be randomly selected from those for which the balance is deemed acceptable. Investigators have to decide what is meant by acceptable balance; this may mean considering balance in individual factors in addition to assessing the overall index.

5.1.8   Blocking

Blocking can be used when all clusters are recruited prior to allocation. In this case all clusters are allocated at the same time. Alternatively it can be used when clusters are recruited sequentially. Here we consider both alternatives.

Using blocking, clusters are divided into blocks, and within each block equal (or as near equal as possible) numbers of clusters are randomised to the intervention and control arms. For example, with a block size of eight, four clusters in each block would be allocated to intervention and four to control. Blocking is used in a stratified design (Section 5.1.4) to ensure that equal or near equal numbers are allocated to each intervention arm from each stratum; without blocking, the advantage of stratification is lost. Often the block is the size of the stratum; if the stratum has an odd number of clusters in it then the numbers in each arm will not be exactly equal, but this will usually still be preferable to a completely randomised design. However, to use a design in which block size is equal to stratum size requires that the number in the stratum is known in advance of the blocking. When clusters are recruited and randomised sequentially this will not be the case and smaller blocks must then be used. It is considered good practice to alter the size of the blocks randomly to lessen the chance of a researcher or cluster professional involved in the trial being able to predict allocation of the next cluster through knowledge of block size and previous allocations. This random assignment of block size is often referred to as random permuted blocks.

Blocking may be used to ensure a pre-specified number of clusters in each arm even when there is no stratification for prognostic or other factors. This may be particularly important in a cluster randomised trial if the intervention being evaluated is costly or time consuming. If blocking is not used, and more clusters than expected end up in the intervention arm, this could have serious resource implications for the trial. If all clusters are to be randomised at the same time, one large block could be used, with block size equal to the number of clusters recruited. However, if recruitment and randomisation are conducted sequentially, using one large block will result in the assignment of the last cluster being predictable. To avoid this predictability, smaller block sizes can be used, and all clusters in an individual block randomised at the same time. One example of this is the Kumasi trial (Table 5.4). In this trial the block sizes were small – only two clusters per block. A pair of clusters was recruited, individual participants within each cluster were recruited, and then the clusters were randomised, one to intervention and one to control. Thus the timing of the intervention was balanced in each block and the field workers would not know the allocation of the last two villages when recruiting participants (Kerry *et al.*, 2005).

Small blocks can also ensure that the number of randomisation units being recruited into the intervention and control arms is fairly even throughout the trial. This is useful to avoid the bias that may occur if, for example, a lot more intervention units than control units are recruited early on and there is a secular trend affecting intervention effectiveness, and also facilitates trial logistics by ensuring resources required for the intervention arm can be distributed evenly over the trial duration.

Unfortunately, blocking cannot be used in conjunction with minimisation. In the OPERA trial described in Section 5.1.10, minimisation resulted in a larger number of clusters than expected in the intervention arm, and a consequent drain on the resources of the trial. Carter and Hood (2008) describe an extension of the method of Raab and Butcher (2001) (Section 5.1.7) which incorporates blocking.

5.1.9   Matched-pair designs

Matching, unlike stratification, is seldom used in individually randomised trials. It is used more often in cluster randomised trials because of the greater chance of imbalance in cluster randomised trials in which complete randomisation is used (see Section 5.1.2), and the fact that clusters can often be identified in advance of a trial so it is easier to approach or select pairs. The principle of matching is that pairs of clusters are constructed so that, within each pair, clusters are as similar as possible in relation to factors that might affect the trial outcomes. It is particularly common for clusters such as towns or communities to be matched; for example, Dietrich *et al.* (1998) used matching in a trial in which the intervention was aimed at encouraging sun protection for children, and the clusters were towns. Matching was also used in the COMMIT trial in which villages were randomised in blocks (Table 5.8). Note that the mechanism for allocation in this trial was similar to that used in the Kumasi trial (Section 5.1.5), but in the Kumasi trial blocking in blocks of two was a device to facilitate trial logistics, while in the COMMIT trial matching was used to balance trial arms in terms of prognostic factors. In the Kumasi trial the blocking was ignored in the trial analysis, but in the COMMIT trial it was not.

Although there can be gains in statistical efficiency from matching (Freedman, Green and Byar, 1990; Freedman *et al.*, 1997), there are also disadvantages. Firstly, if one cluster is lost, the matched cluster cannot be used in a matched analysis. Secondly, if the matching is not effective because the matched clusters are insufficiently similar to each other, then matching can result in decreased rather than increased power (Martin *et al.*, 1993), although this can be dealt with in the analysis by breaking the matches (see Section 6.4.1). Finally, it is not possible to calculate the ICC directly from the trial data (Klar and Donner, 1997) unless it is assumed that the intervention effect is constant across pairs – a rather strong assumption. These disadvantages led Klar and Donner to suggest that stratified rather than

Table 5.8   COMMIT: community-based intervention to increase smoking quit rates.

Aim: To assess whether a community-level, multi-channel, 4-year intervention would increase quit rates among cigarette smokers, with heavy smokers (≥ 25 cigarettes per day) a priority

Location and type of cluster: Communities (20 in United States, 2 in Canada)

Interventions: (i) Control: no intervention (ii) Intervention: each community formed a community board. The intervention focused on public education, healthcare providers, worksite and other organisations, and cessation resources

Primary outcome: Smoking quit rates

Randomisation: Twenty-two communities were matched (in eleven pairs)

Matching factors: (i) Geographic location (state or province) (ii) Size (iii) General socio-demographic factors

---

Source: COMMIT Research Group (1995).

matched designs may be preferable if investigators are not able to achieve a high degree of matching between pairs.

5.1.10   Unequal allocation to intervention arms

There are a number of reasons for unequal allocation to intervention arms in trials. In cluster randomised trials unequal allocation is not common but, when it does occur, the most common reason is to minimise cost. The implementation of an intervention in a cluster randomised trial is frequently expensive and time consuming, and cost savings can therefore be made by allocating a greater number of clusters to the control arm than to the intervention arm. This was the case in the OPERA trial (Table 5.9), in which the allocation ratio was $1.5:1$ (control: intervention). Unfortunately, the use of minimisation resulted in an actual allocation ratio of $1.23:1$, and consequently a greater number of homes in the intervention arm than originally intended.

5.2   Cohort versus cross-sectional designs

A cohort design differs from a cross-sectional design in the specification of which individuals are included in the trial. Most cluster randomised trials have either a

Table 5.9   OPERA: physical activity in residential homes to prevent depression.

Aim: To evaluate the impact on depression of a whole-home intervention to increase physical activity among older people

Location and type of cluster: UK residential and nursing homes for older people

Number of clusters and individual participants: 78 clusters recruited and analysed; 1060 participants recruited

Interventions: (i) Control: depression awareness programme delivered by research nurses (ii) Intervention: depression awareness programme delivered by physiotherapists plus whole-home package to increase activity among older people, including physiotherapy assessments of individuals, and activity sessions for residents

Primary outcomes: Prevalence of depression (Geriatric Depression Scale) at 12 months (outcome at one time point only; cross-sectional design), change in depression score at 12 months in all those present at baseline (repeated measures on same participants; cohort design), change in depression score at 6 months in those depressed at baseline (repeated measures on same participants; cohort design)

Design: Stratification by region and then minimisation of homes after recruitment of individual participants in homes at baseline using allocation ratio within the minimisation program of $1.5:1$ (control intervention). Subsequently further individuals were permitted to join the study

Source: Underwood *et al.* (2011).

cohort or a cross-sectional design, with the latter further divided into single and repeated cross-sectional designs, but sometimes both designs occur within the same trial as we describe later in this section.

In an individually randomised trial, investigators can take outcome measurements on each participant either at the end of the trial, or at more than one time point, for example a baseline measurement followed by the outcome measurement on each participant. The issue of *whom* to take measurements on does not usually arise: measurements are taken on trial participants.

In cluster randomised trials, measurements are taken on individual participants within the clusters recruited into the trial. However, if several measurements are taken over time these can be on the same individuals at each time point or on different individuals at each time point. If repeated measurements are taken on the same individuals at each time point, this is called a *cohort design*. This design is most useful when investigators want to determine how an intervention changes individual-level outcomes. An example of this is the diabetes care from diagnosis trial which evaluated a patient-centred approach to caring for people with diabetes (Table 5.10); consenting patients with newly diagnosed diabetes were followed up for a year, providing baseline and 12-month data on a variety of measures.

If repeated measurements are taken on different individuals at each time point, this is called a *repeated cross-sectional design*. This design is most commonly used when the aim is to determine how an intervention affects some community-level index of health. An example occurs in a trial looking at improving screening for haemoglobin disorders. In this trial a nurse worked within the practice to improve screening (Table 5.11). Screening rates were obtained at baseline and at the end of the intervention period. Clearly it would not have made sense to try and follow up the same individuals for screening after the intervention since they would already have had their screening results from the baseline screening.

Table 5.10   Diabetes care from diagnosis trial.

Aim: To assess the effect of additional training of practice staff in patient-centred care on the current well being and future risk of patients with newly diagnosed type 2 diabetes

Location and type of cluster: UK general practices

Number of clusters and individual participants: 43 clusters recruited, and 41 analysed; 250 individual participants analysed

Interventions: (i) Control: approach to care developed with practices, based on national guidelines and including patient materials (ii) Intervention: as control plus extra training on patient-centred care

Main outcome measures: Quality of life, well-being, haemoglobin A1c and lipid concentrations, blood pressure, body mass index

Data collection: Baseline and one-year data were collected on consenting participants, from clinical notes and by research nurses and project staff

Source: Kinmonth *et al.* (1998).

Table 5.11   Trial to improve screening for carriers of haemoglobin disorders.

Aim: To investigate the effectiveness of improving screening for carriers of haemoglobin disorders in general practice by using a nurse facilitator working with primary care teams and the relevant haematology laboratories

Location and type of cluster: UK general practices

Number of clusters and individual participants: 26 clusters recruited and randomised

Interventions: (i) Control: usual care (ii) Intervention: posters, leaflets, and formal education sessions

Primary outcome: Number of requests for screening tests for haemoglobin disorders

Data collection: The number of requests for screening was obtained from the laboratory at baseline and at the end of the intervention period

---

Source: Modell *et al.* (1998).

In some trials data may be collected using a repeated cross-sectional design, but there may be considerable overlap between those included at the different data collection time points. This may allow some outcomes to be treated as if they come from a cohort design. For example, in the OPERA trial (Table 5.9), investigators measured depression scores (the outcome) at baseline, and then at 6 months and 12 months after the introduction of the intervention. Because of a relatively high rate of death and movement out of the clusters (residential homes), the residents on whom the outcome was measured at 6 and 12 months were not exactly the same individuals as those on whom baseline measurements were taken, although there was considerable overlap. Two outcomes were prevalence of depression at 12 months and remission of depression at 6 months. For the former, a repeated cross-sectional approach to data analysis was used, with prevalence amongst all residents present in a cluster at baseline included as a covariate in the analysis. For remission of depression, however, a cohort approach to data analysis was taken in which only those who were identified as depressed at baseline *and* still present at the 6-month follow-up were included in the analysis.

In some trials some outcomes may be collected on individual participants in a cohort design and others collected at the cluster level in a repeated cross-sectional design. This was the case in the CATCH trial described in Section 3.3 of Donner and Klar (2000).

While the primary reason for selecting a cohort or cross-sectional design should be related to trial aims, there are other considerations when choosing between the two designs, such as availability of outcome data and likely attrition if a cohort design is chosen. These are discussed in Feldman and McKinlay (1994). A cohort design is potentially more statistically efficient than a cross-sectional design, but Donner and Klar (2000) point out that this advantage may be marginal or non-existent in practice and should therefore probably not be used as a reason for choosing one design over the other.

5.3   Parallel designs with more than two arms

5.3.1   Introduction

Parallel designs with more than two arms are less common than those with two arms. The reason for having more than two arms is usually that investigators wish to evaluate more than one active intervention. The simplest way of including more than two arms is to allocate clusters to one more arm than there are active interventions, so that, for example, with two active interventions to evaluate, a trial would have three arms, with the third arm being the control arm. Alternatively a full factorial design can be used. In this section we discuss both options. All of the methods of allocating clusters to intervention arms described for trials with two arms are available for trials with more than two arms.

5.3.2   Trials with one more arm than there are active interventions

One example of a parallel trial with more than two arms is a trial evaluating whether a nutrition manual introduced into physician practices in the United States could enhance nutrition screening, advice/referral, and follow-up for cancer prevention. One intervention arm received a manual, a second intervention arm received the manual and an interactive tutorial, and a control arm received neither (Table 5.12). This type of design, in which one active intervention arm receives the intervention that was implemented in the other active intervention arm plus an extra element, is not uncommon. Alternatively a three-arm trial may compare three quite different

Table 5.12   Different interventions to evaluate methods of improving nutrition-related behaviour of staff.

Aim: To determine the effectiveness of two strategies for promoting the use of the (nutrition) manual in improving nutrition-related behaviour of physicians and office staff

Location and type of cluster: Family practices in the Unites States

Number of clusters and individual participants: 810 practices recruited, and 755 analysed. No information on numbers of individual participants

Interventions: (i) Usual care (ii) Mailing a manual to a physician in the practice (iii) Providing the manual, and training a physician in the practice using an interactive tutorial

Primary outcome: Adherence to recommendations in the manual

Primary comparison: 'We hypothesized that practices with a physician who participated in the in-person tutorial would engage in more nutrition-related behaviours.'

Source: Tziraki *et al.* (2000).

Table 5.13   ASSIST: different interventions to promote secondary prevention of coronary heart disease.

Aim: To assess the effectiveness of three different methods of promoting secondary prevention of coronary heart disease in primary care
Location and type of cluster: UK general practices
Number of clusters and individual participants: 21 clusters recruited and analysed; 1906 participants analysed
Interventions: (i) Audit of notes with summary feedback to primary healthcare team (audit group) (ii) Assistance with setting up a disease register and systematic recall of patients to general practitioner (GP recall group) (iii) Assistance with setting up a disease register and systematic recall of patients to a nurse-led clinic (nurse recall group)
Primary outcome: Adequate assessment of three risk factors: blood pressure, cholesterol and smoking status at follow-up

---

Source: Moher *et al.* (2001).

approaches to achieving changes in outcome. This was the case in the ASSIST trial (Table 5.13).

One of the issues with a three-arm parallel trial is deciding on the primary comparison. Often investigators are primarily interested in the difference between the two active interventions; this was the case in the Tziraki *et al.* (2000) trial. If there is no evidence of a difference between the active interventions, a control arm is useful to identify whether neither active intervention had an effect or whether both had similar effects. In the ASSIST trial (Table 5.13), investigators powered their trial to detect a difference between the audit arm and GP recall arm, although they were also interested in the comparison between nurse recall and audit. The rationale for including three arms in this trial was that the interventions evaluated had been tested before but not compared directly, and their cost effectiveness had not been assessed.

In addition to potentially complicating the analysis by having a variety of possible comparisons, an addition of a third arm in a cluster randomised trial will usually increase the size of the trial by about 50%. Given that these trials are often considerably larger and more complex to conduct than individually randomised trials, there must be good justification for using more than two arms, and investigators should think carefully about this if considering such a trial.

5.3.3   Full factorial designs

An alternative to a trial in which different interventions are compared in the way we have just described is a factorial design. In a factorial design randomised units are divided into arms so that each arm receives a different combination of the various potential interventions. In a full factorial design all possible combinations are represented, but in a fractional factorial design not all possible combinations are represented. Strictly speaking, then, the three-arm trials described in Section 5.3.2 are fractional factorial designs, although this term is almost never used in this context. Recently, fractional factorial designs have been discussed in relation to designing interventions for evaluation in a full trial, and we described these in Chapter 3 (Section 3.6).

The simplest case of a full factorial design and the one most often used in trials, including cluster randomised trials, is a two by two factorial design. In this type of trial there are two interventions; each intervention can be delivered or not. This results in four arms: an arm that receives both interventions, an arm that receives only the first intervention, an arm that receives only the second intervention and an arm that receives neither. These sorts of trials were invented to achieve greater efficiency: potentially, investigators are conducting two independent trials for the price of one. If the two interventions act independently, the sample size needed is equal to that required for whichever intervention evaluation requires the largest sample size.

One example of a factorial cluster randomised trial is a trial investigating the effectiveness of two different interventions aimed at improving attendance for breast screening in general practices failing to meet national targets (Table 5.14). The investigators made a distinction between systematic interventions, such as letters from practitioners, and opportunistic interventions such as prompts to discuss screening when women attended at the general practice. They wished to evaluate the effectiveness and cost effectiveness of both types of intervention, and a factorial trial was an efficient way of doing this.

In the analysis of factorial trials (see Section 6.4.2), comparison is made between those who receive the first intervention and those who do not, ignoring whether or not participants receive the second intervention, and vice versa. The assumption is that whether or not individuals receive the first intervention does not affect the effectiveness of the second intervention and as a corollary, whether or not individuals receive the second intervention does not affect the effectiveness of the first. When this assumption holds good the design is very useful, and investigators do get two trials for the price of one. However, there are situations in which the assumption breaks down, and this can cause problems, which we now describe.

Table 5.14   Two interventions to increase breast screening.

Aim: To examine the effectiveness and cost effectiveness of two interventions based in primary care aimed at increasing uptake of breast screening
Location and type of cluster: UK general practices
Number of clusters and individual participants: 24 practices were recruited and analysed; 6133 women were randomised, and 5732 analysed
Interventions: (i) Control: usual care (ii) General practitioner letter (iii) Flag in women's notes to prompt discussion (iv) Both interventions
Primary outcome: Attendance for screening

Source: Richards *et al.* (2001).

The fundamental problem with a factorial trial occurs when there is an interaction between the interventions being evaluated. Here we illustrate the problem assuming a two by two full factorial trial, but the problem extends to more complex designs. An interaction between two interventions occurs when the effect of one intervention is dependent on whether or not individuals receive the other intervention. There are two different ways that that can happen. An antagonistic interaction means that each intervention works better without the other, so that together they may not do any better than the single interventions by themselves. Alternatively, a synergistic interaction means each intervention is more effective when combined with the other, so that when implemented together they are more effective than might be expected from the action of each separately. One example of a synergistic interaction is a trial evaluating two interventions to reduce blood pressure in Pakistan (Jafar et al., 2009; Table 2.8). In this trial the clusters were communities; one intervention was delivered to households by lay workers and the other intervention was training of general practitioners. When the interventions were delivered together the effect was to decrease systolic blood pressure by 10.8 mm Hg in the combined intervention arm, but by only 5.8 mm Hg in each of the other arms, including the control arm.

Nevertheless, antagonistic interactions are probably more common than synergistic interactions amongst interventions evaluated in cluster randomised trials. Unfortunately, it is antagonistic interactions that cause the more serious problem in factorial trials because they can lead to such trials being underpowered. As an illustration of the effects of an antagonistic intervention, consider a trial in which the mean outcome score for individuals receiving no intervention is 3, for individuals receiving each single intervention 5, and for individuals receiving both interventions 5 (see Table 5.15). In other words, those people who receive both interventions do not see any more improvement in their scores than the people who receive just one or the other. Those receiving neither intervention, however, have a lower outcome score. Based on these results, if investigators were to conduct two separate trials we would expect the difference between the intervention and control arms to be 2 units in each trial. But in the factorial trial, while all of those who receive the first intervention have a mean score of 5, half of those who do not receive this intervention also have a mean score of 5, so the mean difference between those who receive and do not receive the first intervention is no longer 2, but 1. A larger trial is required

Table 5.15   Mean outcome scores for individuals in each arm of hypothetical factorial trial.

	No intervention	Intervention B	Mean score across two arms
No intervention	3	5	4
Intervention A	5	5	5
Mean score across two arms	4	5	

to detect this smaller difference, so the full factorial trial loses some of its advantage. In addition, if there is an antagonistic interaction, investigators need to decide how big this might be before proceeding to calculate the sample size for the full factorial trial. Note that in this example we have illustrated an *additive* interaction on the *linear* scale; other types of interaction are possible.

In drug trials it is plausible that interactions are more common if two drugs act on the same organ in the body. In cluster randomised trials it is often less clear whether interactions might occur, and investigators need to consider this carefully on a trial by trial basis.

Investigators can design trials in which the aim is to detect whether or not there is an interaction, but this requires a much bigger sample size than a trial in which the aim is simply to detect a main effect. As for three-arm trials (Section 5.3.2), ensuring a trial is large enough to detect a realistic interaction is challenging.

Full factorial trials are not possible for all types of intervention. For example, if the aim is to compare interventions that are similar but where one is more intensive than another, it does not make sense to use a full factorial trial. The trial in Table 5.12 is an example of this.

5.3.4   Randomisation at cluster and individual level

Sometimes investigators may wish to evaluate two interventions, of which one must be evaluated using a cluster randomised design, while the other could be evaluated using an individually randomised design. One example of this is the MINT trial that evaluated treatments for whiplash (Table 5.16). An evaluation of the Whiplash Book versus usual advice was carried out using a matched cluster design. Patients with symptoms persisting two weeks after their emergency department attendance were eligible to join an individually randomised trial comparing physiotherapy with further advice. Thus, in this trial only a subset of individuals in clusters were entered into the individually randomised trial, depending on their progress as a result of the cluster-level intervention. In contrast, in some trials the cluster and individual randomisation takes place simultaneously. This was the case in a trial based in residential facilities for older people in which the investigators wished to assess the effectiveness of bright light and melatonin on cognitive and non-cognitive function (Riemersma-van der Lek *et al.*, 2008). Facilities were randomised to bright or dim light, and participants were randomised to melatonin or placebo. In the statistical literature, designs with randomisation at two different levels are referred to as split-plot designs.

5.4   Crossover designs

In a crossover trial all participants (in this case clusters) receive both the active and the control intervention; it is the order in which clusters receive the interventions that is randomised. In the analysis, comparisons are effectively within-participant comparisons; between-participant (cluster) variation is ignored, and as a result

Table 5.16   MINT: two interventions to prevent whiplash.

Aim: To investigate the effectiveness of interventions designed to prevent the
chance of developing whiplash syndrome
Randomisation units: UK National Health Service Acute Trust (cluster-level);
patients with persisting symptoms (individual-level)
Number of clusters: 12 clusters recruited
Interventions:
  Cluster-level: (i) Control: usual advice (ii) Intervention: Whiplash Book
  Individual-level : (i) Control: reinforcement of advice given in emergency
  department (ii) Intervention: physiotherapy
Primary outcome: Neck Disability Index
Randomisation:
  Cluster-level: Trusts matched
  Matching factors: (i) Number of emergency department attendances per year
  (ii) Star rating (iii) Ethnic composition of the surrounding area
  Individual-level: Eligible individuals stratified by emergency department and
  allocated in intervention and control arms (members of the same household are
  assigned to the same intervention, to reduce contamination)

Source: Lamb *et al.* (2007).

Table 5.17   Parenting intervention to improve development in very preterm infants.

Aim: To determine the efficacy of a neonatal parenting intervention for improving
development in very preterm infants
Location and type of cluster: UK neonatal centres
Number of clusters and individual participants: 6 clusters were recruited and
analysed; 195 babies had data analysed
Interventions: Weekly Parent Baby Interaction Programme (PBIP) sessions during
neonatal intensive care unit admission and up to six weeks after discharge
Primary outcome: Bayley scales of infant development
Randomisation: Six clusters, three from each of two regions. For four clusters,
clusters (one from each region) were paired on the basis of deprivation indices,
and the final pair was formed from the third cluster from each region

Source: Johnson *et al.* (2009).

overall variation is reduced and the power of the trial is increased. Thus, as for a
factorial design, the idea behind these trials is to increase the efficiency of the trial
or, working on the same principle, to achieve the same power with a smaller sample
size. For a general introduction to crossover trials see Sibbald and Roberts (1998).

Crossover cluster randomised trials are not very common. One example is a trial
by Johnson *et al.* (Table 5.17): six clinics were arranged into three pairs, and within
each pair one clinic was randomised to receive the intervention first, and one to
receive the control first. Essentially, then, this trial is both matched and crossover:

quite a complicated design. One of the rationales for this design was to increase precision of effect estimates given the limited number of clusters available. The intervention was aimed at parents of preterm babies.

In both periods of the trial, investigators identified mothers within the clinics and followed them up for two years to look at their outcomes. Mothers in the clinics which were receiving the intervention in that period received training.

The major disadvantage of crossover trials is the risk that whatever happens in the first trial period may carry over into the second trial period. This is referred to as the carryover effect, and it can compromise trial results because those who receive the control in the second period will be benefitting from carryover from the intervention; thus any differences between outcomes measured at the end of the control and intervention periods underestimate the effect of the intervention. This means that crossover trials are unsuitable for interventions that produce irreversible change in the first period; for example, in individually randomised trials a crossover design is no good if the intervention being evaluated cures the disease being investigated. When there is potential for short-term carryover, a washout period is introduced between the two trial periods, long enough for any short-term carryover to have disappeared by the time the second trial period begins.

In a cluster randomised trial there is potential for carryover at both cluster and individual level. Irreversible change at the cluster level can be produced in a number of different ways; for example, via education and training for professionals within the cluster. One would normally hope for at least some irreversible changes in behaviour, however small, as a result of education or training, so a crossover trial would not be suitable for evaluating health professional education. Thus, many of the trials used as examples in this chapter, including ELECTRA (Table 5.6) and the Diabetes Manual Trial (Table 5.3), could not have been designed as crossover trials. In the trial by Johnson *et al.*, carryover at the cluster level was avoided because no professionals in the cluster were involved in the intervention. The intervention was delivered direct to individual participants by research nurses who did not belong to the cluster; once they left the cluster, the intervention left with them.

The aim of the intervention in many cluster randomised trials is to produce irreversible change in individual participant behaviour, thus inducing a carryover effect if the *same* individuals are included in both intervention periods. Carryover can be avoided, however, if a repeated cross-sectional design is used (Section 5.2). This was the case in the Johnson *et al.* trial: it was not the same mothers who had outcomes measured on them during the two intervention periods. The investigators also used a three-month washout period which they describe as being instigated to reduce contamination; in other words they allowed recruits from the first period to be discharged before new recruits in the second period were involved in the trial.

Thus, using professionals external to a cluster to deliver the intervention and using a repeated cross-sectional design will reduce the likelihood of carryover in cluster randomised crossover trials. The decision about whom to use to deliver an intervention should, however, be based on an assessment of what would be most effective, and should reflect the most likely delivery strategy to be used in routine practice if the trial shows evidence of effectiveness.

5.5   Further design considerations

5.5.1   Pseudo cluster randomisation

In pseudo cluster randomised trials the majority of individuals (but not all) in intervention clusters receive the intervention, while the majority of individuals (but not all) in control clusters do not (Borm *et al.*, 2005; Teerenstra *et al.*, 2006). The idea is to reduce recruitment bias (Section 2.3) by not informing professionals within a cluster which arm of the trial they are in; while at the same time lessening the chances of contamination by ensuring that within each cluster the majority of individuals are receiving the same intervention. A pseudo cluster randomised design is only suitable for trials in which the intervention is aimed solely at the individual participants (individual-cluster, see Section 2.2.2). The design cannot be used if clusters or professionals within the clusters receive part of the intervention, because they cannot then be kept uninformed about which arm they are in. Moreover, such designs are only likely to achieve the aim of keeping professionals uninformed of which arm they are in when the cluster size is small enough to prevent them guessing by the ratio of intervention to control participants.

5.5.2   Stepped wedge designs

In stepped wedge designs the trial starts with no randomisation units (in our case clusters) in the intervention arm and ends with all units in the intervention arm. The units are gradually included in the intervention arm over time in a random order. The addition of units into the intervention arm takes place at pre-specified time points. One or more clusters may be added at each time point; usually an identical number each time. The number added will depend on the logistics of the trial. Stepped wedge designs are useful when it is necessary to roll out the intervention to all clusters involved in the trial. This may be because a policy decision has been made to do so or because it is felt that the intervention will do more good than harm so that it would be unethical to withhold it from any clusters. Brown and Lilford (2006) and Hussey and Hughes (2007) provide a good introduction to these designs. At the time of writing this is a developing area and there is currently little consensus on how best to analyse stepped wedge designs.

5.5.3   Equivalence and non-inferiority trials

Most cluster randomised trials are designed as superiority trials, to detect a difference in outcomes between trial arms. However, there are a few trials designed as equivalence or non-inferiority trials (Jaffar *et al.*, 2009; Cleveringa *et al.*, 2010). These types of trial may be particularly useful when trial investigators wish to evaluate reorganisation of services but they require larger numbers than superiority trials.

5.5.4   Delayed intervention

A number of trials in this book use a delayed intervention design, for example, the Diabetes Manual trial (Table 5.3) and the IRiS trial (Table 5.7). In these trials the control arm clusters are offered the intervention once the trial period is over. This design may enhance cluster recruitment; clusters may be more willing to participate if they know they will receive an intervention at some point. On the other hand, these designs require further resources in trials which are often already expensive.

5.6   Summary

In this chapter we have introduced a number of possible designs for cluster randomised trials. Although there are several designs to choose from, for trials in health services research the most popular design remains a two-arm parallel trial in which investigators use a method of trying to balance some specific factors between arms. Some aspects of design, such as whether to use more than two arms or whether to use a cohort or cross-sectional design, are largely dictated by the research question that the investigators wish to answer, but logistical factors and statistical considerations can also be influential. For example, unequal allocation was adopted in the OPERA trial to reduce the workload of those who had to deliver the intervention (Section 5.1.10), and the crossover design in the trial to improve development of preterm infants was adopted to increase the power of the study to detect a significant result in a situation where limited clusters were available (Section 5.4). The influence of logistical factors may be greater in cluster randomised trials, which tend to be larger and more expensive than many individually randomised trials.

References

Altman, D.G. (1991) *Practical Statistics for Medical Researchers*, Chapman and Hall, London.

Borm, G.F., Melis, R.J., Teerenstra, S. *et al.* (2005) Pseudo cluster randomization: a treatment allocation method to minimize contamination and selection bias. *Stat. Med.*, **24** (23), 3535–3547.

Brown, C.A. and Lilford, R.J. (2006) The stepped wedge trial design: a systematic review. *BMC Med. Res. Methodol.*, **6**, 54.

Cappuccio, F.P., Kerry, S.M., Micah, F.B. *et al.* (2006) A community programme to reduce salt intake and blood pressure in Ghana [ISRCTN88789643]. *BMC Public Health*, **6**, 13.

Caria, M.P., Faggiano, F., Bellocco, R. *et al.* (2011) The influence of socioeconomic environment on the effectiveness of alcohol prevention among European students: a cluster randomized controlled trial. *BMC Public Health*, **11**, 312.

Carter, B.R. and Hood, K. (2008) Balance algorithm for cluster randomized trials. *BMC Med. Res. Methodol.*, **8**, 65.

Cleveringa, F.G., Minkman, M.H., Gorter, K.J. *et al.* (2010) Diabetes Care Protocol: effects on patient-important outcomes. A cluster randomized, non-inferiority trial in primary care. *Diabet. Med.*, **27** (4), 442–450.

COMMIT Research Group (1995) Community Intervention Trial for Smoking Cessation (COMMIT): I. cohort results from a four-year community intervention. *Am. J. Public Health*, **85** (2), 183–192.

Dietrich, A.J., Tobin, J.N., Sox, C.H. *et al.* (1998) Cancer early-detection services in community health centers for the underserved. A randomized controlled trial. *Arch. Fam. Med.*, **7**, 320–327.

Donner, A. and Klar, N. (2000) *Design and Analysis of Cluster Randomised Trials in Health Research*, Arnold, London.

Eldridge, S., Ashby, D., Feder, G.S. *et al.* (2004) Lessons for cluster randomised trials in the twenty-first century: a systematic review of trials in primary care. *Clin. Trials*, **1**, 80–90.

Evans, S., Royston, P. and Day, S. (2004) Minim: Allocation by Minimisation in Clinical Trials, http://www-users.york.ac.uk/~mb55/guide/minim.htm (accessed May 2011).

Feder, G., Agnew Davies, R., Baird, K. *et al.* (2011) Identification and Referral to Improve Safety (IRIS) of women experiencing domestic violence: a cluster randomised controlled trial of a primary care training and support programme. *Lancet*, Oct 12. [Epub ahead of print]

Feldman, H.A. and McKinlay, S.M. (1994) Cohort versus cross-sectional design in large field trials: precision, sample size, and a unifying model. *Stat Med.*, **13** (1), 61–78.

Freedman, L.S., Green, S.B. and Byar, D.P. (1990) Assessing the gain in efficiency due to matching in a community intervention study. *Stat. Med.*, **9** (8), 943–952.

Freedman, L.S., Gail, M.H., Green, S.B. *et al.* (1997) The efficiency of the matched-pairs design of the Community Intervention Trial for Smoking Cessation (COMMIT). *Control. Clin. Trials*, **18** (2), 131–139.

Griffiths, C., Foster, G., Barnes, N. *et al.* (2004) Specialist nurse intervention to reduce unscheduled asthma care in a deprived multiethnic area: the east London randomised controlled trial for high risk asthma (ELECTRA). *BMJ*, **328** (7432), 144.

Hampshire, A., Blair, M., Crown, N. *et al.* (1999) Action research: a useful method of promoting change in primary care? *Fam. Pract.*, **16** (3), 305–311.

Harmsen, H., Bernsen, R., Meeuwesen, L. *et al.* (2005) The effect of educational intervention on intercultural communication: results of a randomised controlled trial. *Br. J. Gen. Pract.*, **55** (514), 343–350.

Hussey, M.A. and Hughes, J.P. (2007) Design and analysis of stepped wedge cluster randomized trials. *Contemp. Clin. Trials*, **28** (2), 182–191.

Jafar, T.H., Hatcher, J., Poulter, N. *et al.* (2009) Community-based interventions to promote blood pressure control in a developing country: a cluster randomized trial. *Ann. Intern. Med.*, **151** (9), 593–601.

Jaffar, S., Amuron, B., Foster, S. *et al.* (2009) Rates of virological failure in patients treated in a home-based versus a facility-based HIV-care model in Jinja, southeast Uganda: a cluster-randomised equivalence trial. *Lancet*, **374** (9707), 2080–2089.

Johnson, S., Whitelaw, A., Glazebrook, C. *et al.* (2009) Randomized trial of a parenting intervention for very preterm infants: outcome at 2 years. *J. Pediatr.*, **155** (4), 488–494.

Kendrick, T., Burns, T. and Freeling, P. (1995) Randomized controlled trial of teaching general practitioners to carry out structured assessments of their long term mentally ill patients. *BMJ*, **311** (6997), 93–98.

Kerry, S.M., Cappuccio, F.P., Emmett, L. *et al.* (2005) Reducing selection bias in a cluster randomized trial in West African villages. *Clin. Trials*, **2** (2), 125–129.

Kinmonth, A.L., Woodcock, A., Griffin, S. *et al.* (1998) Randomised controlled trial of patient centred care of diabetes in general practice: impact on current wellbeing and future disease risk. *BMJ*, **317** (7167), 1202–1208.

Klar, N. and Donner, A. (1997) The merits of matching in community intervention trials: a cautionary tale. *Stat. Med.*, **16** (15), 1753–1764.

Lamb, S.E., Gates, S., Underwood, M.R. *et al.* (2007) Managing Injuries of the Neck Trial (MINT): design of a randomised controlled trial of treatments for whiplash associated disorders. *BMC Musculoskelet. Disord.*, **8**, 7.

Lasagna, L. (1976) Randomized clinical trials. *N. Engl. J. Med.*, **295**, 1086–1087.

Martin, D.C., Diehr, P., Perrin, E.B. *et al.* (1993) The effect of matching on the power of randomized community intervention studies. *Stat. Med.*, **12** (3–4), 329–338.

Modell, M., Wonke, B., Anionwu, E. *et al.* (1998) A multidisciplinary approach for improving services in primary care: randomised controlled trial of screening for haemoglobin disorders. *BMJ*, **317** (7161), 788–791.

Moher, M., Yudkin, P., Wright, L. *et al.* (2001) Cluster randomised controlled trial to compare three methods of promoting secondary prevention of coronary heart disease in primary care. *BMJ*, **322** (7298), 1338.

Oakeshott, P., Kerry, S.M. and Williams, J.E. (1994) Randomized controlled trial of the effect of the Royal College of Radiologists' guidelines on general practitioners' referrals for radiographic examination. *Br. J. Gen. Pract.*, **44** (382), 197–200.

Peto, R., Pike, M.C., Armitage, P. *et al.* (1977) Design and analysis of randomized clinical trials requiring prolonged observation of each patient. II analysis and examples. *Br. J. Cancer*, **35**, 1–39.

Pocock, S.J. and Simon, R. (1975) Sequential treatment assignment with balancing for prognostic factors in the controlled clinical trial. *Biometrics*, **31**, 103–115.

Raab, G.M. and Butcher, I. (2001) Balance in cluster randomized trials. *Stat. Med.*, **20**, 351–365.

Richards, S.H., Bankhead, C., Peters, T.J. *et al.* (2001) Cluster randomised controlled trial comparing the effectiveness and cost-effectiveness of two primary care interventions aimed at improving attendance for breast screening. *J. Med. Screen.*, **8** (2), 91–98.

Riemersma-van der Lek, R.F., Swaab, D.F., Twisk, J. *et al.* (2008) Effect of bright light and melatonin on cognitive and noncognitive function in elderly residents of group care facilities: a randomized controlled trial. *JAMA*, **299** (22), 2642–2655.

Roberts, C. and Torgerson, D. (1998) Randomisation methods in controlled trials. *BMJ*, **317** (7168), 130.

Scott, N.W., McPherson, G.C., Ramsay, C.R. *et al.* (2002) The method of minimization for allocation to clinical trials: a review. *Control. Clin. Trials*, **23**, 662–674.

Senn, S. (1997) *Statistical Issues in Drug Development*, John Wiley & Sons, Ltd, Chichester.

Sibbald, B. and Roberts, C. (1998) Understanding controlled trials. Cross-over trials. *BMJ*, **316** (7146), 1719–1720.

Sturt, J.A., Whitlock, S., Fox, C. *et al.* (2008) Effects of the Diabetes Manual 1:1 structured education in primary care. *Diabet. Med.*, **25** (6), 722–731.

Taves, D.R. (1974) Minimization: a new method of assigning patients to treatment and control groups. *Clin. Pharmacol. Ther*, **15**, 443–453.

Taves, D.R. (2010) The use of minimization in clinical trials. *Contemp. Clin. Trials*, **31** (2), 180–184.

Teerenstra, S., Melis, R.J., Peer, P.G. *et al.* (2006) Pseudo cluster randomization dealt with selection bias and contamination in clinical trials. *J. Clin. Epidemiol.*, **59** (4), 381–386.

Tziraki, C., Graubard, B.I., Manley, M. *et al.* (2000) Effect of training on adoption of cancer prevention nutrition-related activities by primary care practices: results of a randomized, controlled study. *J. Gen. Intern. Med.*, **15**, 155–162.

Underwood, M., Eldridge, S., Lamb, S. *et al.* (2011) The OPERA trial: protocol for a randomised trial of an exercise intervention for older people in residential and nursing accommodation. *Trials*, **12**, 27.

6

Analysis

In Chapter 5 we introduced a range of possible designs for cluster randomised trials. In this chapter we discuss analysis options for these designs. In Chapter 1 we outlined the importance of accounting for the clustered nature of the data in an analysis of a cluster randomised trial. Most analyses of cluster randomised trials now do this. This reflects an improvement over time: in the past many trials were analysed without accounting for clustering, and even now there is substantial variation between disciplines (Figure 6.1). This chapter focuses on analysis, but we begin with a section on data collection and management, an important precursor to any analysis (Section 6.1). We follow this with an illustration of the consequences of not accounting for clustering in the analysis (Section 6.2). Most of the rest of the chapter (Section 6.3) is concerned with the analysis of two-arm parallel trials which are completely randomised, stratified or minimised; as discussed in Chapter 5, most cluster randomised trials in health services research adopt one of these designs. In Section 6.4 we describe analysis options for other designs, in Section 6.5, avoiding bias in analysis of cluster randomised trials by using intention to treat principles (this is not as straightforward as it is in individually randomised trials) and finally Section 6.6 deals with planning analyses for these trials.

6.1 Data collection and management

For cluster randomised trials, data can be collected at the individual level or the cluster level. Consider, for example, a trial in which clusters are general practices and the outcome measure is prescription rates. In the UK, routine data can provide

A Practical Guide to Cluster Randomised Trials in Health Services Research, First Edition.
Sandra Eldridge and Sally Kerry.
© 2012 John Wiley & Sons, Ltd. Published 2012 by John Wiley & Sons, Ltd.

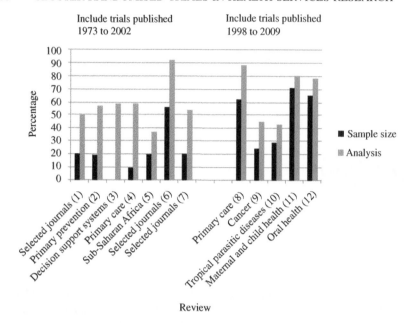

Figure 6.1   Proportion of trials from 12 reviews taking account of clustering in analysis (light grey) and sample size (dark grey).

Included reviews: (1) Donner, Brown and Brasher (1990); (2) Simpson, Klar and Donner (1995); (3) Chuang, Hripcsak and Jenders (2000); (4) Eldridge et al. (2004); (5) Isaakidis and Ioannidis (2003); (6) Puffer, Torgerson and Watson (2003); (7) Varnell et al. (2004); (8) Eldridge et al. (2008); (9) Murray et al. (2008); (10) Bowater, Abdelmalik and Lilford (2009); (11) Handlos, Chakraborty and Sen (2009); (12) Froud et al. (2011).

prescription levels by general practice, while individual patients' medical records can indicate their own prescription levels. Collecting data at an individual level is more time consuming than collecting routine data and, because of data protection considerations, involves governance issues around who collects the data and how. Decisions about the level at which to collect data will depend on the trial in question. For example, in a trial evaluating the impact of teaching general practitioners to carry out structured assessments of their long term mentally ill patients, the investigators measured whether the prescription of psychiatric drugs had changed by accessing the individual medical records of 373 individuals before and after the intervention (Table 6.1). It would not have been possible to assess individual change from practice-level data.

Whether *outcome* data are collected at the individual or cluster level, it would be unusual if no cluster-level data were collected in a cluster randomised trial. These data may be collected before randomisation and used in achieving balanced allocation (Section 5.1.3) or before or after randomisation to use in analyses. In the trial presented in Table 6.1, investigators collected information on the number of partners

Table 6.1   Structured assessments for long term mentally ill patients.

Aim: To assess the impact of teaching general practitioners to carry out structured assessments of their long term mentally ill patients

Location and type of cluster: UK general practices

Number of clusters and individual participants: 16 clusters were recruited and analysed; 440 participants were recruited, and 373 analysed

Interventions: (i) Control: usual care (ii) Intervention: general practitioners were taught a structured assessment schedule to use with patients every six months for two years

Primary outcome: Changes in drug treatments

Method of achieving balanced arms: Minimisation

Analysis: Analysis of covariance at cluster level, with changes in drug treatment in two years prior to intervention as covariate

Source: Kendrick, Burns and Freeling (1995).

in a practice, list size and the number of long term mentally ill patients in the practice before randomisation.

The foregoing discussion suggests that it is almost inevitable that some data will be collected at the individual level and some at the cluster level, and the two sets of data will need to be merged into one for analysis. It is therefore important that the relevant cluster can be easily identified for each individual in the trial. This may sound trivial, but it is sometimes the cause of considerable work trying to reconcile apparently discrepant data. One cause of discrepant data is clusters merging or splitting during the trial. This cannot be prevented. Accurate information must be collected throughout the trial, to enable investigators to deal with any changes appropriately at the analysis stage; it may be more difficult to do this retrospectively at the end of the trial. A clear strategy for handling data from clusters that change structure during the analysis needs to be developed and documented, including how such clusters will be represented in the CONSORT flow chart (Campbell *et al.*, 2004). Ideally, intention to treat principles (Section 6.5) would be followed, but in practice the strategy may depend on data collection options and the allocation status of the clusters. For example, in the IRIS trial (Table 6.13), some included clusters (general practices) merged during the trial period. For two practices originally randomised separately to the same intervention arm it was not possible to separate the data by original practice and they were treated as one practice for the purpose of analysis; while for another included practice that merged with a practice outside the trial it was possible to separate the data from the two practices so that only data from patients in the practice originally included were used in the analysis.

6.2   Analysis – an introduction

In his landmark paper in 1978, Cornfield states that 'Randomisation by cluster accompanied by an analysis appropriate to randomisation by individual is an exercise in self deception, however, and should be discouraged' (Cornfield, 1978). To understand what he meant, consider an extreme example of between-cluster variation in which all members of a single cluster have identical values of the primary outcome but the value of the primary outcome is different for each cluster. In this example, no within-cluster variation exists, so that measuring outcomes from a large number of individuals from a single cluster gives no more information than measuring the outcome on one person from the cluster. In a trial with less extreme between-cluster variation it is still the case that less information is obtained from several individuals in a cluster than from the same number of individuals randomly selected from the general population. Thus, if any degree of clustering is present, analysing a cluster randomised trial as if it were an individually randomised trial deceives the analyst into believing that she or he has as much information from the cluster randomised trial as would be obtained from an individually randomised trial; this is not the case.

6.2.1   Comparing analyses that do and do not take account of clustering

A good illustration of what can happen if a trial is analysed without taking clustering into account comes from a paper by Kerry and Bland (1998) in which they present the results of three different types of analysis on the same data. The data (Table 6.2) are from the trial presented in Table 6.1 and show, for each cluster, the numbers of patients whose drugs had changed in the two-year period after the intervention.

There are a number of ways of comparing changes in drug treatments between intervention and control arms of the trial (Table 6.3). For illustration, Kerry and Bland (1998) first perform an analysis that ignores clustering; a simple comparison of the total proportion of patients who changed in the intervention arm (123/184) and the total number who changed in the control arm (95/189), with confidence intervals (CIs) for the difference between these two proportions calculated in the usual way. This analysis falls into the trap that Cornfield highlights. A better approach is to calculate the proportions who change *in each cluster*, find the mean of those proportions in the two intervention arms, consider the difference between these two means using a *t*-test, and calculate the CIs based on the distribution of cluster proportions. The width of this distribution will reflect the variation between clusters. Using this second analysis, Kerry and Bland obtained wider CIs for the difference in the percentages changing drugs, reflecting the reduced amount of information available from a clustered design. This is an appropriate analysis; it takes account of clustering. However, the estimate of the difference in proportions between the two arms is not the same for this analysis (15.5%) as for the initial (incorrect) analysis (16.6%); if the cluster sizes were identical, then the two differences would be the same, but because of the variability in cluster size they are not. The third analysis that Kerry and Bland conduct weights cluster proportions by cluster size and thus takes account of both clustering and variability in cluster size. The estimate

Table 6.2 Number of patients whose psychiatric drugs were changed for each practice.

Number of patients		Percentage changed
Changed	Total	
Intervention arm		
11	23	47.8
7	12	58.3
23	38	60.5
13	19	68.4
16	23	69.6
15	20	75.0
23	30	76.7
15	19	79.0
123	**184**	
		Mean 66.9
		SD 10.6
Control arm		
4	14	28.6
10	28	35.7
20	48	41.7
4	8	50.0
14	24	58.3
16	27	59.3
16	25	64.0
11	15	73.3
95	**189**	
		Mean 51.4
		SD 15.2

SD = standard deviation.
S. Kerry, J.M. Bland, Trials which randomize practices I: how should they be analysed? *Family Practice*, 1998, 15, by permission of Oxford University Press.

of the difference between the intervention arms is the same as the original estimate, but the CIs are wider.

While the original analysis carried out by Kerry and Bland (1998) ignores clustering altogether, the second and third analyses rely on calculating a summary measure of outcome for each cluster level, and analysing these summary measures. Analysing summary measures from each cluster is referred to as cluster-level analysis, and is one possible way of analysing data from cluster randomised trials.

Kerry and Bland (1998) used a *t*-test of cluster summary measures to test the relevant hypothesis. A straightfoward *t*-test cannot, however, allow for confounding factors. In this trial investigators measured a number of potential confounders

Table 6.3   Summary of analyses conducted on the data from Table 6.2.

Analysis	Effect size estimate (%)	Confidence interval (%)	p-value
Test of the difference between two proportions ignoring clustering (incorrect)	16.6	6.7 to 26.4	0.001
t-test of cluster-level proportions (unweighted)	15.5	1.5 to 29.6	0.033
t-test of cluster-level proportions (weighted by cluster size)	16.6	3.2 to 29.9	0.018

Source: Kerry and Bland (1998).

including, for each of several outcomes, the level of activity for that item in the two years before the intervention. In the trial report these confounders were incorporated into an appropriate cluster-level analysis which we describe in Section 6.3.2.

6.2.2   The intra-cluster correlation coefficient

The reason for the differences between the widths of the CIs in Table 6.3 is the variation in drug change between clusters. This between-cluster variation is usually summarised in a measure referred to as the intra-cluster correlation coefficient (ICC). Because of its importance in cluster randomised trials, Chapter 8 is devoted to the ICC. In particular Section 8.1 covers the definition and interpretation of this quantity.

6.3   Analyses for two-arm, completely randomised, stratified or minimised designs

As described in Chapter 5, the majority of cluster randomised trials in health services research have a parallel design with two arms, with stratified and minimised designs being more common than completely randomised or matched designs. We cover completely randomised, stratified and minimised designs in this section because methods of analysis for these types of cluster randomised trial are similar. We cover matched designs in the next section.

For trials that are stratified, it is generally accepted that analysis should reflect the trial design, and stratification factors should be included as covariates in the analysis, and it has been recommended that minimisation factors also be included in trial analyses (Scott *et al.*, 2002). In addition, investigators using a completely randomised design often wish to include covariates, for example baseline values, in an analysis. Thus analyses of cluster randomised trials that include covariates are far more common than those that do not. Nevertheless, for completeness, the next section covers options for analyses that do not include covariates.

6.3.1 Analyses that do not allow the inclusion of covariates

Most of the analyses described in this chapter can be conducted either with or without covariates. There are, however, some statistical tests appropriate for cluster randomised trials that do not allow the inclusion of covariates. For completely randomised, stratified, and minimised designs, four such tests are a cluster-level, independent-samples t-test; a non-parametric test conducted at the cluster level; a non-parametric test using individual-level data but adjusting for clustering; and, for binary outcomes only, an adjusted chi-squared test.

We presented an example of a cluster-level, independent-samples t-test in Section 6.2, although this was a secondary analysis of trial data conducted for illustrative purposes; in the main trial report authors used an analysis of covariance (Section 6.3.2), not a t-test. An example of a cluster-level t-test in the main report of a cluster randomised trial occurs in Smith et al. (2004). The trial was of structured diabetes shared care amongst general practices in Northern Ireland. An individual-level analysis allowing for clustering and for covariates was also reported for this trial; this use of other analyses alongside cluster-level t-tests is not uncommon. For binary outcomes, the cluster-level summary used in the analysis need not be the proportion, p, for the cluster but could, for example, be the odds $(p/(1-p))$ or logarithm of the odds $(\log(p/(1-p)))$. In fact, a cluster-level t-test can be used for any summary measure of an outcome at cluster level, although investigators should pay attention to the underlying assumptions of a t-test; namely that the summary measures are normally distributed within each arm and that the variances of the distributions are identical in the two arms. A t-test is relatively robust to minor violations of these assumptions but in some cases, features of the data, such as the type of outcome being summarised and unequal cluster size, mean that these assumptions may be seriously violated. As described for the example in Section 6.2, a weighted t-test can be used to deal with unequal cluster sizes. There are two common options for weighting: weighting by cluster size, and inverse variance weighting which takes into account the intra-cluster correlation as well as the cluster size. Although in theory the second type of weighting will provide a more efficient estimate, this will only be the case when the true ICC is known; in most cases it will be an estimate.

Cluster-level non-parametric tests can be conducted in a similar way to cluster-level t-tests using data summarised at the cluster level. Individual-level non-parametric tests adjusted for clustering are a relatively recent development (e.g. Jeong and Hung, 2006; Rosner, Glynn and Lee, 2003; Rosner, Glynn and Lee, 2006).

For binary outcomes, another analysis that does not allow for covariates is an adjusted chi-squared analysis (Donner and Donald, 1988; Donner and Klar, 1994). In this analysis, the usual Pearson chi-squared statistic is adjusted to account for clustering using a formula which incorporates the ICC as a measure of the extent of clustering. If clustering is present, the adjustment results in a reduced chi-squared

Table 6.4 POST: patient and practitioner postal prompts post-myocardial infarction.

Aim: To determine whether postal prompts to patients who have survived an acute coronary event, and to their general practitioners, improve secondary prevention of coronary heart disease

Location and type of cluster: UK general practices

Number of clusters and individual participants: 59 clusters were recruited, and 52 were randomised and analysed; 328 participants were analysed

Interventions: (i) Control: usual care (ii) Intervention: leaflets to patients and letters to practitioners with summary of appropriate treatment based on locally derived guidelines

Primary outcomes: Proportion of patients in whom serum cholesterol concentrations were measured; proportion of patients prescribed β blockers (six months after discharge); and proportion of patients prescribed cholesterol lowering drugs (one year after discharge)

Method of achieving balanced arms: Minimisation

Analysis: Adjusted chi-squared test

Results: See Table 6.10

Source: Feder *et al.* (1999).

statistic, thus reducing the chances of a statistically significant effect. A good example of this analysis is presented in Donner and Klar (1994). This type of analysis was undertaken in the POST trial (Table 6.4). Although the allocation to arms was by minimisation, the minimisation factors could not be included in this analysis.

A permutation test is a further appropriate method for testing hypotheses using cluster-level summary data. The observed effect is first calculated from the cluster-level summaries; this may be, for example, the difference between two means. The same effect is then calculated for every possible way of allocating clusters into the two arms (with the number in each arm identical to the original allocation). An exact *p*-value is then based on the location of the observed effect size within the resulting distribution of effect sizes. The advantage of a permutation test is that, unlike a *t*-test, it does not rely on assumptions about the distribution of the data. A permutation test cannot allow for covariates directly, but the cluster-level summaries which are used in the test can be adjusted to allow for covariates prior to carrying out the test. The performance of adjusted and unadjusted permutation tests is compared in Raab and Butcher (2005). An adjusted permutation test was used to analyse the COMMIT trial (COMMIT Research Group, 1995). This trial had a matched design, and the analysis is described in more detail in Section 6.4.1. Other cluster-level analyses described in this section could also be subject to the same sort of adjustment for covariates in a similar two-stage process. To date, however, most investigators prefer not to use a two-stage process to adjust for covariates. Hayes and Moulton (2009) provide more detail for interested readers.

Cluster-level *t*-tests, non-parametric tests, and permutation tests can be particularly useful in trials in which the number of clusters is small. We discuss this further in Section 6.6. Analyses described in the present section are not common in relation to cluster randomised trials, however. Some analyses such as the cluster-level *t*-test were more popular in the past, but their use has decreased over time, partly because of advances in computing which allow more complex methods to be used more readily. In addition, for most cluster randomised trials investigators wish to include covariates, and the methods described in this section do not allow this unless a two-stage process is adopted. Next, we describe analyses that account for clustering *and* incorporate covariates.

6.3.2   Analysis allowing for the inclusion of covariates at the cluster level only

When investigators wish to incorporate cluster-level covariates but not individual-level covariates into an analysis, analysis of covariance at the cluster level can be used. This type of analysis was used in the trial of structured assessment for long term mentally ill patients that we used as an example in Section 6.2. The covariates were baseline levels of outcome summarised at cluster level. This analysis gave an estimate of the difference between intervention and control in the percentage who changed their psychiatric drugs of 16.6% (95% CI: 2.2 to 31.0%), not dissimilar to the result obtained using a weighted *t*-test without accounting for baseline levels of outcome (Table 6.3). Because measurements before and after the intervention were made on the same individuals (a cohort design – see Section 5.2), it would have been possible to conduct an analysis that incorporated the baseline measurements at the individual level as covariates. However, such individual-level analyses generally require a larger number of clusters than were included in this trial (16 clusters), so a cluster-level analysis was more appropriate. Although minimisation was used in this trial, the minimisation factors were not used as covariates in the analysis; they would be more likely to be included nowadays.

A cluster-level analysis of covariance was also used in a trial evaluating an intervention to implement clinical guidelines in general practice (Table 6.5). Baseline levels of outcomes summarised at the cluster level were included as covariates. In this trial, the baseline levels of outcome could not have been used as individual-level covariates because different individuals had data collected at baseline and follow-up (a repeated cross-sectional design – see Section 5.2). Minimisation was used to achieve balance between intervention and control arms, although, as for the trial in Table 6.1, minimisation factors were not included in the analysis. The analysis of covariance was weighted by cluster size to take account of variability in cluster size. Most outcomes showed some improvement from baseline values in the intervention arm; for asthma-related outcomes there was also an improvement in the control arm. For example, the percentage of patients with diabetes who had their blood glucose measured increased from 56.8 to 75.2% in the intervention arm but remained unchanged at 57.8% in the control arm; while the percentage of patients

Table 6.5   Clinical guidelines introduced with practice-based education.

Aim: To determine whether locally developed guidelines on asthma and diabetes disseminated through practice-based education improve quality of care in non-training, inner-city general practices

Location and type of cluster: UK general practices

Number of clusters: 24 clusters randomised and analysed

Interventions: (i) Intervention: three lunchtime, practice-based education sessions around asthma guidelines (ii) Intervention: three lunchtime, practice-based education sessions around diabetes guidelines

Primary outcomes: Recording of peak flow (for asthma) and blood glucose (for diabetes) in practice-held patient records

Method of achieving balanced arms: Minimisation

Analysis: Analysis of covariance adjusting for baseline levels of outcome

Results:

Adjusted difference in proportions with peak flow measured: 0.7% (95% CI:−15.2 to 16.7%)

Adjusted difference in proportions with blood glucose measured: 20.2% (95% CI: 6.4 to 33.9%)

Source: Feder *et al.* (1995).

with asthma who had their peak flow measured increased from 36.1 to 41.7% in the intervention arm and from 32.9 to 39.5% in the control arm. The difference between peak flow measures at baseline in the two arms is not insubstantial, and such differences are not uncommon in cluster randomised trials in which it is impossible to balance patient characteristics directly through stratification, matching and minimisation. In these circumstances an analysis that controls for baseline levels of outcome is more plausible.

In general, an analysis of covariance is appropriate in the following situations.

- When stratification or minimisation has been used and there are no other covariates; stratification or minimisation factors are used as cluster-level covariates.

- When it is desired to include only covariates measured at the cluster level.

- When some covariates are measured at the individual level but aggregated to the cluster level for analysis; this occurs most frequently when a repeated cross-sectional design (see Section 5.2) is carried out, although, as described above, it may also be used in a cohort design when investigators want to introduce one or two covariates but the number of clusters is relatively small.

While analysis of covariance was common in the past, it is rarely used now. Individual-level analyses adjusted for clustering are much more common and we cover those in the next section.

6.3.3   Analyses allowing for the inclusion of covariates at individual and cluster level

6.3.3.1   Introduction to different models

Analyses in which the individual is the unit of analysis (individual-level analyses) adjusted for clustering can incorporate individual-level covariates such as age, sex and individual baseline characteristics without the need to aggregate these to cluster level, and they are more efficient (in the statistical sense that estimates produced from them are more precise) than some of the analyses described in previous sections when cluster sizes vary. They are now the most common way of analysing cluster randomised trials. Nevertheless, they are often not appropriate when only a small number of clusters is included, as the methods are not then reliable (see Section 6.6). They can be used without covariates or with only cluster-level covariates, but, as described in the previous sections, there are also other options for analysis when investigators do not wish to include individual-level covariates.

The standard way of incorporating covariates into the analysis of *any* trial is to use a regression model appropriate to the structure of the data. For example, linear regression is usually used for continuous outcomes, logistic regression for binary outcomes, Poisson regression for rates and counts, and Cox's proportional hazards or other suitable regression models for time-to-event data. The same basic types of analysis are used for clustered data, but analyses need to be adjusted for the effect of clustering. Adjustment can be carried out in two distinct ways – using a cluster-specific model or a population-averaged model. These two models produce estimates of effects that have different interpretations.

A population-averaged effect answers the question: if an individual in the population moves from control to intervention arm, what will the effect be, on average? A cluster-specific effect, by contrast, answers the question: if an individual stays in the same cluster but moves from the control to intervention arm, what will the effect be, on average? Many researchers take the view that the first of these two questions is the more sensible to ask in relation to a cluster randomised trial, because in most trials the primary aim is to assess the impact of an intervention on individual participants. In these cases a population-averaged analysis is more appropriate. However, if the main aim of a trial is to assess impact on clusters, a cluster-specific analysis may be more appropriate.

Because the two effects are answering different questions, investigators should be careful to choose and interpret them appropriately. For linear and Poisson regression, the effects being estimated by population-averaged and cluster-specific models are essentially identical (Sections 6.3.3.2 to 6.3.3.6 and 6.3.3.12). They differ for logistic regression (Sections 6.3.3.7 to 6.3.3.11), but any difference is likely to be small in cluster randomised trials in health services research because it is dependent on the extent of clustering, which is usually relatively small in these trials. The following sections are organised according to the type of outcome (continuous, binary, time-to-event, count). We begin with continuous outcomes – these are the most straightforward. Binary outcomes, however, are the most popular type of primary outcome in cluster randomised trials.

Table 6.6   Continuous outcomes by cluster and arm for 12 clusters.

Arm	Cluster	Outcomes
1	1	5,6,6,6,7
1	2	5,5,7,7,8
1	3	6,6,7,8,8
1	4	5,5,6,6,6
1	5	5,7,7,8,9
1	6	6,7,8,9,10
2	7	5,5,5,5,6
2	8	6,6,6,7,7
2	9	3,4,5,5,6
2	10	4,5,5,5,6
2	11	4,4,4,5,6
2	12	4,5,5,5,6

6.3.3.2   Continuous outcomes – population-averaged and cluster-specific models

Table 6.6 shows outcome data from a small hypothetical trial in which 12 clusters, each with 5 members, were randomised to intervention or control arms. The intervention arm is coded 1, and the control arm is coded 2.

To estimate the population-averaged effect from these data we estimate the effect of an individual moving from the control arm to the intervention arm, by ignoring the clustering and simply calculating the mean in each arm (6.70 in the intervention arm and 5.13 in the control arm). The difference between the two means (1.57) gives us the population-averaged effect.

However, for the cluster-specific model we want to estimate what the effect would be for an individual who stays in the same cluster, but moves from the control to the intervention arm. To do this we make two assumptions: first, that the distribution of cluster means is identical in both the intervention and control arms (usually a normal distribution with identical variance in each arm), and second that the intervention effect is the same for every cluster. The second assumption implies that to estimate the cluster-specific effect it is simply necessary to estimate the difference between the mean of the distribution of cluster means in the intervention arm (6.70) and the mean of the distribution of cluster means in the control arm (5.13). In the case of this example, with a continuous outcome and equal sized clusters, it is straightforward to see that this is mathematically identical to the population-averaged effect.

If the cluster sizes in a trial are not equal, slightly different estimates of this effect may be obtained due to the different estimation procedures that the two models use. Nevertheless, the true effects will still be identical.

So far we have considered a simple example, without covariates, to illustrate the difference between population-averaged and cluster-specific effects. To generalise the example and to clarify how covariates are introduced into population-averaged and cluster-specific models, we present these two contrasting models algebraically. We begin with the simplest case in which the models are fitted without covariates, only a single predictor that represents the effect of the intervention. This can easily be expanded to the case of multiple covariates as we show below. In the expressions below, i represents clusters and j represents individuals. A population-averaged model can then be written as

$$Y_{ij} = \alpha + \beta x_{ij} + e_{ij} \tag{6.1}$$

where

Y_{ij} indicates the value of an outcome for the jth individual in the ith cluster

α = constant

β = effect size

x_{ij} indicates intervention arm. When there are only two arms, x_{ij} takes the value 1 when the ith cluster is in the intervention arm, and 0 when ith cluster is in the control arm

e_{ij} = residual for jth individual in the ith cluster

In a population-averaged model, the residuals within a cluster, e_{ij}, are correlated. To illustrate this, consider the hypothetical example presented in Table 6.5, in which $\alpha = 5.13$, and $\beta = 1.57$. The residuals are the differences between the observed outcome for an individual, Y_{ij}, and the outcome predicted for that individual, $\alpha + \beta x_{ij}$. For a control cluster the predicted outcome will be 5.13 (since $x_{ij} = 0$), and, for an intervention cluster, $5.13 + 1.57$. Rewriting Equation 6.1 for an individual in a control cluster

$$e_{ij} = (Y_{ij} - 5.13)$$

and for an individual in an intervention cluster

$$e_{ij} = (Y_{ij} - 5.13 - 1.57)$$

Thus, the residuals only differ from Y_{ij} by a constant. If clustering is present, the Y_{ij} in each cluster will be correlated, and therefore so will be the e_{ij}.

By contrast, for a cluster-specific model, the algebraic specification contains an extra term, μ_i, which represents the mean effect of being in cluster i; that is the difference between the mean outcome Y_i for cluster i and the constant α: $\mu_i = Y_i - \alpha$, where

$$Y_i = \sum_{j=1}^{n_i} \frac{Y_{ij}}{n_i}$$

and n_i is the number of individuals in cluster i.

Thus, the cluster-specific model is

$$Y_{ij} = \alpha + \beta x_{ij} + \mu_i + e_{ij} \tag{6.2}$$

and, using the same example, for this model, residuals for the control arm are

$$e_{ij} = [Y_{ij} - (Y_i - 5.13) - 5.13] = Y_{ij} - Y_i$$

and similarly for the intervention arm.

Assuming that there is the same degree of clustering within each cluster, the residuals within a cluster are then uncorrelated. This distinguishes these residuals from the correlated residuals in a population-averaged model. Usually it is assumed that the residuals, e_{ij}, within each cluster are normally distributed with the same mean and variance. This is written $e_{ij} \sim N(0, \sigma_w^2)$, where σ_w^2 then represents the within-cluster variance.

It is also usually assumed that μ_i are normally distributed: $\mu_i \sim N(0, \sigma_b^2)$, where σ_b^2 represents the between-cluster variance as previously. The μ_i are *random* effects, in contrast to α and β which are *fixed* effects. This type of model is often referred to as a *mixed effects* model because it contains both fixed and random effects. The reason for using a random rather than a fixed effect for clusters is that separate effects for each cluster are not of interest in a cluster randomised trial, in the same way that separate effects for each individual are not of interest in an individually randomised trial. The clusters are assumed to be a random sample of clusters that could have been included in the trial, all of which will have different μ_i values. It is most sensible to estimate the distribution of μ_i values, that is estimate σ_b^2, rather than individual μ_i values for each cluster; σ_b^2 is also often of interest in its own right or to estimate the ICC. Throughout this chapter we refer to models of the type reflected in Equation 6.2, which contain fixed effects and random effects, as mixed effects models, although the terms random effects model, hierarchical model and multilevel model are also used in this context. Strictly, these terms are not interchangeable, but for a cluster randomised trial a sensible mixed effects model will also be a multilevel model and will also be hierarchical. We prefer the term mixed effects model because it is immediately obvious that two different types of effect must be incorporated, and for cluster randomised trials that is the key feature which then makes these models multilevel or hierarchical.

Equations 6.1 and 6.2 can easily be extended to include further covariates, by including further x_{ij} representing the covariates and further β values representing the effects of these covariates. In summary, then, the three elements of a population-averaged model are the constant, a set of fixed effects which includes the intervention effect, and the residuals. A cluster-specific model is similar but includes an extra random effect term representing the cluster-specific effects. The residuals in a cluster-specific model are uncorrelated; while those in a population-averaged model are correlated. The models can become more complex with the addition of further random effects, including those that allow for different effects of the intervention in different clusters, but we do not discuss more complex models here because in general they have little relevance in cluster randomised trials.

At the beginning of this section we illustrated the difference in the way that effect size is estimated by the two types of model. Because of the differences in correlation structure between the cluster-specific and population-averaged models, the precision of effect estimates is also estimated differently. We now briefly describe the usual methods of fitting these models and estimating the precision of effect estimates. For population-averaged models we describe generalised estimating equations, and for cluster-specific models, the fitting of mixed models.

6.3.3.3   Continuous outcomes – generalised estimating equations

Generalised estimating equations (GEEs) (Liang and Zeger, 1986) are usually used to fit population-averaged models for cluster randomised trials. Using this method, the processes of estimating the effect and its precision are carried out separately. The correlation between observations within clusters is treated as a nuisance parameter, estimated from residuals, and used to correct the precision of estimates. Different correlation structures can be assumed in the modelling. When analysing cluster randomised trials, the usual assumption is that responses of cluster members are equally correlated with each other, referred to as the assumption of exchangeability. Without further information about cluster members this is an appropriate assumption. Using GEEs, inferences about model parameters can be made in two ways: either based on explicit modelling of variances in the data via the specified correlation structure, or relying on methods of estimating variances which are robust to misspecification of the correlation structure (Diggle *et al.*, 2002). Variance estimators based on the specified correlation structure are often referred to as 'model-based' to distinguish them from robust variance estimators. The advantage of model-based estimators is that they are more efficient if the correlation structure is correctly specified. On the other hand, robust estimators are consistent (in the statistical sense that as the sample size increases they will converge to the true value) even if this structure is misspecified. Robust variance estimators are due to Huber (1967), and more recently in the context of GEEs to Zeger and Liang (1986), and are also called sandwich estimators since the estimator can be written as an approximate correlation matrix 'sandwiched' between two similar expressions of matrix algebra. The papers by Liang and Zeger provide more detail (Liang and Zeger, 1986; Zeger and Liang, 1986). Robust estimators are almost always used in the analysis of cluster randomised trials. Strictly speaking, in this situation, the estimation process is semi-robust since it relies on correct specification of the mean, rather than being robust to the misspecification of the mean as well as the correlation structure. A non-technical introduction to GEEs is provided by Hanley *et al.* (2003).

Generalised estimating equations were used in the analysis of the Diabetes Manual trial (Table 6.7). Two of the factors used for minimisation (Section 5.1.6) were also used as covariates in the analysis. The third minimisation factor was the mean baseline value of HbA1c in each cluster; in the analysis, individual baseline value of HbA1c was used as a covariate. Other covariates used were practice geographic location, patient age, sex and socio-demographic status and a dummy variable indicating whether the patient had been recruited before or after a minor

Table 6.7   Diabetes Manual trial: manual and structured care to improve outcomes.

Aim: To determine the effects of the Diabetes Manual on glycaemic control, diabetes-related distress and confidence to self-care of patients with type 2 diabetes

Location and type of cluster: UK general practices

Number of clusters and individual participants: 48 practices randomised and analysed; 245 individual participants recruited, and 202 analysed

Interventions: (i) Control: usual care (ii) Intervention: education to nurses, followed by one-to-one structured education to patients via a self-completed manual and nurse support, and audiotapes

Primary outcome: HbA1c level

Method of achieving balanced arms: Minimisation

Analysis: Population-averaged models with robust standard errors using GEEs with adjustment for practice self-assessed quality of diabetes care, geographic location, value of outcome at baseline, age, gender, socio-economic status, and whether patient was recruited before or after protocol change

Result: Adjusted mean difference in HbA1c at six months: −0.08% (95% CI: −0.28 to 0.11%)

Source: Sturt *et al.* (2008).

protocol amendment. An exchangeable correlation structure was used, although this is not specified in the trial publication. An estimate of the ICC was produced directly from the analysis (Table 6.7). There was no significant difference at the 5% level between intervention arms in the primary outcome, HbA1c, but there was a significant difference in a secondary outcome, self-efficacy. It is not unusual to see changes in process or mediating outcomes in a cluster randomised trial alongside very little change in clinical outcomes.

Generalised estimating equations are now a popular method for analysing cluster randomised trials. In order to use GEEs, a trial must include a sufficient number of clusters. It is difficult to specify precisely how many this should be, but it has been shown that the method performs well when there are around 50 or more clusters and poorly if there are fewer than 10 clusters unless distributional assumptions are fully met (Feng, McLerran and Grizzle, 1996). There were 48 clusters in the Diabetes Manual trial (Table 6.7). In a trial with fewer clusters (Goud *et al.*, 2009), investigators used a jackknife method recommended by Long and Ervin (2000) to compensate for the small number of clusters, although they report that this did not make a substantial difference to the results. We describe this trial in Section 6.6. Other methods for compensating for small numbers of clusters and variation in cluster sizes in GEEs are becoming available. We now turn to analysis using cluster-specific models.

6.3.3.4   Continuous outcomes – mixed effects models

As described in Section 6.3.3.2, an appropriate cluster-specific model for a cluster randomised trial with a continuous outcome is a linear mixed effects model with the cluster treated as a random effect. The model is fitted to estimate the cluster-specific effect of the intervention on an outcome and the variance of the distribution of cluster means (σ_b^2) and within-cluster variance (σ_w^2) for this outcome. The precision of the effect estimate correctly adjusted for clustering can then be expressed as a combination of these two variances. When covariates are included, the effect estimate and variances will be adjusted for these covariates. Furthermore, the model will provide estimates of the precision of each included covariate adjusted for clustering and the effect of all other covariates and the intervention effect. Many methods are available for fitting mixed effects models in both general and bespoke statistical software packages. Common methods of fitting are maximum likelihood or restricted maximum likelihood. Unrestricted maximum likelihood estimates of variance components are known frequently to be biased downwards unless there are a large number of clusters. Restricted maximum likelihood has been developed more recently and tends to produce less biased estimates. It is also less computationally intensive. Both methods are widely available in software such as MLwiN (Rasbash *et al.*, 2005), SAS (www.sas.com) and Stata (Statacorp, 2009).

Mixed effects models are now very popular for analysing cluster randomised trials. One example is the trial of an intervention designed to improve intercultural communication that we described in Section 5.1.2. Table 6.8 shows the difference between the level of mutual understanding in intervention and control arms at the end of the intervention period controlling for baseline levels; this difference is small and not-significant at the 5% level. In the trial report, the analysis of this trial is described as multilevel regression analysis. The report contains no details of either the fitting procedures, for example whether unrestricted or restricted maximum likelihood was used, or the software used. This is not unusual, but if authors do provide this it is informative for statistically minded readers, and

Table 6.8   Educational intervention to improve intercultural communication.

Aim: To assess the effectiveness of an educational intervention on intercultural communication aimed to decrease inequalities in care provided between western and non-western patients

Location and type of cluster: Dutch general practitioners

Number of clusters and individual participants: 38 clusters were recruited, and 35 analysed; 986 individual participants were analysed

Interventions: (i) Control: (details not specified) (ii) Intervention: educational intervention to patients (12-minute videotape in waiting rooms) and for general practitioners (2.5 days of training spread over 2 weeks)

Primary outcome: Mutual understanding between patients and general practitioners (on a validated scale ranging from −1 to +1)

Method of achieving balanced arms: Complete randomisation

Analysis: Mixed effects linear regression with adjustment for baseline values

Results: Adjusted mean difference at six months: 0.01 (95% CI: −0.103 to 0.129)

Source: Harmsen *et al.* (2005).

provides a more secure basis for interpretation. Often, a mixed effects model for a cluster randomised trial will include more covariates than were included in this trial, and will include them at both individual and cluster level.

As for GEEs, the use of mixed effects models requires a sufficient number of clusters. Snijders and Bosker (1999) suggest that at least 10 clusters are necessary. However, as with many statistical techniques for which minimum numbers are suggested, this does not mean that the method is always suitable for trials with more than 10 clusters. Performance will also depend on other factors such as how closely the assumptions of the model are met, size of clusters and variability in cluster size. Many of those working in this area would recommend including more clusters. Furthermore, since it is generally agreed that the number of units analysed in a regression model should be at least 10 times the number of predictor variables to ensure model stability, trials should ideally have at least 30 or 40 clusters in order to allow for the inclusion of 2 or 3 covariates at cluster level in addition to the intervention effect. Nevertheless, linear mixed effects models are less biased than GEEs when the number of clusters is small.

6.3.3.5   Continuous outcomes – other methods of analysis

Spiegelhalter (2001) extended the cluster-specific mixed effects formulation given in Section 6.3.3.2 from a Bayesian perspective, allowing the incorporation of external evidence about parameters and relaxing some of the distributional and other assumptions. He concluded that Bayesian methods can be useful but could also lead to different results depending on the prior distributions used for the variance estimates. Prior distributions are used in a Bayesian analysis to quantify what the analyst believes about the parameter on which the prior is placed. For example, we may believe that an ICC cannot take negative values; an appropriate prior distribution will then reflect this. A Bayesian analysis produces the intervention effect as a posterior distribution which reflects both the prior distribution of the parameter and the data collected in the trial. In terms of priors for variance estimates, a prior distribution can be placed on either the ICC or between-cluster variance, and the prior for the alternate parameter can then be derived. There has been some work developing priors for ICCs, and we discuss this further in Chapter 8 (Section 8.3.4). Bayesian analyses have been little used in analysing cluster randomised trials, but they have the potential to provide more precise estimates if reliable methods of estimating and fitting appropriate informative prior distributions can be found. There are a small number of recent methodological papers in this area, but none focuses on continuous outcomes apart from the paper by Spiegelhalter.

6.3.3.6   Continuous outcomes – comparison of methods

Murray *et al.* (2006) compared the performance of permutation tests and mixed effects models for continuous clustered data, and concluded that there was little difference in their performance except when normality assumptions are violated and the ICC is larger than 0.01, when the permutation test performs better, with the mixed effects method being less powerful. ICCs are often larger than 0.01 in cluster randomised trials in health services research.

6.3.3.7   Binary outcomes – population-averaged and cluster-specific models

In Section 6.2.1 we calculated a population-averaged effect for the binary outcome 'whether individuals had their drugs changed or not'. This effect was presented as a difference between two proportions $(123/184) - (95/189)$. Calculating differences between proportions is one way of summarising binary outcomes, but it is commonly recognised that, to take account of covariates in estimating an effect for a binary outcome, it is necessary to transform the outcome onto the logistic scale. Effect estimates are then calculated on this scale. The logistic transformation of a proportion, p, is $\log (p/(1 - p))$, often referred to as the log odds, or logit of p. Transformation of data onto the logistic scale causes a difference between effect estimates from population-averaged and cluster-specific models (Neuhaus, Kalbfleisch and Hauck, 1991). In fact, Neuhaus *et al.* showed that if clustering is present, the effect being estimated by the cluster-specific model is always further from the null than the effect being estimated by the population-averaged model. We illustrate this with a hypothetical example.

Table 6.9 shows a hypothetical example of binary outcome data from a trial with equal sized clusters. As for continuous outcomes, it is easier to demonstrate the difference between population-averaged and cluster-specific effects using equal sized clusters, but the same principles apply when cluster sizes are unequal. Consider first the number of positive responses in each intervention arm overall (18 in the intervention arm and 11 in the control arm), and transformation onto the logistic scale (by taking the natural logarithm of the overall odds in each arm):

Table 6.9   Binary outcomes by cluster and arm for 12 clusters.

Arm	Cluster	Outcomes
1	1	1,1,1,1,0
1	2	1,1,1,1,0
1	3	1,1,1,0,0
1	4	1,1,1,1,0
1	5	1,0,0,0,0
1	6	1,1,0,0,0
2	7	1,0,0,0,0
2	8	1,0,0,0,0
2	9	1,1,0,0,0
2	10	1,0,0,0,0
2	11	1,1,1,1,0
2	12	1,1,0,0,0

log(18/12) and log(11/19). The absolute difference between these two gives the population-averaged effect on the logistic scale (0.4055 − −0.5465 = 0.9520), and it is easy to show that taking the exponent of such an effect gives an estimate of an odds ratio (2.591), in this case the population-averaged odds ratio. This can also be obtained more simply by calculating the overall odds ratio [(18/12) / (11/19)].

To estimate the cluster-specific effect we use an identical process to that carried out for continuous outcomes, except that the process is conducted on the logistic scale. We assume that the log odds (log $[p/(1 − p)]$) from each cluster are identically distributed in the intervention and control arms. We calculate the mean of the cluster log odds in each arm and find the difference. This gives the cluster-specific effect on the logistic scale, in this case 1.059, and taking the exponent gives the cluster-specific odds ratio (2.883). This is not the same as the population-averaged effect. The difference between the two effects depends on the extent of clustering. If clustering is not present the two effects will be the same. Algebraically, a population-averaged model for binary outcomes can be written as:

$$\text{logit } \pi_{ij} = \alpha + \beta x_{ij} \tag{6.3}$$

$$Y_{ij} \sim \text{binomial}(1, \pi_{ij})$$

where most notation follows from Section 6.3.3.2, and π_{ij} is expected probability of 'success' for individual j in cluster i (where success is defined as the binary outcome taking the value 1 and failure as the binary outcome taking the value 0).

In this model, no residuals are specified on the logistic scale. The residuals are instead specified on the linear scale, and residuals within clusters are correlated in a similar fashion to the residuals for continuous outcomes estimated from a population-averaged model (Section 6.3.3.2).

The cluster-specific model for a binary outcome is given by

$$\text{logit } \pi_{ij} = \alpha + \beta x_{ij} + \mu_i \tag{6.4}$$

$$Y_{ij} \sim \text{binomial}(1, \pi_{ij})$$

As for continuous outcomes, a random effect, μ_i, is introduced which represents the effects of the clusters. Further covariates can be introduced into Equations 6.3 and 6.4 as described for continuous outcomes in Section 6.3.3.2.

When population-averaged and cluster-specific models are fitted to estimate effect sizes and precision of odds ratios, the discrepancy between the effects obtained under each model may also depend on the methods of fitting and other factors such as the validity of assumptions made about the distribution of the cluster log odds in each arm (usually assumed normally distributed), the number of clusters, and the variation in cluster size.

Table 6.10 shows the results of population-averaged and cluster-specific analyses for the POST trial (Table 6.4) calculated using Stata software (Statacorp, 2009), and compares these with results from the adjusted chi-squared analysis presented in the trial report. The overall odds ratio calculated directly from the overall odds

Table 6.10   Effect sizes, precision and ICC for the outcome 'whether prescribed β blockers or not' from the POST trial, using different methods of analysis.

Analysis	Estimated odds ratio	95% confidence interval	Estimated ICC
Adjusted chi-squared	1.69	0.90 to 3.00	0.050
Population-averaged regression	1.66	0.96 to 2.85	0.029
Cluster-specific regression	1.68	0.93 to 3.03	—

in the two intervention arms is 1.69. This is also the odds ratio calculated using the adjusted chi-squared analysis, although the estimate has been rounded up in the trial report. The estimate from the population-averaged model is 1.66, slightly lower than the overall odds. A priori we would have expected the odds ratio from the population-averaged model to be equal to 1.69; the fact that it is not is due to the estimation procedures used in Stata; most likely in this case caused by unequal cluster sizes. The estimate from the cluster-specific model is higher than that from the population-averaged model as expected, but the difference is small. The ICC value for the adjusted chi-squared analysis was calculated using analysis of variance (Section 8.4.1). Again the discrepancy between this ICC estimate and that for the population-averaged model is most likely due to different estimation procedures. In spite of this, the confidence intervalss for these two methods are very similar. We do not present an ICC for the cluster-specific model because an equivalent ICC cannot be produced directly from a logistic-normal cluster-specific model (see Section 8.4.3).

6.3.3.8   Binary outcomes – generalised estimating equations

Generalised estimating equations for continuous outcomes were outlined in Section 6.3.3.3. The principles are the same for analyses of binary outcomes except that an effect is estimated on the logistic scale, while residuals have a binomial distribution on the linear scale. The function used to transform the data onto the analysis scale (in this case the logit function, $\log [p/(1 - p)]$, and the error structure (in this case binomial) must be specified when fitting the model. The function used to transform the data is referred to as the link function. Trial publications usually report an estimate of the odds ratio for these types of analysis. Odds ratios are estimated as the exponent of the effect estimate on the logistic scale.

In the DESMOND trial (Table 6.11), investigators used GEEs to estimate the effect of group education for diabetes on the proportions who smoked. Several individual-level covariates were included in the model. Although stratified randomisation was used, the stratification factors were not included as covariates. At the end of the trial period, 11% of participants in the intervention arm smoked: a decrease of 3% from baseline; whereas in the control arm the percentage smoking remained unchanged at 16%. Information about smoking status was obtained from

Table 6.11   DESMOND: diabetes education and self-management.

Aim: To evaluate the effectiveness of a structured group education programme on biomedical, psychosocial and lifestyle measures in people with newly diagnosed type 2 diabetes

Location and type of cluster: UK general practices

Number of clusters and individual participants: 207 clusters; 824 individuals recruited, and 562 provided information on smoking status

Interventions: (i) Control: guidelines pack plus resources to provide extra time with patients (ii) Intervention: group education programme delivered by healthcare professionals with quality assurance to ensure consistency

Relevant outcome: Smoking status (yes/no)

Method of achieving balanced arms: Stratification

Analysis: Robust GEEs with exchangeable correlation structure, logit link and binomial error distribution, with adjustment for age, sex and baseline value of the outcome variable

Results: Adjusted odds ratio of not smoking at 12 months: 3.56 (95% CI: 1.11 to 11.45)

Source: Davies *et al.* (2008).

a questionnaire administered at baseline and follow-up points; at 12 months only 74% of those recruited responded to the questionnaire. As in the clinical guidelines trial presented in Table 6.5, there was a considerable difference in baseline smoking level between the arms; again analyses that adjust for baseline levels may appear more plausible.

Generalised estimating equations were also used in the ELECTRA trial (Table 6.12). However, in an analysis of the effect of the intervention on the proportion of participants with asthma attending their general practice for unscheduled care, the ICC estimated from the model was negative. When this happens it is more appropriate to present an analysis unadjusted for clustering (see Section 6.6).

As for continuous outcomes (Section 6.3.3.3), a reasonably large number of clusters is required when using a GEE approach to analysing binary data from cluster randomised trials. The DESMOND trial included 207 clusters and the ELECTRA trial included 44.

6.3.3.9   Binary outcomes – mixed effects models

As described in Section 6.3.3.7, for binary outcomes an appropriate cluster-specific model for a cluster randomised trial is a mixed effects model with the cluster treated as a random effect. The difference between such a model for continuous outcomes (Section 6.3.3.1) and a model for binary outcomes is that for the latter the effect of the intervention is estimated on the logistic scale, while the residuals are estimated on the linear scale (Section 6.3.3.7). As a result of the two different scales involved, the fitting of mixed effects models for binary outcomes differs from the fitting for continuous outcomes. It is more complex, and methods are either computationally

Table 6.12   ELECTRA: asthma liaison nurses to reduce unscheduled care.

Aim: To determine whether asthma specialist nurses, using a liaison model of
   care, reduce unscheduled care in a deprived multiethnic setting
Location and type of cluster: UK general practices
Number of clusters: 44 clusters randomised and analysed; 324 participants
   recruited, and 319 analysed
Interventions: (i) Control: a visit promoting standard asthma guidelines; patients
   were checked for inhaler technique (ii) Intervention: patient review in a
   nurse-led clinic and liaison with general practitioners and practice nurses
   comprising educational outreach, promotion of guidelines for high risk asthma,
   and ongoing clinical support
Primary outcome: Unscheduled care for acute asthma over one year, and time to
   first unscheduled attendance
Analysis: GEEs adjusting for baseline levels of outcome and using link functions
   and error structures appropriate to the type of outcome
Method of achieving balanced arms: Minimisation
Results:
Adjusted incident rate ratio for number of attendances for unscheduled care
   during year of intervention: 0.91 (95% CI 0.66 to 1.26)
Adjusted odds ratio of attending for unscheduled care during year: 0.62 (95% CI
   0.38 to 1.01)

Source: Griffiths *et al.* (2004).

intensive (e.g. Gauss–Hermite Quadrature or Markov chain Monte Carlo) or approximate (e.g. Penalised Quasi-likelihood). Different software uses different methods.

Mixed effects models are now a popular method of analysing data from cluster randomised trials, but effect estimates produced by these models have a different interpretation from the effect estimates produced by GEEs (Section 6.3.3.1). Ideally, a choice between these two methods should be based on the trial aims. Mixed effects models do, however, offer an advantage in terms of flexibility; including the ease with which further random effects can be introduced into the analysis. For example, a trial investigating the impact of a school-based prevention programme on alcohol use was conducted in several regions in different European countries. In the analysis, investigators included a random effect for regional centre as well as one for school (Caria *et al.*, 2011). In a trial involving two interventions to improve function in older people living in residential homes, Riemersma-van der Lek *et al.* (2008) also used a model with several random effects (see Section 6.4.2).

There is more literature on the minimum numbers of clusters required for mixed effects analyses of binary outcomes than for mixed effects analyses of continuous outcomes. A recent paper by Austin (2010) summarises previous work in this area, and in keeping with the previous research suggests that 10 clusters are the minimum required. This paper also suggests that most estimation procedures used for fitting these types of model perform poorly in terms of estimating variance components when there are fewer than five individuals per cluster, regardless of the number of clusters. There were, however, some differences in the performance of different estimation procedures.

6.3.3.10   Binary outcomes – other methods of analysis

Bayesian methods have been suggested for analysing binary data from cluster randomised trials. Turner, Omar and Thompson (2001) extended the model presented in Equation 6.3. Thompson *et al.* suggested a method for analysing binary outcomes from these trials on the absolute risk scale (Thompson, Warn and Turner, 2004). Ma *et al.* (2009) compared a Bayesian analysis with several other analyses of the Community Hypertension Assessment Trial (CHAT). They found that the results obtained were robust to the analyses used, although the Bayesian analyses produced the widest CIs and a logistic regression ignoring clustering was inappropriate. Alternative models to the logistic-normal specification of a cluster-specific model could be used (e.g. a beta-binomial model), but we are not aware of any examples of their use for analysing empirical trials.

6.3.3.11   Binary outcomes – comparison of methods

Austin (2007) compares the performance of the *t*-test, the Wilcoxon rank-sum test, the permutation test at cluster level, an adjusted chi-square test, a logistic-normal mixed effects model, and GEEs for analysing clustered binary data using simulation, and concludes that the power of the tests is very similar. The numbers and sizes of clusters used in the simulation and level of intra-cluster correlation were similar to that encountered in cluster randomised trials in health services research. The simulated variation in cluster size (using a Poisson distribution) is likely to underestimate actual variation in cluster size in most of these trials, however. Omar and Thompson (2000) compare the use of different methods including a cluster-specific model fitted using a logistic mixed effects model, and a population-averaged model fitted using GEEs with a logit link, for analysing a trial with 26 clusters and variable cluster sizes. A GEE approach produced a higher statistical significance for the intervention effect compared to that obtained from a mixed effects model and a summary statistic method. The authors suggest that the GEE approach may have been unreliable because of the relatively small number of clusters.

6.3.3.12   Count outcomes

In cluster randomised trials in health services research count outcomes are usually the number of events an individual experiences during the duration of the trial, for example the number of exacerbations of a condition. Commonly, the length of follow-up for each individual is fixed and the events are counted over this fixed period. When the length of time over which events are counted differs from individual to individual this must be accounted for in the analysis.

The standard way of analysing counts or rates is to use Poisson regression. The method results in an incident rate ratio, a measure of the relative incidence of an event in the intervention arm compared to the control arm. GEEs or mixed effects models can be used to account for clustering. The principles of these methods have been described in previous sections.

Generalised estimating equations were used to analyse the number of attendances for unscheduled asthma care per participant in the ELECTRA trial (Table 6.12). Participants had, on average, 1.98 attendances for unscheduled asthma care in the intervention arm and 2.36 in the control arm during the trial period. Using GEEs with a log link, a Poisson error structure, and number of unscheduled attendances in the year prior to the intervention as a covariate, resulted in an incident rate ratio of 0.91 (95% CI 0.66 to 1.26).

Mixed effects Poisson regression was used to analyse data from the IRIS trial (Table 6.13). The outcomes were numbers of women identified as victims of domestic violence and the numbers of women referred to advocacy services in each cluster. These numbers and total numbers of eligible women were provided by each cluster. Because the total number of women varied from cluster to cluster, this was controlled for in the analysis in the same way that the length of time might be controlled for in an analysis where the length of time over which data were collected varies from individual to individual. GEEs could not be used to analyse the data because this necessitates the direct estimation of within-cluster correlation to account for clustering; this is not possible if there is only a single measure per cluster. However, a mixed effects model which fits a random effect representing the effect of individual clusters could be used. This accounts for the variation between

Table 6.13   IRIS: training to increase identification and referral of victims of domestic violence.

Aim: To test the effectiveness of a training and support programme for general practice teams targeting identification of women experiencing domestic violence, and referral to specialist domestic violence advocates

Location and type of cluster: UK general practices

Interventions: (i) Control: usual care (ii) Intervention: multidisciplinary training sessions in each practice, electronic prompts in the patient record and referral pathway to a named domestic violence advocate, as well as feedback on referrals and reinforcement over the course of a year

Primary outcome: Number of recorded referrals of women aged over 16 years to advocacy services based in specialist domestic violence agencies recorded in the general practice records

Method of achieving balanced arms: Minimisation

Analysis: Mixed effects Poisson regression models with random effect for practice, adjusted for minimization factors

Results: Adjusted incident rate ratio for number of recorded referrals: 22.0 (95% CI 11.5 to 42.4)

Source: Feder *et al.* (2011).

clusters over and above that expected if the data at cluster level followed a strict Poisson distribution. Thus, another way of thinking of this model is that the distribution of numbers of women identified (or referred) per practice follows an over-dispersed Poisson distribution. The random effect is then taking account of this over-dispersion. Model-based or robust estimators can be used to estimate the random effect structure. The difference between these two estimators was introduced in Section 6.3.3.

Outcomes that are counts or rates are more common in large, community-intervention trials in low-income countries than in trials in health services research. Bennett *et al.* (2002) provide an overview of methods for the analysis of incidence rates in cluster randomised trials orientated towards large community-intervention trials in these countries. Durán Pacheco *et al.* (2009) discuss the performance of some of these methods, again orientated towards large community-intervention trials. Many of the methods have been well used in this field.

6.3.3.13 Time-to-event outcomes

The standard method for analysing time-to-event data is a Cox's proportional hazards model. The model assumes that the hazard ratio (the ratio of the chance of an event happening in one arm to the chance of it happening in the other arm) is constant over time. Other models can be used which require more stringent assumptions than the Cox's proportional hazards model; namely that in addition to a constant hazard ratio, the distribution of events follows a specific form. Details about Cox's proportional hazards and other models can be found in relevant textbooks (e.g. Kalbfleisch and Prentice (2002)). Similar approaches to analysis can be used as have been described in the rest of this chapter. For example, in the ELECTRA trial (Table 6.12), time to first unscheduled care and time to first review were analysed using a GEE approach to account for clustering, assuming an underlying Weibull distribution for the hazard rate. The Weibull distribution was chosen because it gave the best fit to the observed data. Models for time-to-event data in which a random effect is introduced are often referred to as frailty models. As for other types of outcome, cluster-level analyses can be used if data are summarised and weighted appropriately.

6.4   Analyses for other designs

6.4.1   Matched designs

Matched cluster randomised trials can be analysed using paired (matched) versions of the *t*-test and non-parametric tests on data summarised at the cluster level. Stiell, Clement and Grimshaw (2009) used a paired *t*-test in a 12-centre, matched cluster randomised trial implementing the Canadian C-Spine Rule (Table 6.14); Hickman *et al.* (2008) used a Wilcoxon signed-rank test in a matched cluster randomised trial of an intervention aiming to increase the uptake of hepatitis C virus testing among

Table 6.14   Evaluating the implementation of the C-Spine Rule.

Aim: To evaluate the effectiveness of an active strategy to implement the
   validated Canadian C-Spine Rule into multiple emergency departments
Location and type of cluster: Canadian university and community emergency
   departments in hospitals
Number of clusters and individual participants: 12 clusters recruited and
   analysed; routine data from 11 824 individual participants analysed
Interventions: (i) Control: usual care (ii) Intervention: strategies within emergency
   departments to implement the Canadian C-spine Rule, a clinical decision rule
   for selective ordering of cervical spine imaging
Primary outcomes: Referral for diagnostic imaging
Method of achieving balanced arms: Matching
Recruitment and data collection: There was no recruitment; data were collected
   from routine records
Analysis: t-tests including weighted tests, and random effects meta-analysis
Results: Intervention arm showed reduction of 12.8% in imaging, and control arm
   showed 12.5% increase; this difference was significant at the 5% level
   ($p < 0.001$), but no further data are reported

Source: Stiell, Clement and Grimshaw (2009).

injecting drug users; and an adjusted (to allow for covariates) permutation test was
used for analysis of the COMMIT trial (Commit Research Group, 1995).

Other methods that have been advocated are meta-analysis techniques (Thompson, Pyke and Hardy 1997), and mixed effects models similar to those described in
Section 6.3 for non-matched designs (Nixon *et al.*, 2000). Meta-analysis has been
widely used, and was also used in the trial presented in Table 6.14. The use of mixed
models is less widespread. In some circumstances, such trials can be analysed as if
they had not been matched. This can be more efficient statistically, but has disadvantages (Donner *et al.*, 2007).

Cluster-level analyses and permutation tests are used more widely for matched
designs than for completely randomised designs. This is partly because matched
designs tend to be used when the number of clusters is relatively few, so that
individual-level analyses are less suitable.

6.4.2   Parallel trials with more than two arms

We include in this section trials with one more arm than there are active interventions,
full factorial trials, and trials in which randomisation has been conducted at the
cluster and individual level. The design of these trials was described in Section 5.3.

Dependent on the number of clusters and other features of the trial, trials with
one more arm than there are interventions can be analysed using mixed effects
models, GEEs, permutation tests or analysis of covariance; these techniques were
all described in Section 6.3. To avoid issues of multiple comparisons, cluster-level

Table 6.15 ASSIST: different interventions to promote secondary prevention of coronary heart disease.

Aim: To assess the effectiveness of three different methods of promoting secondary prevention of coronary heart disease in primary care

Location and type of cluster: UK general practices

Number of clusters and individual participants: 21 clusters recruited and analysed; 1906 participants analysed

Interventions: (i) Audit of notes with summary feedback to primary healthcare team (audit group) (ii) Assistance with setting up a disease register and systematic recall of patients to general practitioners (GP recall group) (iii) Assistance with setting up a disease register and systematic recall of patients to a nurse-led clinic (nurse recall group).

Primary outcome: Adequate assessment of three risk factors: blood pressure, cholesterol, and smoking status

Analysis: Analysis of covariance, adjusting for baseline values, weighting by number of patients in the practice

Results: Adjusted difference in assessment of all three risk factors: nurse recall cf. audit 33% (95% CI 19% to 46%); GP recall cf. audit 23% (10% to 36%)

Source: Moher *et al.* (2001).

t-tests and non-parametric equivalents are best replaced with the comparable tests appropriate for more than two groups. For example, one-way analysis of variance at the cluster level can be used instead of several cluster-level *t*-tests, and a cluster-level Kruskal–Wallis test instead of several cluster-level Mann–Witney U tests.

In Section 5.3 we introduced two trials with more than two arms. In the ASSIST trial (Table 6.15), one-way analysis of variance was conducted at cluster level using cluster-level means for continuous outcomes and cluster-level proportions for binary outcomes. The analysis was weighted by the cluster size to account for variation in this size. The investigators also conducted an analysis using a mixed effects model to incorporate individual-level covariates, but they found that this made no material difference to the results and this analysis is not reported in the trial publication. When an analysis of variance showed statistically significant results at the pre-specified 5% significance level, the authors compared pairs of arms using *t*-tests, a standard procedure when using this type of analysis. Given this two-stage approach to identifying the arms that differed significantly in relation to each outcome, they did not need to adjust for multiple comparisons. This is an appropriate strategy when investigators are potentially interested in comparisons between any two arms, but as discussed in Section 5.3.2, it is important to decide whether this is the case or whether there is a comparison between two of the arms which is of primary interest, in which case a different analysis strategy could be employed.

Peters *et al.* (2003) (Table 6.16) used a number of the methods described in this chapter to analyse a trial with a factorial design. They used three cluster-level and five individual-level methods to estimate the odds ratio of attendance for breast

Table 6.16   Two interventions to increase breast screening.

Aim: To examine the effectiveness and cost effectiveness of two interventions based in primary care aimed at increasing uptake of breast screening

Location and type of cluster: UK general practices

Number of clusters and individual participants: 24 clusters recruited and analysed; 6133 women randomised; 5732 analysed

Interventions: (i) Control (ii) General practitioner letter (iii) Flag in women's notes to prompt discussion (iv) Both interventions

Primary outcome: Attendance for screening

Analysis in main trial report: Mixed effects logistic regression adjusting for stratification factors

Results:

Proportions attending for screening:

   Control 55% (897/1621)

   Letter 64% (1097/1703)

   Flag 65% (752/1151)

   Letter + flag 68% (854/1257)

Adjusted odds ratio flag cf. control: 1.43 (95% CI 1.14 to 1.79)

Adjusted odds ratio letter cf. control: 1.31 (95% CI 1.05 to 1.64)

Source: Richards *et al.* (2001); Peters *et al.* (2003).

screening, its standard error, and associated *p*-value. The outcome was based on the number attending for breast screening in each of the clusters out of the numbers of invited women for whom data were available (5732). Probably as a result of the relatively small number (24) of large clusters (mean cluster size 239), there were some not-insubstantial differences between the results for the different methods. Peters *et al.* highlight, in particular, the computational instability of the mixed effects model; a problem known to occur when clusters are large and the intra-cluster correlation is relatively large.

It is good practice to adjust the effect of one intervention for the effect of the other in the analysis in a factorial trial. In an individually randomised trial with equal numbers in each of the intervention arms, adjusted and unadjusted analyses will give identical effect estimates, although the adjusted analysis will usually give more precise estimates. However, in a cluster randomised trial with clusters of varying sizes, equal numbers of clusters in each intervention arm does not mean equal numbers of individuals, and effect estimates for the adjusted and unadjusted analyses may then differ.

In Chapter 5 (Section 5.3.4) we described a trial of the effect of bright light (cluster randomisation) and melatonin (individual randomisation) (Riemersma-van der Lek *et al.*, 2008). In this trial the investigators also collected data at a number of time points. The model they used for analysis was a multilevel model with three levels: cluster, individual, and time point, with random effects introduced for cluster and time.

6.4.3   Crossover, stepped wedge and pseudo cluster randomised designs

The design of crossover cluster randomised trials was discussed in Section 5.4. The analysis of such trials must account for within-period correlation as well as within-cluster correlation (aka between-cluster variation). Using appropriate individual-level analyses, a multilevel modelling approach is necessary to incorporate within-period correlation. While a multilevel model for a cluster randomised trial usually requires the inclusion of a random effect to represent clusters, in a crossover trial this is not strictly necessary because there are measurements pertaining to intervention and control within each cluster; thus the intervention effect is estimated *within* clusters. Clusters can be represented by a fixed effect instead. Using cluster-level analyses, data are summarised at cluster level as for analyses in previous sections of this chapter. Analysts must make sure that a summary measure adequately captures data from both time periods, and that any analyses are correctly weighted. We have covered the principle of weighting in Section 6.3.1. An appropriate cluster summary measure is the difference between the mean outcome in the cluster in the first time period and the mean outcome in the cluster in the second time period.

Turner *et al.* (2007) used simulation to compare the performance of two individual-level and three cluster-level analyses appropriate for these trials. The individual-level analyses used a multilevel modelling approach; one incorporating a random effect for cluster and the other incorporating fixed effects for clusters. Clusters were weighted differently in each of the three cluster-level analyses: equally, by cluster size, and using inverse variance weights. The comparison of performance was motivated by the authors' involvement in the cluster randomised crossover trial to improve development in preterm babies introduced in Section 5.4. One of the rationales for using a crossover design for this trial was to increase the statistical power given that only a small number of clusters were available. In the comparison of methods, Turner *et al.* therefore simulated data for trials with relatively small numbers of clusters. Size of clusters and ICC values used in the simulation were fairly typical of cluster randomised trials in health services research. Turner *et al.* found that three methods appeared to perform well in all situations.

Because of the additional complications of design and analysis, crossover designs are not common amongst cluster randomised trials. In addition, as described in Section 5.4, sometimes a crossover design is impossible in such trials. Nevertheless, there are potential gains in efficiency from crossover designs, and they may be particularly useful when other methods of improving efficiency such as stratification, matching and adjusting for covariates are unable to achieve the desired power.

There are similarities between a stepped wedge design and the more conventional crossover design in the sense that, at each time period, each cluster receives either the active or the control intervention but not both, and that over the period of the trial all clusters receive both interventions. One difference is that the clusters always cross over in the same direction, from control to intervention. Nevertheless, issues pertaining to the analysis of these trials are similar to the issues for crossover trials. These are discussed in detail by Hussey and Hughes (2007), who also use simulation to explore the performance of the different methods.

Pseudo cluster randomised designs are similar to crossover and stepped wedge designs, in that each cluster receives both the active and control interventions, but in these trials some individuals within a cluster receive the intervention at the same time as other individuals within the cluster receive the control intervention. Teerenstra *et al.* (2007) compared mixed effects models, GEEs and *t*-tests for the analysis of these trials.

6.5   Intention to treat and missing values

Most cluster randomised trials are designed to detect evidence of the effectiveness of an intervention (see Section 5.5.3). If trial results suggest evidence of effectiveness, practices or policies may be changed. In these circumstances it is seen as desirable to err on the side of caution and avoid conducting analyses that might overestimate effectiveness. Intention to treat analyses are important in this respect, because of the potential for upward bias in the estimate of effect size if these types of analyses are not used. Two principles should be followed in a strict intention to treat analysis, although in practice the term 'intention to treat' is used rather loosely by the research community (see also Section 10.4.16). The first principle is that participants should be analysed in the intervention arm to which they were allocated, regardless of the treatment they received, and the second is that all participants should be included in the analysis whether or not they provided outcome data. These two principles aim to preserve the balance in the characteristics of participants between arms that results from randomisation.

The principle that participants should be included in the analysis whether or not they provide outcome data can only be adhered to if investigators are willing to impute data (Altman, 2009); that is, to assign data values to those for whom data are not available. A description of methods of imputation is outside the scope of this book, but there have been several recent publications in this area (Ma *et al.*, 2011; Birhanu *et al.*, 2011). In cluster randomised trials, intention to treat principles should ideally be applied at cluster level and at individual level. As with many aspects of cluster randomised trials this is not quite as straightforward as it seems at first. The principle of analysing clusters in the arm to which they were randomised is relatively easy to adhere to, but including clusters that provide no data in an analysis is more problematic because of the difficulty of inferring information at individual level for such clusters.

The extent to which analysts can adhere to the principle of analysing individual participants in the arm to which they were allocated depends on the design of the trial, including recruitment procedures and outcome collection. For example, in the OPERA trial (Table 6.17), individual participants who contributed to outcome data collection were all recruited at an earlier time point and exposed to the intervention in the intervening period. Thus, it was possible to identify, for each participant, the cluster, and hence the intervention arm, to which they had originally been allocated.

Table 6.17   OPERA: physical activity in residential homes to prevent depression.

Aim: To evaluate the impact on depression of a whole-home intervention to
   increase physical activity among older people

Location and type of cluster: UK residential homes and nursing for older people

Number of clusters and individual participants: 78 clusters randomised and
   analysed; 1060 participants recruited

Interventions: (i) Control: depression awareness programme delivered by research
   nurses (ii) Intervention: depression awareness programme delivered by
   physiotherapists plus whole-home package to increase activity among older
   people, including physiotherapy assessments of individuals, and activity
   sessions for residents

Primary outcomes: Prevalence of depression (Geriatric Depression Scale) at 12
   months (outcome at one time point only; cross-sectional design), change in
   depression score at 12 months in all those present at baseline (repeated
   measures on same participants; cohort design), and change in depression score
   at 6 months in those depressed at baseline (repeated measures on same
   participants; cohort design)

Recruitment and data collection: Recruitment of those resident in residential
   home prior to randomisation; recruitment of residents joining the home during
   the trial period; collection of outcome data at 6 months and 12 months post-
   randomisation on all those resident in the home at data collection time point

Analysis: For cohort design: clusters and individuals analysed in the intervention
   arm to which they were initially allocated; no clusters dropped out, individuals
   for whom outcome data were not available were not included in the primary
   analysis but were included in a sensitivity analysis

Source: Underwood *et al.* (2011).

Some participants changed homes during the trial period; where outcome data were
available they were analysed in the arm to which they had originally been allocated.
By contrast, in the IRIS trial (Table 6.13) there was no recruitment of individuals.
The intervention was delivered to the practices and after a year data were collected
from the practice records. Anonymised data were collected on all women registered
with the practice at the 12-month data collection time point. Without consent from
individuals, which the researchers did not have in this trial, there was no possibility
of identifying which practices individual women had been registered with at the
start of the trial period. Thus, if a woman moved between practices during the trial
period her data were analysed in the practice she ended up in, not the practice in
which she was allocated. While strictly this breaks intention to treat principles, the
more important issue to consider is the extent to which this is likely to cause bias,
and in particular an overestimate in effect size – a result that intention to treat is
designed to minimise. For IRIS this would occur only if there was some systematic
difference in the numbers of women who switched from intervention to control
practices or vice versa during the intervention period. This seems unlikely, and thus

the fact that intention to treat was not followed strictly is probably not important. In different contexts, others have argued that in practice we need pragmatic applications of intention to treat principles, and this may be one example. Jo, Asparouhov and Muthén (2008) describe a method for allowing for between cluster variation in non-compliance in intention to treat analyses for cluster randomised trials.

6.6   Analysis planning

In this chapter we have described a number of methods of analysing cluster randomised trials, distinguishing between methods that allow for the inclusion of covariates and the methods that do not, and illustrating the use of the methods for different types of outcome and design. Throughout the chapter we have also discussed the influence of the number of clusters, the size of clusters and variable cluster size on the reliability and performance of some methods. The amount of intra-cluster correlation will also influence reliability and performance, but we have discussed this less often because, for most cluster randomised trials in health services, intra-cluster correlation is relatively small. We recommend that investigators consider all of these aspects of their trial before deciding on an analysis strategy.

In relation to covariates, the decision is more complex than simply deciding which covariates to use. For potential covariates measured at the individual level, investigators must decide whether to use these at the individual level in an analysis or summarise and use them at cluster level. This decision should be influenced by clinical reasoning about whether the action of the covariate is most plausibly at cluster or individual level, but it may also be dictated by other factors. For example, in the trial presented in Table 6.1, the number of clusters involved made a cluster-level analysis more sensible than an individual-level analysis, and all covariates were therefore incorporated at the cluster level. In addition, covariates at the individual level can only be introduced in a repeated cross-sectional design if investigators use an analysis in which *all* individuals are included with time point and allocation specified as fixed effects in the model and the intervention effect estimated as an interaction. This is not commonly done.

In terms of options for type of analysis, with over 40 clusters, and with cluster sizes that are not extremely small or, extremely large or extremely variable, investigators can choose from a range of analyses presented in this chapter. With fewer than 10 clusters options are much more limited, with GEEs, mixed effects models and adjusted chi-squared tests unlikely to produce reliable results. When between 10 and 40 clusters are involved, other factors may have a stronger influence on the performance of methods, and we recommend that investigators refer to relevant methodological literature before deciding on an analysis. New literature on the performance of methods such as GEEs and mixed effects models is appearing all the time; we have included reference to some of this literature in this chapter but our references are by no means exhaustive and we have usually presented only headline results. In some cases, investigators may wish to introduce into their analysis plan more flexibility about the type of analysis they use than is usually the case for individually randomised trials. For example, for a trial in cardiac rehabilitation which involved only 21 clusters, Goud *et al.* (2009) describe an analysis using GEEs. In addition to the standard GEE analysis, they also used a method of jackknifing to allow for the relatively small number of clusters involved. This second analysis was not presented in the trial publication, however, because it gave very similar results to the more straightforward analysis. When there is some doubt about the reliability of the preferred analysis, an explicit analysis strategy that details the preferred analysis, and a secondary analysis that is likely to be more robust in the presence of the particular features of the trial, may be the best way forward. If both analyses give similar results then only the preferred analysis need be presented. Yudkin and Moher (2001) also advocate this type of flexible approach to the analysis of cluster randomised trials, particularly when the number of clusters is small, but it may also be a useful approach when, for example, cluster sizes are very small or trials have other features that make investigators unsure about the suitability of their preferred analysis.

Flexibility in analyses undertaken and presented in publications may be needed for another reason. In the ELECTRA trial (Table 6.12), the binary outcome denoting whether or not an individual attended for unscheduled care during the trial period was analysed using GEEs. This analysis produced a negative ICC of −0.0056. When GEEs produce negative ICCs, the estimate of intervention effect will have narrower confidence intervals than the comparable analysis not adjusting for clustering. In this trial, the odds ratio from the GEEs was 0.61 (95% CI 0.38 to 0.99), while the odds ratio from ordinary logistic regression was 0.62 (95% CI 0.38 to 1.01). An analysis that produces more precise estimates than would be obtained from an analysis ignoring clustering is counterintuitive. It is also generally assumed that ICCs cannot be negative in most cluster randomised trials. Therefore the investigators presented the second of these results in their publication. In general it is useful to employ an explicit analysis strategy that specifies that an analysis not adjusting for clustering will be used when the ICC is found to be negative. This does, of course, necessitate the calculation of the ICC, which should also form part of the analysis plan, and not only for this reason. We discuss the estimation and interpretation of ICCs further in Chapter 8 (Section 8.4), and the CONSORT recommendations to present these in trial reports in Chapter 10 (Section 10.4.17).

6.7 Summary

In this chapter we have described the analyses most commonly used in cluster randomised trials in health services research, highlighting the factors that are likely to determine choice of analysis. We have not specifically included a section on ordinal outcomes, but the principles of analysing these types of outcomes, which relatively rare in cluster randomised trials, are similar to those that apply to continuous and binary outcomes. We have also described less common analyses, namely cluster-level analyses and Bayesian analyses, because both offer potential advantages which may currently be overlooked.

Because this book attempts to be a practical guide, we have deliberately avoided the use of equations except where these illustrate the basic principles, and refer readers interested in a more algebraic treatment of the subject to some of the literature referenced in the chapter. We hope that this strategy makes this chapter accessible to those without substantial mathematical knowledge. In the following chapter we cover sample size calculations. Sample size calculations should be dependent on choice of analysis to a greater extent than is often acknowledged in empirical research.

References

Altman, D.G. (2009) Missing outcomes in randomised trials: addressing the dilemma. *Open Med.*, **3**, e51–e53.

Austin, P.C. (2007) A comparison of the statistical power of different methods for the analysis of cluster randomization trials with binary outcomes. *Stat. Med.*, **26** (19), 3550–3565.

Austin, P.C. (2010) Estimating multilevel logistic regression models when the number of clusters is low: a comparison of different statistical software procedures. *Int. J. Biostat.*, **6** (1), Article 16. doi: 10.2202/1557-4679.1195

Bennett, S., Parpia, T., Hayes, R. *et al.* (2002) Methods for the analysis of incidence rates in cluster randomized trials. *Int. J. Epidemiol.*, **31** (4), 839–846.

Birhanu, T., Molenberghs, G., Sotto, C. *et al.* (2011) Doubly robust and multiple-imputation-based generalized estimating equations. *J. Biopharm. Stat.*, **21** (2), 202–225.

Bowater, R.J., Abdelmalik, S.M. and Lilford, R.J. (2009) The methodological quality of cluster randomised controlled trials for managing tropical parasitic disease: a review of trials published from 1998 to 2007. *Trans. R. Soc. Trop. Med. Hyg.*, **103** (5), 429–436.

Campbell, M.K., Elbourne, D.R., Altman, D.G. (2004) CONSORT statement: extension to cluster randomised trials. *BMJ*, **328** (7441), 702–708.

Caria, M.P., Faggiano, F., Bellocco, R. *et al.* (2011) The influence of socioeconomic environment on the effectiveness of alcohol prevention among European students: a cluster randomized controlled trial. *BMC Public Health*, **11**, 312.

Chuang, J.H., Hripcsak, G. and Jenders, R.A. (2000) Considering clustering: a methodological review of clinical decision support system studies. *Proc. AMIA Symp.*, **2000**, 146–150.

COMMIT Research Group (1995) Community Intervention Trial for Smoking Cessation (COMMIT): I. cohort results from a four-year community intervention. *Am. J. Public Health*, **85** (2), 183–192.

Cornfield, J. (1978) Randomization by group: a formal analysis. *Am. J. Epidemiol.*, **108** (2), 100–102.

Davies, M.J., Heller, S., Skinner, T.C. *et al.* (2008) Effectiveness of the diabetes education and self management for ongoing and newly diagnosed (DESMOND) programme for people with newly diagnosed type 2 diabetes: cluster randomised controlled trial. *BMJ*, **336** (7642), 491–495.

Diggle, P.J., Heagerty, P., Liang, K.Y. *et al.* (2002) *Analysis of Longitudinal Data*, Oxford University Press, New York.

Donner, A. and Donald, A. (1988) The statistical analysis of multiple binary measurements. *J. Clin. Epidemiol.*, **41** (9), 899–905.

Donner A, Taljaard M, Klar N. (2007) The merits of breaking the matches: a cautionary tale. *Stat Med.* **26** (9), 2036–2051.

Donner, A. and Klar, N. (1994) Methods for comparing event rates in intervention studies when the unit of allocation is a cluster. *Am. J. Epidemiol.*, **140** (3), 279–289.

Donner, A., Brown, K.S. and Brasher, P. (1990) A methodological review of non-therapeutic intervention trials employing cluster randomization, 1979–1989. *Int. J. Epidemiol.*, **19**, 795–800.

Durán Pacheco, G., Hattendorf, J., Colford, J.M. Jr. *et al.* (2009) Performance of analytical methods for overdispersed counts in cluster randomized trials: sample size, degree of clustering and imbalance. *Stat. Med.*, **28** (24), 2989–3011.

Eldridge, S.M., Ashby, D., Feder, G.S. *et al.* (2004) Lessons for cluster randomised trials in the twenty-first century: a systematic review of trials in primary care. *Clin. Trials*, **1**, 80–90.

Eldridge, S., Ashby, D., Bennett, C. *et al.* (2008) Internal and external validity of cluster randomised trials: systematic review of recent trials. *BMJ*, **336** (7649), 876–880.

Feder, G., Griffiths, C., Highton, C. *et al.* (1995) Do clinical guidelines introduced with practice based education improve care of asthmatic and diabetic patients? A randomised controlled trial in general practices in east London. *BMJ*, **311**, 1473–1478.

Feder, G., Griffiths, C., Eldridge, S. *et al.* (1999) Effect of postal prompts to patients and general practitioners on the quality of primary care after a coronary event (POST): randomised controlled trial. *BMJ*, **318**, 1522–1526.

Feder, G., Agnew Davies, R., Baird, K. *et al.* (2011) Identification and Referral to Improve Safety (IRIS) of women experiencing domestic violence: a cluster randomised controlled trial of a primary care training and support programme. Oct 12. [Epub ahead of print]

Feng, Z., McLerran, D. and Grizzle, J. (1996) A comparison of statistical methods for clustered data analysis with Gaussian error. *Stat. Med.*, **15** (16), 1793–1806.

Froud, R., Eldridge, S., Diaz Ordaz, K. *et al.* (2011) Quality of cluster randomised controlled trials in oral health: a systematic review of reports published between 2005 and 2009. *Community Dent. Oral Epidemiol.*, in press.

Goud, R., de Keizer, N.F., ter Riet, G. *et al.* (2009) Effect of guideline based computerised decision support on decision making of multidisciplinary teams: cluster randomised trial in cardiac rehabilitation. *BMJ*, **338**, b1440. doi: 10.1136/bmj.b1440

Griffiths, C., Foster, G., Barnes, N. *et al.* (2004) Specialist nurse intervention to reduce unscheduled asthma care in a deprived multiethnic area: the east London randomised controlled trial for high risk asthma (ELECTRA). *BMJ*, **328** (7432), 144.

Handlos, L.N., Chakraborty, H. and Sen, P.K. (2009) Evaluation of cluster-randomized trials on maternal and child health research in developing countries. *Trop. Med. Int. Health*, **14** (8), 947–956.

Hanley, J.A., Negassa, A., Edwardes, M.D. *et al.* (2003) Statistical analysis of correlated data using generalized estimating equations: an orientation. *Am. J. Epidemiol.*, **157** (4), 364–375.

Harmsen, H., Bernsen, R., Meeuwesen, L. *et al.* (2005) The effect of educational intervention on intercultural communication: results of a randomised controlled trial. *Br. J. Gen. Pract.*, **55** (514), 343–350.

Hayes, R.J. and Moulton, L.H. (2009) *Cluster Randomised Trials*, Chapman & Hall, Boca Raton.

Hickman, M., McDonald, T., Judd, A. *et al.* (2008) Increasing the uptake of hepatitis C virus testing among injecting drug users in specialist drug treatment and prison settings by using dried blood spots for diagnostic testing: a cluster randomized controlled trial. *J. Viral Hepat.*, **15** (4), 250–254.

Huber, P.J. (1967) The behaviour of maximum likelihood estimators under nonstandard conditions, in *Proceedings of the Fifth Berkeley Symposium on Mathematical Statistics and Probability* (eds L.M. LeCam and J. Neyman), University of Califormia Press, pp. 221–233.

Hussey, M.A. and Hughes, J.P. (2007) Design and analysis of stepped wedge cluster randomized trials. *Contemp. Clin. Trials*, **28** (2), 182–191.

Isaakidis, P. and Ioannidis, J.P. (2003) Evaluation of cluster randomized controlled trials in sub-Saharan Africa. *Am. J. Epidemiol.*, **158**, 921–926.

Jeong, J.H. and Jung, S.H. (2006) Rank tests for clustered survival data when dependent subunits are randomized. *Stat. Med.*, **25** (3), 361–373.

Jo, B., Asparouhov, T. and Muthén, B.O. (2008) Intention-to-treat analysis in cluster randomized trials with noncompliance. *Stat. Med.*, **27** (27), 5565–5577.

Kalbfleisch, J.D. and Prentice, R.L. (2002) *The Statistical Analysis of Failure Time Data*, 2nd edn, John Wiley & Sons, Inc., Hoboken, NJ.

Kendrick, T., Burns, T. and Freeling, P. (1995) Randomised controlled trial of teaching general practitioners to carry out structured assessments of their long term mentally ill patients. *BMJ*, **311** (6997), 93–98.

Kerry, S.M. and Bland, J.M. (1998) Trials which randomize practices I: how should they be analysed? *Fam. Pract.*, **15** (1), 80–83.

Liang, K.Y. and Zeger, S.L. (1986) Longitudinal data analysis using generalized linear models. *Biometrika*, **73**, 13–22.

Long, J.S. and Ervin, L.H. (2000) Using heteroscedasticity consistent standard errors in the linear regression model. *Am. Stat.*, **54**, 217–224.

Ma, J., Thabane, L., Kaczorowski, J. *et al.* (2009) Comparison of Bayesian and classical methods in the analysis of cluster randomized controlled trials with a binary outcome: the Community Hypertension Assessment Trial (CHAT). *BMC Med. Res. Methodol.*, **9**, 37.

Ma, J., Akhtar-Danesh, N., Dolovich, L. *et al.* (2011) Imputation strategies for missing binary outcomes in cluster randomized trials; CHAT investigators. *BMC Med. Res. Methodol.*, **11**, 18.

Moher, M., Yudkin, P., Wright, L. *et al.* (2001) Cluster randomised controlled trial to compare three methods of promoting secondary prevention of coronary heart disease in primary care. *BMJ*, **322** (7298), 1338.

Murray, D.M., Hannan, P.J., Pals, S.P. *et al.* (2006) A comparison of permutation and mixed-model regression methods for the analysis of simulated data in the context of a group-randomized trial. *Stat. Med.*, **25** (3), 375–388.

Murray, D.M., Pals, S.L., Blitstein, J.L. *et al.* (2008) Design and analysis of group-randomized trials in cancer: a review of current practices. *J. Natl. Cancer Inst.*, **100** (7), 483–491.

Neuhaus, J.M., Kalbfleisch, J.D. and Hauck, W.W. (1991) A comparison of cluster-specific and population-averaged approaches for analyzing correlated binary data. *Int. Stat. Rev.*, **59**, 25–35.

Nixon, R., Prevost, T.C., Duffy, S.W. *et al.* (2000) Some random-effects models for the analysis of matched-cluster randomised trials: application to the Swedish two-county trial of breast-cancer screening. *J. Epidemiol. Biostat.*, **5** (6), 349–358.

Omar, R.Z. and Thompson, S.G. (2000) Analysis of a cluster randomized trial with binary outcome data using a multi-level model. *Stat. Med.*, **19** (19), 2675–2688.

Peters, T.J., Richards, S.H., Bankhead, C.R. *et al.* (2003) Comparison of methods for analysing cluster randomized trials: an example involving a factorial design. *Int. J. Epidemiol.*, **32** (5), 840–846.

Puffer, S., Torgerson, D. and Watson, J. (2003) Evidence for risk of bias in cluster randomised trials: review of recent trials published in three general medical journals. *BMJ*, **327**, 785–789.

Raab, G.M. and Butcher, I. (2005) Randomization inference for balanced cluster-randomized trials. *Clin. Trials*, **2** (2), 130–140.

Rasbash, J., Charlton, C., Browne, W.J. *et al.* (2005) *MLwiN Version 2.02*, Centre for Multilevel Modelling, University of Bristol.

Richards, S.H., Bankhead, C., Peters, T.J. *et al.* (2001) Cluster randomised controlled trial comparing the effectiveness and cost-effectiveness of two primary care interventions aimed at improving attendance for breast screening. *J. Med. Screen.*, **8** (2), 91–98.

Riemersma-van der Lek, R.F., Swaab, D.F., Twisk, J. *et al.* (2008) Effect of bright light and melatonin on cognitive and noncognitive function in elderly residents of group care facilities: a randomized controlled trial. *JAMA*, **299** (22), 2642–2655.

Rosner, B., Glynn, R.J. and Lee, M.L. (2003) Incorporation of clustering effects for the Wilcoxon rank sum test: a large-sample approach. *Biometrics*, **59** (4), 1089–1098.

Rosner, B., Glynn, R.J. and Lee, M.L. (2006) Extension of the rank sum test for clustered data: two-group comparisons with group membership defined at the subunit level. *Biometrics*, **62** (4), 1251–1259.

Scott, N.W., McPherson, G.C., Ramsay, C.R. *et al.* (2002) The method of minimization for allocation to clinical trials: a review. *Control. Clin. Trials*, **23** (6), 662–674.

Simpson, J.M., Klar, N. and Donner, A. (1995) Accounting for cluster randomization: a review of primary prevention trials, 1990 through 1993. *Am. J. Public Health*, **85**, 1378–1383.

Smith, S., Bury, G., O'Leary, M. *et al.* (2004) The North Dublin randomized controlled trial of structured diabetes shared care. *Fam. Pract.*, **21** (1), 39–45.

Snijders, T. and Bosker, R. (1999) *Multilevel Analysis: An Introduction to Basic and Advanced Multilevel Modelling*, Sage Publications Inc., Thousand Oaks, CA.

Spiegelhalter, D.J. (2001) Bayesian methods for cluster randomized trials with continuous responses. *Stat. Med.*, **20** (3), 435–452.

StataCorp (2009) *Stata Statistical Software: Release 11*, StataCorp LP, College Station, TX.

Stiell, I.G., Clement, C.M. and Grimshaw, J. (2009) Implementation of the Canadian C-Spine Rule: prospective 12 centre cluster randomised trial. *BMJ*, **339**, b4146. doi: 10.1136/bmj.b4146

Sturt, J.A., Whitlock, S., Fox, C. *et al.* (2008) Effects of the Diabetes Manual 1 : 1 structured education in primary care. *Diabet. Med.*, **25** (6), 722–731.

Teerenstra, S., Moerbeek, M., Melis, R.J. *et al.* (2007) A comparison of methods to analyse continuous data from pseudo cluster randomized trials. *Stat. Med.*, **26** (22), 4100–4115.

Thompson, S.G., Pyke, S.D. and Hardy, R.J. (1997) The design and analysis of paired cluster randomized trials: an application of meta-analysis techniques. *Stat. Med.*, **16** (18), 2063–2079.

Thompson, S.G., Warn, D.E. and Turner, R.M. (2004) Bayesian methods for analysis of binary outcome data in cluster randomized trials on the absolute risk scale. *Stat. Med.*, **23** (3), 389–410.

Turner, R.M., Omar, R.Z. and Thompson, S.G. (2001) Bayesian methods of analysis for cluster randomized trials with binary outcome data. *Stat. Med.*, **20** (3), 453–472.

Turner, R.M., White, I.R., Croudace, T. (2007) Analysis of cluster randomized cross-over trial data: a comparison of methods. *Stat. Med.*, **26** (2), 274–289.

Underwood, M., Eldridge, S., Lamb, S. *et al.* (2011) The OPERA trial: protocol for a randomised trial of an exercise intervention for older people in residential and nursing accommodation. *Trials*, **12**, 27.

Varnell, S.P., Murray, D.M., Janega, J.B. *et al.* (2004) Design and analysis of group-randomized trials: a review of recent practices. *Am. J. Public Health*, **94**, 393–399.

Yudkin, P.L. and Moher, M. (2001) Putting theory into practice: a cluster randomized trial with a small number of clusters. *Stat. Med.*, **20** (3), 341–349.

Zeger, S.L. and Liang, K.Y. (1986) Longitudinal data-analysis for discrete and continuous outcomes. *Biometrics*, **42**, 121–130.

7

Sample size calculations

As described in Chapter 1, sample sizes for cluster randomised trials usually need to be inflated over and above the sample size required for an individually randomised trial designed to answer the same research question. This is because individuals within the same cluster will have a tendency to be more similar in their outcomes than a random sample of individuals from all clusters. The greater this effect, the greater will be the increase in sample size required.

This chapter begins with an overview of the additional factors influencing sample size that need to be considered in cluster randomised trials compared with individually randomised trials (Section 7.1), and gives formulae for taking these into account for simple two-arm trials with equal numbers of participants per cluster (Section 7.2). However, trials with unequal numbers of individuals per cluster are very common, and adaptations to sample size calculations to accommodate this are described in Section 7.6. Logistical factors may make it attractive to carry out a trial in a small number of clusters, but this has drawbacks for the power of the study. Sections 7.4 and 7.5 describe some of the reasons why the numbers of clusters might be restricted, and implications for such restriction. Most of the formulae described in this chapter use the intra-cluster correlation coefficient (ICC) as the measure of between-cluster variability. Other measures are described and compared in Section 7.7. In particular the ICC is not suitable when the outcome is expressed as a rate, and a formula based on the coefficient of variation of the outcome is given in Section 7.3.

The final sections of the chapter, Sections 7.8 and 7.9, deal with other designs, such as matched pairs. Analysis of these designs was described in Chapter 6.

A Practical Guide to Cluster Randomised Trials in Health Services Research, First Edition.
Sandra Eldridge and Sally Kerry.
© 2012 John Wiley & Sons, Ltd. Published 2012 by John Wiley & Sons, Ltd.

Theoretically these designs will improve the power of the study. However, in many cases, the information, such as the stratum-specific rates for the outcome variable, is not available at the design stage, so we have described modifications to sample size calculations only for those designs where relevant additional information is likely to be available.

7.1   Factors affecting sample size for cluster randomised designs

In common with all randomised trials, a sample size calculation should be carried out at the design stage to ensure that the study has a high chance of detecting, as statistically significant, a worthwhile effect if it exists. There are several standard texts on sample size calculations (Altman, 1991; Machin *et al.*, 2009; Bland, 2000; Petrie and Sabin, 2009) which give full explanations of power, 'clinically important difference', whether one-tailed or two-tailed tests are appropriate, and how to estimate the underlying variability in the primary outcome. In this chapter we focus on those additional factors which need to be considered for cluster randomised trials (Table 7.1); namely the between-cluster variation in the primary outcome, the number of participants per cluster who will contribute to the final analysis and how much that number varies between clusters. The first of these, the between-cluster variability in the primary outcome, lies outside the investigator's control, while the number of participants per cluster is usually within the investigator's control and may be influenced by a desire to decrease the sample size required.

7.1.1   Measuring between-cluster variation in an outcome variable

In this book we concentrate on sample size calculations which use the ICC to estimate between-cluster variability, although the ICC cannot be used for rates. A common alternative measure of the between-cluster variation is the between-cluster coefficient of variation of the outcome. Trials in low-income countries often have outcomes expressed as rates, and this coefficient of variation is a convenient way to estimate between-cluster variability in those trials. Researchers in primary care and health services research usually use the ICC. We compare the two methods in Section 7.7. One advantage of using the ICC is that there is considerable literature to guide researchers working in primary care as to the likely values, both through published values of ICCs for specific outcomes (Hannan *et al.*, 1994; Kelder *et al.*, 1993; Murray and Short, 1995; Murray *et al.*, 2004; Reading, Harvey and Mclean, 2000; Smeeth and Ng, 2002; Ukoumunne *et al.*, 1999; Verma and Le, 1996) and through factors which affect the value of the ICC (Adams *et al.*, 2004; Gulliford *et al.*, 2005; Campbell, Fayers and Grimshaw, 2005). Estimating the ICC for use in a sample size calculation will be discussed in more detail in Section 8.3, although we give some examples here.

Table 7.1   Factors affecting sample size[a] requirements for cluster randomised trials.

Type of factor	Factors affecting sample size requirements in all trials	Extra factors in cluster randomised trials
Outside an investigator's control	Underlying variability in primary outcome	Between-cluster variation in primary outcome
Within an investigator's control, but should not be influenced by desire to decrease sample size required	Clinically important difference Significance level Whether to use a one-tailed or two-tailed test	

Within an investigator's control and can be influenced by a desire to decrease sample size required	*Related to design:*
	    Whether to use stratification or matching
	    Relative number of individuals in different intervention arms
	Related to analysis:
	    Type of analysis[c]
	    Measurement of primary outcome
	    Use of repeat measures
	Related to execution:
	    Loss to follow-up[b]
		Related to design:
		Cluster size
		Variability in cluster size[b]

[a]Sample size recruited.
[b]These factors may sometimes be only partially within an investigator's control, and sometimes not within an investigator's control at all.
[c]Choice depends on other factors as well as desire to increase efficiency.

7.1.2   Definition of cluster size

The power of a study is determined by the number of individuals analysed in each cluster as opposed to the number approached or recruited. We will denote the number analysed in each cluster by m. The natural cluster size (Section 1.3.2) is often much larger. A trial to reduce baby walker use (Table 7.2) randomised practices and recruited 1174 women from 46 clusters; an average of 26 per cluster. As only 1008 women completed the final questionnaire, the average cluster size for the analysis was 22 although the number recruited was higher.

Table 7.2   Promoting child safety by reducing baby walker use.

Aim: To evaluate the effectiveness of an educational package provided by midwives and health visitors to reduce baby walker possession and use

Location and type of cluster: UK groups of general practices sharing a health visitor (between one and four practices)

Interventions: (i) Control: usual care (ii) Intervention: trained midwives and health visitors delivered an educational package to mothers to be, at 10 days postpartum and 3–4 months later, to discourage baby walker use or encourage safe use for those who already had baby walkers

Primary outcome: Possession and use of a baby walker

Difference to be detected: Reduction from 50% in control to 40% in intervention arms

Number of clusters analysed: 46

Number of individuals analysed: 1008

7.1.3   Variability in cluster size

Rarely does a cluster randomised trial analyse the same number of participants per cluster. Even in trials where this is planned and the same number of participants from each cluster is selected at baseline, it is common for some participants not to be followed up. Patients may die or move away from the practice. Although this is less likely when the outcome data are obtained from routine general practitioner records, in most cases it will lead to a small imbalance in the cluster sizes at the analysis stage.

Not all trials plan to recruit the same number of individuals per cluster. In these trials an important source of variability in the analysed cluster size is the variability in natural cluster size. In the clinical guidelines trial described in Section 6.3.2 (Feder *et al.*, 1995), the number of patients selected was directly proportional to the number of practitioners, and hence large practices would contribute more patients. Finally, when collecting incident cases there may be additional random variability in the number of cases diagnosed during the course of the study. In the diabetes care from diagnosis trial (Kinmonth *et al.*, 1998; Section 5.2), incident cases were recruited and the number of patients per practice varied from 1 to 22.

In Sections 7.2 to 7.4 we will assume, for simplicity, that there are the same number of individuals per cluster, m. If the variability in cluster size is small then the average cluster size could be used instead of m in the formulae given. In Section 7.6 we present a more appropriate method for calculating sample sizes required when cluster sizes vary considerably.

7.1.4   Clinically important difference

While common to both individually randomised trials and cluster randomised trials, estimating the minimally important difference for complex interventions needs careful consideration to avoid over-optimistic estimates of the difference that could be achieved. Investigators may be tempted to base their sample size simply on what might be considered a clinically worthwhile change, without considering whether or not this is achievable. Careful consideration of the available literature on individual components of the intervention may reveal that the expected benefit is smaller than could be detected within funding available or with the available clusters. In this case it is not worth investing time and money in a large, expensive trial. For example, this was the case in a proposed trial of a falls prevention programme discussed in Section 4.2.2 (Eldridge *et al.*, 2005).

On the other hand, preventive strategies and public health promotion interventions may produce only small changes in risk factors in the whole population which lead to important changes for a number of individuals. For example, a small reduction in average blood pressure in the whole population may lead to an important reduction in the number of individuals requiring antihypertensive treatment or suffering from strokes or heart attacks. This phenomenon was first described in 1985 by Geoffrey Rose (Rose, 1985) in 'Sick individuals and sick populations'. Thus the criteria for minimally important differences usually applied to treatment trials will be inappropriate for many cluster randomised trials.

7.1.5 Sample size formulae for individually randomised trials

In Section 7.2 we show how sample sizes for trials can be inflated to adjust for clustering. The first step in this process is to calculate the sample size for an individually randomised trial designed to detect the same sized effect. Here we give the basic formulae for completeness, but we strongly recommend using a statistical package such as Stata (www.stata.com) to carry out the calculations. The minimum sample size can then be calculated easily and with less chance of mistakes. If the trial is not feasible at this stage, then it is not sensible to proceed further.

If the outcome is continuous then the number of subjects required in each arm for an individually randomised trial can be calculated as

$$N = \frac{2(z_{\alpha/2} + z_{\beta})^2 (\sigma^2)}{(\mu_1 - \mu_2)^2} \tag{7.1}$$

where $z_{\alpha/2}$ and z_{β} are the standard normal values corresponding to the upper tail probabilities of $\alpha/2$ and β respectively; α is the two-sided significance level, and $1 - \beta$ is the power; μ_1 and μ_2 are the means in the two arms; and σ is the standard deviation of the outcome.

For trials involving proportions, the variance of the outcome will depend on the value of π_1 and π_2, the expected proportions in each arm. The number of subjects required in each arm is given by

$$N = \frac{(z_{\alpha/2} + z_{\beta})^2 (\pi_1(1 - \pi_1) + \pi_2(1 - \pi_2))}{(\pi_1 - \pi_2)^2} \tag{7.2}$$

For trials involving rates, the variance of the outcome will depend on the values of λ_1 and λ_2, the expected rates in each arm. The number of person years required in each arm is given by

$$N = \frac{(z_{\alpha/2} + z_\beta)^2 (\lambda_1 + \lambda_2)}{(\lambda_1 - \lambda_2)^2} \qquad (7.3)$$

7.2 Calculating sample size using the intra-cluster correlation coefficient

This method (Donner, Birkett and Buck, 1981) involves multiplying the sample size needed for an equivalent (in terms of other design features) individually randomised trial, by what has variously been called the design effect or the variance inflation factor.

The design effect can be expressed as

$$Deff = 1 + \rho(m-1) \qquad (7.4)$$

where ρ denotes the ICC, and m is the size of each cluster.

Trials which randomise general practices using clinical or other patient outcomes, such as blood pressure or cholesterol level, typically have ICCs of 0.05 or less. Using Equation 7.4, if the ICC is 0.01, then a trial with 20 participants per cluster would need only 20% more participants than an individually randomised trial to detect the same intervention effect. However as the number analysed in each cluster, m, increases, so the design effect increases and the design becomes statistically inefficient; that is, the variance of the estimate of treatment effect is very large compared with designs with fewer subjects per cluster (Dodge, 2003).

Equation 7.4 assumes that all clusters within the trial have the same number of individuals in the analysis; that clusters are randomised using simple random allocation (with no stratification, blocking or matching); that outcomes are continuous or binary; and that the intervention effect is to be quantified as the difference between means or proportions. It also assumes that the ICC is the same in the intervention and control arms of the trial. These assumptions are discussed in Section 7.7. Chapter 8 gives more details on estimating the ICC for use in a sample size calculation, and a useful definition is given in Section 8.1.1.

7.2.1 Increasing the number of clusters to allow for a clustered design

Increasing the number of clusters is the most efficient way of increasing the sample size to allow for a clustered design. The number of clusters, k, is given by the formula

$$k = N(1 + \rho(m-1))/m \qquad (7.5)$$

where N is the sample size required for an individually randomised trial designed to detect the same effect size.

The steps to adjust the sample size for clustering are illustrated using the trial described in Table 7.2.

1. Calculate N.
   For this trial, 776 mothers (388 per arm) were required to detect a 10% fall in baby walker possession from 50 to 40% with 80% power and 5% significance.

2. Obtain an estimate of ρ.
   A previous study reported this as 0.017.

3. Consider how many individuals could be recruited and followed up, m, from each cluster.
   This was chosen to be 23.

4. Calculate the sample size required as $N_c = N \times Deff$.
   The number of clusters recruited is then N_c/m.
   $Deff = 1 + (0.017 \times 22) = 1.374$.
   $N_c = 776 \times 1.374 = 1066$.
   Number of clusters required $= 1066/23 = 46$.
   In order to allow for 10% loss to follow-up in the participants, but assuming all clusters would contribute some participants to the final analysis, 1173 participants were recruited from 46 clusters, approximately 26 per cluster. Box 7.1 gives the sample size statement from the trial report illustrating how this information can be presented.

7.2.2 Increasing cluster size to allow for a clustered design

If the number of clusters is fixed then the sample size can be increased by increasing the cluster size. Rearranging Equation 7.5 gives

$$m = \frac{N(1-\rho)}{(k-\rho N)} \tag{7.6}$$

To detect a 10% difference in baby walker possession, based on 50% of mothers in the control arm owning a walker, 80% power and a two-sided 5% significance level, 388 mothers per arm were required. The design effect was calculated as 1.374, based on an intra-class correlation coefficient of 0.017 (from a previous primary care child injury study in Nottingham [reference]) and an average cluster size of 23 participants. Allowing for up to 10% losses to follow-up, 1173 participants were required.

Source: Kendrick *et al.* (2005).

Box 7.1   Baby walker trial; sample size statement

Table 7.3   ELECTRA: asthma liaison nurses to reduce unscheduled care.

Aim: To determine whether asthma specialist nurses, using a liaison model of
   care, reduce unscheduled care in a deprived multiethnic setting
Location and type of cluster: UK general practices
Interventions: (i) Control: a visit promoting standard asthma guidelines; patients
   were checked for inhaler technique (ii) Intervention: patient review in a
   nurse-led clinic, and liaison with general practitioners and practice nurses
   comprising educational outreach, promotion of guidelines for high risk asthma
   and ongoing clinical support
Primary outcome: Proportion of patients receiving unscheduled care for acute
   asthma over one year
Difference to be detected: 90% in control arm to 75% in intervention arm
Number of clusters: 44 (fixed)
Target number of individuals: 290
Average target cluster size: 6.6
Number of individuals analysed: 319

Source: Griffiths *et al.* (2004).

The steps are illustrated using data from the ELECTRA trial (Table 7.3), although
this was not the method of determining sample size actually used in planning this trial.
All general practices in the area around one large teaching hospital were randomised.
Patients were identified from hospital accident and emergency (A&E) department or
general practice out-of-hours services when they attended for unscheduled asthma
care. For illustration, we assume the number of patients recruited could be increased
by increasing the recruitment period, but that the number of practices was fixed.

1. Calculate the sample size, N, required for an individually randomised trial
   employing simple random allocation, as before.
   *$N = 226$ patients (113 per arm), the number required to detect a decrease in
   proportion of patients receiving unscheduled care from 90 to 75% with 80%
   power and 5% significance.*

2. Obtain an estimate of ρ.
   This was assumed to be 0.05, based on previous studies.

3. Consider how many clusters could be recruited to the study, k.
   This was all 44 practices in one London borough.

4. Calculate the number of patients per cluster using Equation 7.6.
   $m = 226 \times (1 - 0.05) / (44 - (0.05 \times 226)) = 6.6$.
   Total number of patients $= 6.6 \times 44 = 290$.

Although both of the examples shown above use outcomes measured as proportions, the same method can be used for adjusting for clustering when the outcome
is continuous and means are being compared.

7.3   Sample size calculations for rates

Community trials in low-income countries for the control of infectious diseases or to reduce infant mortality often have outcomes that are expressed as a rate per person years. The sample size relates to the number of person years of follow-up, and consequently it is not possible to estimate the ICC. The coefficient of variation method of calculating sample sizes was developed by Hayes and Bennet (1999), mainly for studies of infectious diseases involving rates, although it can also be applied to means and proportions (Section 7.7.2). The between-cluster coefficient of variation of the outcome is the ratio of the between-cluster standard deviation to the overall mean. Thus, the coefficient of variation is $cv = \sigma_{b1}/\lambda_1 = \sigma_{b2}/\lambda_2$, where λ_1 is the event rate in the intervention arm and σ_{b1} the standard deviation of the event rate between clusters in the intervention arm, while λ_2 and σ_{b2} refer to the control arm.

The total number of person years required per intervention arm, N_c, is given by the number of person years for an individually randomised trial, N, multiplied by the design effect,

$$N_c = N \times Deff$$

where

$$Deff = 1 + \frac{cv^2(\lambda_1^2 + \lambda_2^2)t}{\lambda_1 + \lambda_2} \tag{7.7}$$

and t is the number of person years per cluster.

The number of clusters required, k, is N_c/t.

For a fixed number of clusters, the number of person years required per cluster is given by

$$t = \frac{N}{k - cv^2 N\left(\lambda_1^2 + \lambda_2^2\right)/(\lambda_1 + \lambda_2)} \tag{7.8}$$

Alternatively the number of clusters could be estimated directly by

$$k = \frac{(z_{\alpha/2} + z_\beta)^2 \left(\dfrac{(\lambda_1 + \lambda_2)}{t} + cv^2(\lambda_1^2 + \lambda_2^2) \right)}{(\lambda_1 - \lambda_2)^2} \tag{7.9}$$

In addition to rates expressed as per person years, these formulae can also be applied to the rate per number of individuals when this is low, such as neonatal mortality rate.

The Ekjut project (Table 7.4) in rural India assumed the neonatal mortality rate in the control clusters would be 58 per 1000 live births, and the study was powered

Table 7.4   Ekjut project: participatory women's group to improve birth outcomes and maternal depression.

Aim: To see whether a community mobilisation through participatory women's groups might improve birth outcomes and maternal depression
Location and type of cluster: Indian rural communities, with a mean population of 6338 per cluster (range 3605–7467)
Interventions: (i) Control: no intervention (ii) Intervention: a facilitator convened 13 groups every month to support participatory action and learning for women, and facilitated the development and implementation of strategies to address maternal and newborn health problems
Primary outcome: Neonatal mortality rate and maternal depression scores
Number of clusters: 36
Required cluster size: 270 births per cluster

Source: Tripathy *et al.* (2010).

to detect a fall of 25%. In this case the number of person years is replaced by the number of live births.

Using Equation 7.9, with $\lambda_1 = 0.058$, $\lambda_2 = 0.0435$, $z_{\alpha/2} = -1.96$ (corresponding to 5% significance level), $z_\beta = 0.84$ (corresponding to 80% power), $cv = 0.15$, and $t = 270$ live births per cluster, 18 clusters per arm would be required. Allowing for 10% loss to follow-up, 300 live births per cluster would be required. It was anticipated that over a year there would be approximately 324 births per cluster; so the study would have slightly more power than 80%.

7.4   Restricted number of clusters

The design effect in the ELECTRA trial was relatively small (Section 7.2.2), requiring an increase of 28% in the number of participants per cluster compared to an individually randomised trial. This was because the availability of a reasonably large number of clusters meant that the number of subjects per cluster was fairly small. In other circumstances a smaller number of clusters with more participants per cluster cannot be avoided. The following sections describe some of the reasons that the number of available clusters might be limited.

7.4.1   Administrative reasons

There may be administrative reasons for a limited number of clusters; for example if the trial is to be conducted within an administrative district or specific umbrella organisation, it may be difficult or impossible to involve those outside that district or organisation. If separate approvals are required for each organisation or geographical area to participate, then reducing the number of organisations or areas

Table 7.5   Chronic care clinics for common geriatric syndromes.

Aim: To determine whether a new model of primary care can improve outcomes
of common geriatric syndromes in frail older adults
Location and type of cluster: US primary care physician practices
Interventions: (i) Control: usual care (ii) Intervention: half-day chronic care
clinics every three to four months, including visit with physician and nurse,
pharmacist visit and patient self-management/support group for six to eight
patients
Primary outcome: Quality of life – SF36 measure
Number of clusters analysed: 9
Number of individuals analysed: 142

Source: Coleman *et al.* (1999).

reduces the investigator time spent obtaining the necessary permissions for the
research. In the United States, healthcare services are often organised under the
umbrella of funding organisations and, particularly when the intervention is some
sort of reorganisation of healthcare services, it may be logistically easier to intervene
simply within one funding organisation. A trial conducted amongst frail older adults
who received their healthcare from a large Health Maintenance Organization in
western Washington State (Table 7.5) randomised only nine primary care practices,
all of those available within that Health Maintenance Organization.

In the x-ray guidelines trial (Oakeshott, Kerry and Williams, 1994; Section
1.3.1), practices referring patients to one hospital radiology department were randomised. As data were being collected in the department, practices referring to other
hospitals could not be included.

7.4.2   Few clusters are available

Community-wide interventions are likely to involve large clusters, such as counties
or regions. This will restrict the number of clusters available. The COMMIT trial
described in Section 3.1 (Gail *et al.*, 1992) tested such an intervention to reduce
smoking. The intervention aimed to change community attitudes and policies
towards smoking, as well as helping individual smokers quit. Twenty two communities of between 52 000 and 167 000 residents were randomised.

7.4.3   Cost or other practical difficulties of delivering
the intervention

Where the intervention, or the research to evaluate it, is costly to implement, it
may be necessary to restrict the number of intervention clusters. In the ASSIST

Table 7.6   ASSIST: different interventions to promote secondary prevention of coronary heart disease.

Aim: To assess the effectiveness of three different methods of promoting
   secondary prevention of coronary heart disease in primary care
Location and type of cluster: UK general practices
Interventions: (i) Audit of notes with summary feedback to primary healthcare
   team (audit group) (ii) Assistance with setting up a disease register and
   systematic recall of patients to general practitioner (GP recall group)
   (iii) Assistance with setting up a disease register and systematic recall of
   patients to a nurse-led clinic (nurse recall group)
Primary outcome: Adequate assessment of 3 risk factors, blood pressure,
   cholesterol and smoking status at follow-up
Number of clusters: 21
Number of individuals: 1906 had outcome assessment
Difference to be detected: Rise from 35% in the audit only group to 55% in the
   GP recall group. It was assumed that nurse recall would be more effective than
   GP recall

Source: Yudkin and Moher (2001).

trial (Table 7.6), investigators had committed themselves to auditing all the patient notes in each practice as a service to the general practices. Because of the amount of work involved, they did not then have the resources to include more practices in the trial.

7.4.4   Minimum number of clusters required

Having a limited number of clusters can, however, present problems. As the number of available clusters decreases then, to recruit the same number of individuals in total, investigators must recruit more per cluster. This, in turn, puts up the design effect, requiring even more individuals to be recruited. If, for example, the ELECTRA trial had been restricted to only 12 clusters, a total of 3782 patients would have been required, many more than the actual 290 from 44 clusters. Moreover, if we further reduce the number of clusters to 10, Equation 7.6 gives a negative value. If k is less than ρN, then it is impossible to conduct the trial without increasing the number of clusters.

This problem of limited number of clusters becomes acute either when the number required without taking clustering into account is very large, or when the total number of clusters is very small. Figure 7.1 shows the minimum number of clusters required for different values of the ICC and different sample sizes. When the number of individuals required for an individually randomised trial is 3000, a cluster randomised trial with as many as 100 clusters will not have sufficient power unless the ICC is less than 0.033.

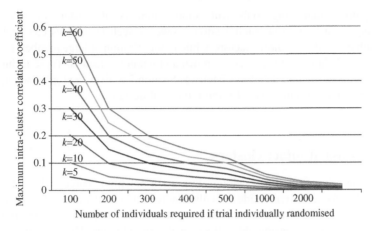

Figure 7.1   Maximum intra-cluster correlation coefficient values for a feasible trial given a limited number of clusters (k).

7.5   Trials with a small number of clusters

Unless there is a substantive reason for doing so, the practice of recruiting small numbers of clusters should be avoided. In addition to the difficulty in achieving the required power, these trials may be difficult to analyse (see Chapter 6), there is a risk of considerable loss of power if one cluster drops out, and it is difficult to balance the characteristics of clusters between different intervention arms.

7.5.1   Adjustment to sample size calculations when number of clusters is small

Sample size calculations shown above are based on the normal distribution and are only appropriate when the number of clusters is large; often assumed to be more than 30. In the Kumasi trial (Cappuccio *et al.*, 2006; Table 5.4), values for the *t*-distribution were used instead of the normal distribution in sample size calculations. However, since the degrees of freedom for the *t*-test depends on the number of clusters, which is what investigators are trying to estimate, this can be a lengthy, iterative process. Snedecor and Cochran (1980) suggest adding one cluster per arm for significance tests at 5% and 10%, and two to three clusters per arm for a significance level of 1% when there are fewer than 30 clusters. Other authors have also adopted this approach (Hayes and Moulton, 2009; Donner and Klar, 2000).

7.5.2   Balance between the arms in cluster characteristics

Randomisation will lead to balance between trial arms in terms of cluster characteristics only if a large number of clusters are randomised. To ensure balance, investigators conducting trials with small numbers of clusters often employ matching, stratification or minimisation. However such techniques can deal only with imbalance due to known factors, while randomisation of large numbers of units will lead to balance with respect to known and unknown factors. These techniques were discussed in more detail in Chapter 5. Section 7.8 gives the formulae required for calculating the sample size for these types of design.

7.5.3   Loss of intact clusters

In any trial, drop outs post-randomisation are a potential source of bias. If those responsible for a cluster decide to withdraw from the study, all participants from that cluster will be withdrawn, whether or not the participants wish to continue, and this may have considerable effect on the sample size. However the risk of clusters dropping out of a trial is in general small, and a review of cluster randomised trials published between 1997 and 2000 (Eldridge *et al.*, 2004) found that, in trials which recruited fewer than 20 clusters and reported adequate information to be able to judge drop-out rates, none lost any clusters to the analysis. It may be easier to keep track of and support clusters, and to keep all clusters on board as far as the analysis is concerned, where the number of clusters is small. As long as investigators have procedures in place to combat it, loss of clusters is unlikely to be a substantial problem in practice. Even amongst trials with a large number of clusters there is evidence that very few trials lose more than 10% of clusters before analysis.

7.6   Variability in cluster size

Formulae above assume that equal numbers of subjects are recruited in each cluster. If the variability in cluster size is small then the average cluster size, $\bar{m}$, can be used instead of m in Equations 7.4 and 7.5. Alternatively, the maximum cluster size could be used. This is likely to work well when allowing for losses to follow-up or failure to achieve a target sample size in some clusters, but where there are a few very large clusters it is likely to give overly large estimates of the required sample size (Guittet, Ravaud and Girandeau, 2006).

If the numbers per cluster are known in advance then the design effect can be estimated as

$$Deff = 1 + \rho(m_a - 1) \text{ where } m_a = \frac{\sum m_i^2}{\sum m_i} \tag{7.10}$$

where m_i is the number of individuals in the ith cluster (Donner, Birkett and Buck, 1981).

This formula is strictly only applicable to methods of analysis that give equal weight to each individual such as cluster-level analyses weighted by cluster size. This would be appropriate for individual-cluster interventions (see Section 2.2.2) where the trial aims to estimate the effect of the intervention on the population as a whole; for example, in the Ekjut project (Table 7.4), the aim was to reduce neonatal mortality in the population. Kerry and Bland (2001) give a formula for analyses that give equal weight to each cluster. This weighting would be appropriate for professional-cluster interventions (Section 2.2.2) when the focus of the intervention is to improve the knowledge or practice of the health professional. An alternative is to weight each cluster by the inverse of its variance, giving more weight to clusters with lower variance in order to reduce the overall variance of the effect size. Cluster-level analyses using minimum variance weights or other individual-level analyses such as maximum likelihood estimation for mixed effects models (Section 6.3.3) will be more powerful. van Breukelen, Candel and Berger (2008) show that, using such a model, the increase in variance of the intervention effect due to variation of cluster sizes rarely exceeds 20% and can be compensated for by sampling 25% more clusters. This approximation does not apply to increasing the cluster size instead of increasing the number of clusters. The next section describes a formula that allows for increasing the number of clusters or increasing the number of individuals per cluster to allow for variation in cluster size, which is an adaptation of Equation 7.10. It therefore strictly applies to methods of analysis that give equal weight to each individual, and will be conservative for other types of analysis.

7.6.1   Using coefficient of variation in cluster size for estimating sample size

While Equation 7.10 is relatively straightforward to use, actual cluster sizes are often not known in advance. In this case it may be possible to estimate the mean and standard deviation of the cluster size for the population from which the clusters will be sampled. The coefficient of variation of the *cluster sizes*, cv_c, can then be estimated (note: this is not to be confused with the between-cluster coefficient of variation of the *outcome* used in Section 7.3)

$$cv_c = \frac{s_c}{\bar{m}}$$

where s_c is the standard deviation of cluster sizes and $\bar{m}$ is the average cluster size. The design effect can then be calculated by the formula (Eldridge, Ashby and Kerry, 2006)

$$Deff = 1 + \left(\left(cv_c^2 + 1 \right) \bar{m} - 1 \right) \rho \tag{7.11}$$

7.6.2   Estimating coefficient of variation in cluster size

The coefficient of variation in cluster size can be estimated from other trials involving similar clusters, modelling sources of variation or estimating the standard deviation from the minimum and maximum expected cluster sizes.

UK primary care trials often involve the randomisation of practices. The main source of variability in cluster size is the number of patients on the practice list. List sizes may be available locally for the target population of practices. For example, Kerry and Bland (2001) used nationally collected data on practice list size (NHS Executive, 1997). Using these data, the coefficient of variation of cluster size is 0.65 (Eldridge, Ashby and Kerry, 2006). The ELECTRA trial (Table 7.3) recruited patients attending A&E departments for unscheduled asthma care. Smaller practices are likely to have fewer patients attending A&E than larger practices, so list size is likely to be a major determinant in the variability in cluster size. The coefficient of variation in cluster size in the final trial sample was 0.64, similar to that obtained from national data (Eldridge, Ashby and Kerry, 2006).

Kendrick, Burns and Freeling (1995) recruited only practices with three or more partners to a trial of structured assessment for patients with long term mental illness. The coefficient of variation in cluster size from this trial was 0.42 (Eldridge, Ashby and Kerry, 2006). Since smaller practices were excluded, the coefficient of variation would be expected to be smaller than when all practices were included. An estimate could have been obtained in advance using national data and excluding smaller practices; for example those with fewer than 5000 patients.

The ELECTRA calculations in Section 7.2.2 and in Griffiths *et al.* (2004) do not allow for variability in cluster size.

Using $cv_c = 0.65$ from UK national data, then

$$Deff = 1 + ((0.65^2 + 1) \times 6.6 - 1) \times 0.05 = 1.42$$

This compares with 1.28 when variability in cluster size is ignored. Allowing for variability in cluster size, the trial would need to recruit 48 practices, 24 per arm.

Alternatively, keeping the number of practices fixed at 44, but allowing for variability in cluster size, the average number of patients required per practice can be calculated as

$$\bar{m} = \frac{N(1-\rho)}{(k - \rho N(1 + cv_c^2))} \tag{7.12}$$

For the ELECTRA trial this is 7.7, and the total sample size required would be 338. The trial recruited 345 individuals of whom 319 were included in the final analysis (Table 7.3)

7.6.3   Small clusters arising from incident cases

If a trial recruits incident cases then there will be additional variability in cluster size due to random variability in numbers of patients diagnosed. In a trial to assess

Table 7.7   Average cluster size and expected percentage of practices lost to the study when recruiting incident cases, based on practice list size in England and Wales (1995).

Proportion of population diagnosed during study	Average expected number of cases per cluster	Expected percentage of practice lost to the study	Clusters with at least one case			
			Expected Range	$\bar{m}$	s_c	cv_c
0.0002	1.1	0.41	1 to 6	1.8	1.12	0.62
0.0003	1.6	0.29	1 to 8	2.3	1.52	0.66
0.0005	2.8	0.16	1 to 11	3.3	2.22	0.67
0.0008	4.4	0.08	1 to 16	4.8	3.32	0.69
0.0010	5.5	0.05	1 to 19	5.8	4.03	0.69
0.0012	6.6	0.04	1 to 22	6.9	4.77	0.69
0.0016	8.7	0.02	1 to 28	8.9	6.19	0.70
0.0020	11.0	0.01	1 to 34	11.1	7.52	0.68
0.0030	16.5	0.00	1 to 49	16.5	11.05	0.67
0.0040	22.0	0.00	2 to 63	22.0	14.46	0.66
0.0060	32.9	0.00	3 to 91	32.9	21.38	0.65

Source: adapted from Kerry and Bland (2001).

the effectiveness of guidelines to improve the management of chlamydia infection (Oakeshott and Kerry, 1999), incident cases were identified and their management assessed, blind to intervention status, at the end of the trial. Since the incidence of chlamydia infection is relatively low, some clusters did not diagnose any cases. Kerry and Bland (2001) used the national practice list sizes in 1995 (NHS Executive, 1997) to estimate how many clusters were likely to be lost, and the distribution of cluster sizes for the remaining clusters using different incidence rates. The probability that a cluster will not identify a case, and the resulting average cluster size and cv_c is shown in Table 7.7, which is adapted from Kerry and Bland (2001).

When the average number of cases per practice is expected to be less than five, there is a high chance of some clusters failing to recruit any patients. Consequently the average cluster size for the remaining clusters is increased. There is a small increase in the coefficient of variation and then a decrease as cluster sizes increase, but cv_c does not rise above 0.71. This is illustrated in Figure 7.2 (Eldridge, Ashby and Kerry, 2006). The loss of clusters, increase in cluster size for the analysis and increase in coefficient of variation will all increase the number of clusters investigators needed to approach. This will be important if the ICC is fairly high. In the chlamydia guidelines trial, the ICC was 0.29, and the design effect was increased from 1.36 ignoring the variability in cluster size to 1.67 taking account both of variability in list size and random variability in number of cases identified (Kerry and Bland, 2001).

It is fairly straightforward to calculate the number of clusters required for a given value of the expected average cluster size. If, on the other hand, we wish to calculate the required cluster size, Equation 7.12 can be used to calculate $\bar{m}$, but some itera-

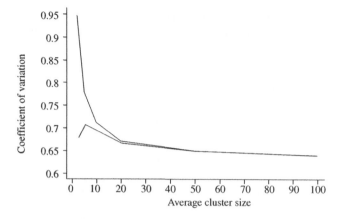

Figure 7.2   Expected coefficient of variation of cluster size by average cluster size for trials randomising UK general practices, where incident cases are being recruited. S.M. Eldridge, D. Ashby, S. Kerry, Sample Size for cluster randomized trials: effect of coefficient of variation of cluster size and analysis method, International Journal of Epidemiology, 2006, 35, 5 by permission of Oxford University Press.

tion will be required to allow for clusters lost to the analysis, as this will in turn depend on the cluster size.

7.6.4   Variable cluster size for rates

Since the above formulae use the design effect, they cannot be used when the outcome is expressed as a rate. In Equation 7.9, t is number of person years of follow-up per cluster, and assumed to be the same for all clusters. If cluster sizes vary, t can be replaced by, t_h, the harmonic mean of the number of person years per cluster.

7.7   Comparison of different measures of between-cluster variability

In this section we compare formulae for sample size for different measures of between-cluster variation. These formulae will not always give the same results, as they use slightly different assumptions about how the between-cluster variance varies between intervention and control arms of the study; we discuss the effect of these assumptions on sample size calculations for means in Section 7.7.3 and for proportions in Section 7.7.4.

7.7.1   Estimating sample size using between-cluster variance

Instead of using the ICC, the variability of the outcome between clusters can be estimated directly using the between-cluster variance σ_b^2. If the effect is summarised as the difference between two means, then the number of clusters required per arm can be expressed as

$$k = \frac{2(z_{\alpha/2} + z_\beta)^2 \left(\sigma_b^2 + \dfrac{\sigma_w^2}{m} \right)}{(\mu_1 - \mu_2)^2} \tag{7.13}$$

where $z_{\alpha/2}$ and z_β are the standard normal values corresponding to the upper tail probabilities of $\alpha/2$ and β respectively, and μ_1 and μ_2 are the means in the two arms.

Kerry and Bland (1998) illustrate the use of this formula for a proposed trial using a behavioural intervention in general practice to lower blood cholesterol concentrations. Using data from a previous study, σ_b^2 was estimated to be 0.0046 mmol/l and σ_w^2 to be 1.28 mmol/l. The trial was designed to detect a difference of 0.1 mmol/l using a 5% significance level and 90% power. Using Equation 7.13, 63 practices would be required in each arm if 50 patients were recruited per practice: 126 practices in total. The number of practices could be reduced to 16 in each arm if the number of patients per practice was increased to 500.

This formula is equivalent to using the design effect (Equation 7.4), and assumes that the between-cluster variance is the same in the intervention and control arms. A more general formula is given by

$$k = \frac{(z_{\alpha/2} + z_\beta)^2 \left(\sigma_{b1}^2 + \sigma_{b2}^2 + \dfrac{2\sigma_w^2}{m} \right)}{(\mu_1 - \mu_2)^2} \tag{7.14}$$

where σ_{b1}^2 and σ_{b2}^2 denote the between-cluster variance within the intervention and control arms.

For trials comparing proportions, the within-cluster variance will depend on the value of π_1 and π_2, the expected proportions in each arm. The number of clusters per arm is given by

$$k = \frac{(z_{\alpha/2} + z_\beta)^2 \left(\sigma_{b1}^2 + \sigma_{b2}^2 + \dfrac{(\pi_1(1 - \pi_1) + \pi_2(1 - \pi_2))}{m} \right)}{(\pi_1 - \pi_2)^2} \tag{7.15}$$

For trials involving rates, the within-cluster variance will depend on the value of λ_1 and λ_2, the expected rate in each arm. The number of clusters per arm is given by

$$k = \frac{(z_{\alpha/2} + z_\beta)^2 \left(\sigma_{b1}^2 + \sigma_{b2}^2 + \dfrac{(\lambda_1 + \lambda_2)}{t} \right)}{(\lambda_1 - \lambda_2)^2} \tag{7.16}$$

7.7.2   Estimating sample size using between-cluster coefficient of variation in outcome

Although Hayes and Bennet (1999) originally developed the method of calculating the sample size using the coefficient of variation for rates (Section 7.3), the same method could be applied to means and proportions. For means, the coefficient of variation is σ_b/μ. If we assume that the coefficient of variation is the same in both arms ($cv = \sigma_{b1}/\mu_1 = \sigma_{b2}/\mu_2$) and that the within-cluster variance, σ_w^2, is the same in both arms, then rearranging Equation 7.14, the number of clusters per arm can be calculated by

$$k = \frac{(z_{\alpha/2} + z_\beta)^2 \left(\dfrac{2\sigma_w^2}{m} + cv^2(\mu_1^2 + \mu_2^2) \right)}{(\mu_1 - \mu_2)^2} \tag{7.17}$$

For proportions assuming the cv is the same in both arms of the study, the number of clusters required in each arm is given by

$$k = \frac{(z_{\alpha/2} + z_\beta)^2 \left(\dfrac{(\pi_1(1-\pi_1) + \pi_2(1-\pi_2))}{m} + cv^2(\pi_1^2 + \pi_2^2) \right)}{(\pi_1 - \pi_2)^2} \tag{7.18}$$

7.7.3   Comparison of measures of between-cluster variability for means

In sample size calculations for continuous outcomes it is often assumed that the variance between individuals is the same in both arms of the trial. For a cluster randomised trial, if we also assume that the variance between clusters is the same in both arms, then the ICC will also be the same in both arms. In this case the cv will not be the same in both arms, as μ_1 and μ_2 are different. Equations 7.4 and 7.17 will therefore always give different answers.

Hayes and Moulton (2009) suggest that, when the intervention effect can be considered to be constant across all clusters, the variability between clusters is likely to be the same, and therefore the ICC will be constant. In the cholesterol example, from Section 7.7.1, it might be reasonable to assume that if the intervention was effective, the average cholesterol from patients in the intervention practices would be 0.1 mmol/l lower than from those in the control arm. The sample size assuming constant ICC might be most appropriate. However, the assumptions used in the sample size calculation should also be those used in the analysis. For example, the usual assumption in a linear mixed model is that the ICC is constant.

If, on the other hand, we expect the reduction in cholesterol to be proportional to the mean, Hayes and Moulton (2009) suggest the between-cluster standard deviation would also reduce proportionately, so that the cv would be the same in both arms of the trial. For instance, in the cholesterol example, if there is a 10%

fall in cholesterol, then practices in the intervention arm with a mean of 7 mmol/l at baseline would be expected to have a fall of 0.7 mmol/l, while practices with a mean of 5 mmol/l at baseline would be expected to have a fall of 0.5 mmol/l. The sample size assuming the coefficient of variation is constant might be most appropriate.

7.7.4   Comparison of measures of between-cluster variability for proportions

In the previous section we showed that using the ICC or using the cv to calculate the sample size will give different answers. For proportions there is an additional complication that the within-cluster variance will also vary with the value of the outcome (see Section 8.1.1). We can write

$$cv = \frac{\sigma_b}{\pi} \quad \text{and} \quad \rho = \frac{\sigma_b^2}{\pi(1-\pi)}$$

Rearranging these formulae gives two expressions for the between-cluster variance

$$\sigma_b^2 = \pi^2 cv^2 \tag{7.19}$$

$$\sigma_b^2 = \rho\pi(1-\pi) \tag{7.20}$$

For a fixed value of ρ or cv, the assumed between-cluster variance can be calculated for different values of π. In order to compare the effect of assuming that either the coefficient of variation or the ICC is constant across intervention arms, we will estimate what happens to the variance between clusters under each assumption. First of all we will look at what happens when the value of π is small, similar to those situations for which the coefficient of variation method was developed, and then extend across the whole range of values between 0 and 1, covering values likely to be found in primary care trials.

As an example we use values of the ICC from the falls prevention pilot study (Table 7.8) and calculate the corresponding value of the cv for the control arm. Trial investigators planned to use a multifaceted intervention to reduce the risk of falling among older people. To detect a difference between the proportion with a fracture in the control arm of 0.006 and in the intervention arm of 0.0048, a sample size of 58 478 people aged over 65 would be required in each arm if the trial was individually randomised, with 80% power and 5% significance. The ICC was estimated for Primary Care Trusts to be 0.000224, and the number of older people per cluster was estimated to be 20 000. Using Equation 7.4, the design effect is 5.5 and the number of clusters required is 16.0.

For any value of the ICC and π, the corresponding value of the coefficient of variation can be calculated, and vice versa, using the formulae

Table 7.8   Pilot study for a falls prevention programme.

Aim: To assess whether a falls prevention programme would reduce the rate of hip fractures in older people

Location and type of cluster: UK Primary Care Trusts (approximately 100 000 patients each – see Section 4.2.2 for more detail)

Interventions: (i) Control: usual care (ii) Intervention: identification of older people at risk of falling and referral to a falls clinic

Primary outcome: Fractured neck of femur

Cluster size: 20 000 approximately

Intra-cluster correlation coefficient 0.000224

Difference to be detected: 6 per 1000 to 4.8 per 1000

Source: Eldridge *et al.* (2001; 2005).

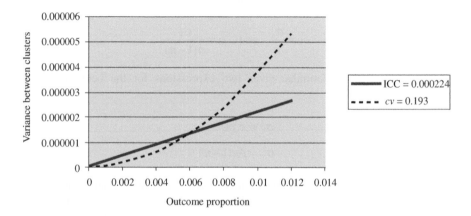

Figure 7.3   The relationship of the variance between clusters and outcome proportion, π, when the ICC is fixed or the coefficient of variation is fixed, and π is very small.

$$\rho = cv^2 \left(\frac{\pi}{1-\pi} \right) \quad \text{or} \quad cv = \sqrt{\frac{\rho(1-\pi)}{\pi}}$$

If the ICC is 0.000224 and the value of π is 0.006, then the coefficient of variation is 0.193. Using Equation 7.18, the number of clusters required per arm is 14.9; slightly lower than using the ICC.

Figure 7.3 shows the variance between clusters, σ_b^2, for different values of π, assuming that ICC remains constant at 0.000224, or assuming the *cv* remains constant at 0.193. The two lines cross when π is 0.006, the value of the outcome in the control arm. As π decreases the variance between clusters decreases when either the *cv* or the ICC is constant, but the decrease is steeper when *cv* is constant. When the effect of intervention is to reduce π, the sample size calculated using Equation 7.18 (*cv* constant) will always be less than when using Equation 7.4 (ICC constant), but the difference may not be very great. When the intervention is designed to increase π, the different assumptions have a greater effect on the variance, and sample sizes based on the coefficient of variation will be larger.

When π is small, as in Figure 7.3, it seems sensible that the between-cluster variance should decrease as π decreases, since π cannot be less than zero. Thus although the two methods give different answers, they are unlikely to be very different, and both approaches seem reasonable. However, when the purpose of the intervention is to increase π, unless there is good evidence that the intervention will have a marked increase on the variability between clusters, using the design effect method that keeps the ICC constant is probably the better option. Using Equation 7.18 which keeps the cv constant is likely to overestimate the variance between clusters in the intervention arm and hence the sample size will be overestimated.

Cluster randomised trials in health services research tend to have outcomes with prevalences towards the middle of the range, between 0.2 and 0.8, and interventions may aim to increase or decrease π. Figure 7.4 shows the relationship between σ_b^2 and π across the whole range of possible values of π, when the ICC is set at 0.05, a fairly common value in primary care, and when the cv is constant, taking values corresponding to an ICC of 0.05 and π equal to 0.2, 0.4, 0.6, and 0.8. When the ICC is fixed, the variance between clusters is lower for extreme values of π and highest when π is 0.5. When the coefficient of variation is fixed, the variance changes are more marked and the variance always increases as π increases. For values of π over 0.5 this is somewhat counterintuitive. As π tends towards unity, the between-cluster variance is likely to decrease as π cannot be greater than 1.

The ASSIST trial (Table 7.6) aimed to increase the proportion of patients with adequate cardiovascular risk assessment from 35% to 55%. If the trial was individually randomised, 93 patients per arm would be required to detect this difference with

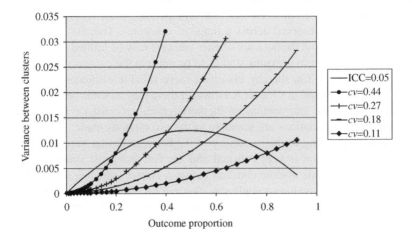

Figure 7.4   The relationship of the variance between clusters and outcome proportion, π, when the ICC is fixed at 0.05 or the coefficient of variation is fixed, across the whole range of π.

80% power using a 5% significance level. With 100 patients per cluster and an ICC of 0.05, the design effect would be 5.95 and 554 patients per arm would be required using Equation 7.4. The equivalent cv in the control arm, when $\pi = 0.35$, is 0.3047. Using Equation 7.18, 866 patients per arm would be required; far more than using the ICC formula. The between-cluster standard deviation was 0.107, or 10.7% in the control arm. If the ICC remained constant, this increases by a small amount to 11.1% in the intervention arm, using Equation 7.19, whereas it increases to 16.5% when the cv remains constant, using Equation 7.20. One element of the intervention was discussion of guidelines, in order to reduce variability in practice; Equation 7.18 is therefore likely to overestimate the required sample size.

An associated complication of using the coefficient of variation is that it is sensitive to whether the outcome is expressed as the proportion of 'successes' or the proportion of 'failures'. Thomson, Hayes and Cousens (2009) suggest that, where the outcome is expected to be greater than 50% in the control arm and the intervention aims to increase proportion, it would be better to reverse the direction of the outcome; for example, to assess the proportion of inappropriate referrals rather than the proportion of appropriate referrals. This is not an issue if the ICC is used as a measure of between-cluster variance, as the relationship between σ_b^2 and π is then symmetrical about $\pi = 0.5$. Another consideration in choosing between different methods is whether the outcome is to be analysed as the difference in proportions, odds ratios or relative risks. For a fuller discussion see Thomson, Hayes and Cousens (2009).

Equations 7.14, 7.15 and 7.16 allow the components of variance to be modelled explicitly and the between-cluster variance to vary between the intervention and control arms. This has been recommended by Thomson, Hayes and Cousens (2009) as an alternative to making assumptions about constant ICC or constant cv. However, the between-cluster variance needs to be estimated for each outcome specifically and is measured in the units relevant to each outcome, while ICCs are ratios, and patterns have been observed across a range of outcomes. Therefore at the design stage information about the between-cluster variance may be limited. Using the ICC allows information from previous studies to be put into the context of other known information about ICCs, thereby obtaining more reliable estimates. This will be discussed in more detail in Chapter 8. However there may be some benefit in modelling the effect of the intervention on the between-cluster variance to see whether the sample size calculations are sensitive to the assumptions made.

In summary, owing to the instability of the between-cluster variance when the coefficient of variation is kept constant and the fact that most standard software procedures for analysis assume constant between-cluster variance, we recommend using the ICC for calculating sample size required for all trials where outcomes are expressed as proportions, unless the outcome proportion is very low.

7.8 Matched and stratified designs

Matched and stratified designs were described in Chapter 5, Sections 5.1.4 and 5.1.9. The power of the trial using stratification (or matching) is determined by the between-cluster variance within strata (or within matched pair), but only if analysed in a way which takes account of the stratification (or matching). Matching is simply an extreme form of stratification with two clusters per stratum, so matching is likely to have a greater effect on the sample size required than stratification, provided that investigators have been able to find appropriate factors on which to match. If σ_{bm} is the standard deviation of the outcome between clusters within strata then, if matching is effective, the value of σ_{bm} for matched pairs will usually be less than for stratified designs, which will in turn be less than σ_b, the between-cluster standard deviation for a completely randomised design.

In this section we present the formulae for sample size for the difference between two means and the difference between proportions, and then discuss the practical application of these formulae. We show how other researchers have dealt with lack of information on the effectiveness of matching, and give some general guidance on the likely effectiveness of stratification (or matching).

7.8.1   Matched and stratified designs comparing means

For detecting the difference between two means the same formula can be used whether there are two members of each stratum (matched design) or more. Adapting Equation 7.13, the number of clusters per arm is given by

$$k = \frac{2(z_{\alpha/2} + z_{\beta})^2 \left(\sigma_{bm}^2 + \dfrac{\sigma_w^2}{m} \right)}{(\mu_1 - \mu_2)^2} \qquad (7.21)$$

For a matched design this will also be the number of pairs. The addition of two clusters per arm will be required if the number of clusters is small, to compensate for the loss of degrees of freedom induced by matching (Snedecor and Cochran, 1980; see also Section 7.5.1). Since fewer degrees of freedom are lost in a stratified design, the addition of two clusters would be conservative. Alternatively, for a stratified design, values from the t-distribution can be used instead of $z_{\alpha/2}$ and z_{β}, but this will involve some iteration if determining the number of clusters with fixed size (Watson *et al.*, 2004).

7.8.2   Matched and stratified designs comparing proportions

For a matched or stratified design and a binary outcome, adapting Equation 7.15 the number of clusters in each arm is given by

$$k = \frac{(z_{\alpha/2} + z_{\beta})^2 \left(2\sigma_{bm}^2 + \dfrac{(\pi_1(1-\pi_1) + \pi_2(1-\pi_2))}{m} \right)}{(\pi_1 - \pi_2)^2} \qquad (7.22)$$

If the outcome is to be an odds ratio calculated for each stratum and then combined to give an overall average effect, the formula is more complicated. Donner and Klar

(2000) give a formula which depends on the stratum-specific success rates and incorporates variable cluster size, so that either the number of subjects or the number of clusters remains constant from stratum to stratum.

7.8.3   Matching correlation

The matching correlation, ρ_m, is the correlation between the intervention and control cluster means for each matched pair. It is related to the two measures of between-cluster variance, σ_{bm}^2 and σ_b^2 by $\rho_m = 1 - \dfrac{\sigma_{bm}^2}{\sigma_b^2}$. In studies where the between-cluster variance within pairs is not known, an estimate of between-cluster variance across all clusters allows a conservative sample size to be calculated ignoring the matching. The effect of different values of the matching correlation, usually unknown, can then be assessed.

In the PRISM trial (Table 7.9), 21 clusters were eligible and willing to participate, of which 16 were selected in matched pairs. The matching factors, number of births, geographic size and 'similar ratings of community infrastructure and activity', were chosen from a number of factors as they were most closely related to the rates of depression prior to the study. The researchers (Watson *et al.*, 2004) reported that the data were 'too sparse' to give a reliable estimate of between-cluster variance, but when clusters were grouped into pairs the standard deviation of rates of depression between clusters was halved; that is $\sigma_{bm}/\sigma_b = 0.5$. This gives a value of ρ_m of 0.75. Using a form of Equation 7.22 adapted to allow for variable cluster size, and using values from the *t*-distribution instead of the normal distribution, Watson *et al.* (2004) estimated the relationship between the between-cluster variance and match-

Table 7.9   PRISM: program of resources, information and support for mothers.

Aim: To determine whether a whole-community approach to improving support for mothers in the 12 months after birth would decrease the rate of postnatal depression

Location and type of cluster: Local government areas in Victoria, Australia with between 300 and 1500 births per annum

Interventions: (i) Control (ii) Primary care and community-based strategies embedded in existing services; information for new mothers and community development officer

Primary outcome: Depression at six months as measured by the Edinburgh Postnatal Depression Scale

Cluster size: 800

Between-cluster standard deviation 1.5 to 3%

Difference to be detected: 16.9 to 13.9%

Source: Watson *et al.* (2004).

ing correlations assuming the trial would recruit 800 women in each of 8 matched pairs. They demonstrated that the trial would be large enough if the matching correlation was 0.3 and when the between-cluster standard deviation was 0.015 or 1.5%. If the study was unmatched, approximately 1200 mothers per cluster would be required. If the between-cluster standard deviation was as high as 0.03, or 3%, then an unmatched study would not be feasible without recruiting more clusters as the ICC would be too high (see Section 7.4.4), but the matched trial would have sufficient power provided the matching correlation was 0.7.

Gail *et al.* (1992) carry out a similar sensitivity analysis in estimating the power of the COMMIT study (see Section 7.4.2). The sample size calculation is based on analysis using a paired *t*-test. Advance estimates of appropriate between-cluster (in this case community) variances were obtained from a previous trial randomising individuals, and the sample size calculations are carried out assuming both that matching will be as good as randomising individuals, and that matching will be completely ineffective. As expected, larger sample sizes are required for the case of ineffective matching, highlighting the effect of the closeness of matching on the sample size requirements.

7.8.4   Strength of relationship between stratification factors and outcomes

The PRISM study investigators tried a number of factors to create matched pairs; they chose those factors most associated with the outcome at baseline, and chose only those clusters that could form well matched pairs. This is likely to produce better matches than those achieved when all available or willing clusters are matched and there is no information is available on baseline values of the outcome variable. Few cluster randomised trials in health services research are able to use baseline values of the outcome variable to identify closely correlated factors. More commonly, cluster-level factors such as number of partners in the practice, the way the practice is organised, the computer system or the way the practice is funded are chosen.

The diabetes care from diagnosis trial (Table 7.10) stratified general practices by the hospital to which they usually referred patients, the practice list size and whether or not diabetes care was organised using a practice-based system . Table 7.11 shows correlations between some outcomes and stratification factors in the trial. The strongest correlation is −0.13 between systolic blood pressure and practice size. It can be shown that this would result in a reduction in observed variance at the cluster level of 1.7% in a balanced design and a smaller reduction in an unbalanced design. This is therefore the maximum effect of stratification with one factor.

7.8.5   Cluster size as a stratification factor in primary care

Many trials use either cluster size or a measure which relates to cluster size as a stratification factor (Section 5.1.3). We have shown that variable cluster size leads

Table 7.10   Diabetes care from diagnosis trial.

Aim: To assess the effect of additional training of practice staff in patient centred care, on the current well-being and future risk of patients with newly diagnosed type 2 diabetes

Location and type of cluster: UK general practices

Interventions: (i) Control: approach to care developed with practices, based on national guidelines and including patient materials (ii) Intervention: as control plus extra training on patient centred care

Main outcome measures: Quality of life, well-being, haemoglobin A1c and lipid concentrations, blood pressure, body mass index

Stratification factors: Stratified by district general hospital, practice list size >10 000, and style of diabetes care – personal or practice-based organisation

---

Reproduced by permission of Michael J. Campbell.

Table 7.11   Correlations between stratifying factors and potential outcomes in the diabetes care from diagnosis trial.

Type of stratification factor	Stratification factor	Outcome	Correlation (95% confidence interval)
Cluster feature	Practice organisation of diabetes care	Body mass index	0.10 (−0.22 to 0.41)
		Weight	0.12 (−0.20 to 0.42)
		Systolic blood pressure	−0.12 (−0.42 to 0.20)
		Diastolic blood pressure	−0.00 (−0.32 to 0.32)
Cluster size	Practice size	Body mass index	0.10 (−0.23 to 0.40)
		Weight	−0.03 (−0.34 to 0.29)
		Systolic blood pressure	−0.13 (−0.43 to 0.19)
		Diastolic blood pressure	−0.03 (−0.35 to 0.29)

to a reduction in power, and the design effect is given in Equation 7.11. If cluster size is the only stratification factor (so that stratification reduces the variation in cluster size within strata) and the ICC is the same across all strata and is not reduced by the stratification, then the design effect accounting for stratification becomes

$$Deff = \frac{\sum_{s=1}^{S} \bar{m}_s}{\sum_{s=1}^{S} \frac{\bar{m}_s}{1 + \left((1 + cv_{cs}^2)\bar{m}_s - 1\right)\rho}} \qquad (7.23)$$

where there are S strata and the subscript s refers to the stratum number.

In trials randomising general practices, for example, the cluster sizes are often related to the number of patients registered with the practice. Although the actual cluster sizes might not be known in advance, the value of cv_{cs} may be assumed to be proportional to the list size. Using Equation 7.23 and data from UK primary care on average list sizes, it can be shown that the maximum reduction in sample size when using two strata of equal numbers of practices is 18%, and the maximum reduction using four strata is 25%. Maximum reductions occur with very large average clusters sizes and large ICCs.

7.8.6   Summary of the effect of stratification on power

If matching is not very effective, then it is possible for the potential gain in power from matching to be outweighed by the effect on the analysis of reducing the number of degrees of freedom. Klar and Donner (1997) show that, when there are 2 strata and 12 clusters per arm, a correlation of 0.11 between stratification factor and cluster-specific outcome is necessary to ensure increased efficiency from stratification. This break-even correlation increases to 0.17 with 8 clusters per arm. The situation is even worse for matching, when a correlation between cluster-level matching factors and a cluster-level outcome needs to be over 0.2 when the number of pairs is 25 or more, and about 0.35 when the number of pairs is 10.

It seems unlikely from the previous sections that any form of stratification can substantially reduce the required sample size of a cluster randomised trial in primary care. This is likely to hold for trials in other areas of health services research unless baseline data on the outcome are available and there is good reason to believe this predicts the outcome. For fuller discussion of trials in low-income countries see Hayes and Moulton (2009). Even when baseline data might be available at the randomisation stage, the impact is difficult to predict in advance, because of uncertainties in estimating the required parameters. The most useful function of stratification in these trials is to ensure balance in various factors between intervention and control arms. Since these factors exist at cluster level and therefore often relate to cluster characteristics and not individual characteristics, this does not guarantee balance in important patient prognostic factors between the trial arms, but it does provide some face validity regarding lack of bias in a trial. The best course of action is to carry out stratification primarily to balance intervention arms and ignore any effect of stratification on precision in calculating sample sizes. If stratification is effective, this strategy will result in a conservative sample size estimate. Although many trials use stratification (see Section 5.1.4), we could not find any examples of trials in which stratification was used *and* accounted for in the sample size, except the WHO antenatal trial (Villar *et al.*, 1998) described in Donner and Klar (2000).

7.9 Sample size for other designs

7.9.1 Unequal numbers in each arm

Most of the examples in this chapter are trials in which investigators have intended to recruit equal numbers of clusters and subjects to each arm of the trial. If the trial is designed to have more clusters in one arm than another, for example to reduce costs if the intervention is expensive, then the trial will require a larger sample size than one where the arms are of equal size. This is true whether or not the trial is cluster randomised. If the average cluster size is the same in each arm, then the design effect will be the same whether or not the arms have the same number of clusters and, following the calculation of sample size required for a trial with unequal sized arms in the normal way (Bland, 2000), Equation 7.4 and its variants (Equations 7.5, 7.6, 7.11 and 7.12) can be used to adjust for clustering.

7.9.2 Block randomisation

Block randomisation (Section 5.1.8) of clusters is usually carried out to ensure that there are equal numbers of clusters in each arm. Although it is normally used with stratification, it can be used alone. It also aids even allocation throughout the trial, which may be useful to control workload if one intervention is more resource intensive than another. Which block the cluster falls into is unlikely to be related to the outcome, so blocking is unlikely to increase power and can be ignored in the sample size calculations.

7.9.3 Minimisation

Although Equations 7.21 and 7.22 account for stratification, these are rarely used as it is difficult to obtain estimates for the within-strata variability between clusters. Minimisation adds another layer of complexity, and even if appropriate sample size formulae were available it would be unlikely that researchers would have sufficient information at the design stage to make use of them.

7.9.4 Cohort versus cross-sectional studies

Most randomised trials follow the same individuals over the course of the trial; often described as a cohort design (Section 5.2). If the primary outcome is change from baseline in some quantity, then the standard deviation of the change should be used for the sample size. Ideally, the ICC used would also be for the change outcome, although this may be difficult to estimate and the ICC for the outcome itself could be used instead.

Where repeated cross-sectional studies are used, the outcome may be change from baseline at the cluster level, or outcome measured at follow-up with baseline cluster measures as covariates in a mixed model or generalised estimating equation. Knowledge of the correlation between the outcomes at baseline and follow-up within cluster would be required in order to take the repeat measures into account in the sample size calculations, or an estimate of the standard deviation between two cross-sectional surveys in the same cluster.

Equations 7.21 and 7.22 can be adapted to a repeated cross-sectional design, where σ_{bm} now represents the standard deviation between the two cross-sectional samples in the same cluster, rather than the standard deviation between two clusters within the same matched pair.

Assuming that the same number of subjects will contribute data at baseline and follow-up, the number of clusters per arm is given by

$$k = \frac{2(z_{\alpha/2} + z_\beta)^2 \left(\sigma_{bm}^2 + \dfrac{2\sigma_w^2}{m} \right)}{(\mu_1 - \mu_2)^2}$$

for a difference of means, and

$$k = \frac{2(z_{\alpha/2} + z_\beta)^2 \left(\sigma_{bm}^2 + \dfrac{(\pi_1(1 - \pi_1) + \pi_2(1 - \pi_2))}{m} \right)}{(\pi_1 - \pi_2)^2}$$

for a difference of proportions.

7.9.5   More than two intervention arms

Since cluster randomised trials are often resource intensive and face challenges recruiting sufficient numbers of clusters, most cluster randomised trials compare two arms, one an intervention and the other a control arm. Where more than two arms are used, the comparisons of interest need to be carefully specified and the trial powered to detect these. In the ASSIST trial (Table 7.6), 21 practices were randomised to 3 different arms: audit only, audit plus GP recall or audit plus nurse recall. The trial was powered to detect an increase in the percentage of patients adequately assessed for coronary heart disease risk, from 35% in the audit only arm to 55% in the GP recall arm. It was assumed that the nurse recall would be more effective than the GP recall, and therefore the study would also be able to detect a benefit of nurse recall compared with audit alone. The study also had sufficient power to detect an increase from 55% in the GP recall to 75% in the nurse recall arm. If a study is powered only to detect a difference between the two arms thought

Table 7.12   Two interventions to increase breast screening.

Aim: To examine the effectiveness and cost effectiveness of two interventions
   based in primary care aimed at increasing uptake of breast screening
Location and type of cluster: UK general practices
Interventions: (i) Control (ii) General practitioner (GP) letter (iii) Flag in women's
   notes prompting discussion by health professionals (iv) Both interventions
Primary outcome: Attendance for screening
Difference to be detected: 50% without the intervention to 58.5 to 60% for either
   intervention
*Number of clusters:*24
Standard deviation between clusters: 7.7%

Source: Richards *et al.* (2001).

to be the most different, then it is unlikely to have sufficient power to detect differences between the other arms.

7.9.6   Factorial designs

A factorial design is an efficient way of testing two interventions against their appropriate controls simultaneously. The effect of each intervention can be analysed separately using all the randomised units. If the design is a 2×2 factorial, then half the participants will be in each arm for both interventions.

In Section 5.3.3 and 6.4.2 we introduced a 2×2 factorial trial to improve attendance for breast cancer screening testing two interventions (Table 7.12): a systematic approach (general practitioner letter) and an opportunistic intervention (flag in the women's notes prompting discussion by health professionals). Twenty-four practices were randomised to one of four arms: one of the two interventions, neither or both interventions. The primary analysis was to compare those practices receiving each intervention with those not receiving that intervention. The sample size calculations were performed as a simple comparison of two arms; that is, GP letter versus no GP letter and flag in notes versus no flag in notes.

The researchers assumed that 252 women in each cluster would be available for outcome assessment and that the standard deviation between clusters was 7.7%. Using Equation 7.15, the number of practices required to detect an increase from 50% without the flag to 60% with the flag is 10.8, with 80% power at the 5% significance level and assuming that $\sigma_{b1} = \sigma_{b2}$. The study recruited a total of 24 practices, 12 with the flag and 12 without; so the power to detect this difference was greater than 80%. The sample calculations are the same for GP letter versus no GP letter.

This trial did not test the effect of the interaction between the two interventions; that is, is an opportunistic intervention more effective in the presence of the systematic intervention? If the research team had wished to test the interaction between the interventions, then the sample size would have needed to be larger. Section 5.3.3

describes the implications of different types of interactions on the design of the study, but we are not aware of any cluster randomised trials that have been powered to look for interactions.

7.9.7 Crossover trials

In a crossover trial, each cluster is randomised to receive an intervention for a set period, then, after a washout period, to receive the alternative intervention. If there is no carryover effect and no period effect, the implications for sample size are the same as in a matched design, where the ICC for matched pairs is replaced by the ICC between different time periods within a cluster. No period effect means that the effect of the intervention is the same whether applied in the first or second time period. Giraudeau, Ravaud and Donner (2008) give a more general formula, for use when these assumptions cannot be made.

7.10 Summary

Samples sizes for cluster randomised trials will always be greater than for an equivalent trial randomising individuals, but if the outcome is to be expressed as a mean or proportion, a useful first step is to calculate the sample size in the usual way ignoring the clustering. The sample size can then be inflated to allow for clustering using the design effect, which incorporates the ICC as a measure of the between-cluster variation. Cluster randomised trials with large cluster sizes or high ICCs will need to be inflated more than those with small cluster sizes and small ICCs. Cluster randomised trials will be more powerful if clusters are the same size, but we have presented a modification to the design effect to allow for variable cluster size, which is fairly straightforward to use. For outcomes expressed as rates an alternative sample size formula based on the coefficient of variation of the outcome measure has been presented.

References

Adams, G., Gulliford, M.C., Ukoumunne, O. *et al.* (2004) Patterns of intra-cluster correlation from primary care research to inform study design and analysis. *J. Clin. Epidemiol.*, **57** (8), 785–794.

Altman, D.G. (1991) *Practical Statistics for Medical Research*, Chapman & Hall, London.

Bland, M. (2000) *An Introduction to Medical Statistics*, 3rd edn, Oxford University Press.

van Breukelen, G.J.P., Candel, M.J. and Berger, M.P. (2008) Relative efficiency of unequal cluster sizes for variance component estimation in cluster randomized and multicentre trials. *Stat. Methods Med. Res.*, **17**, 439–458.

Campbell, M.K., Fayers, P.M. and Grimshaw, J.M. (2005) Determinants of the intracluster correlation coefficient in cluster randomized trials: the case of implementation research. *Clin. Trials*, **2** (2), 99–107.

Cappuccio, F.P., Kerry, S.M., Micah, F.B. *et al.* (2006) A community programme to reduce salt intake and blood pressure in Ghana (ISRCTN88789643). *BMC Public Health*, **6**, 13.

Coleman, E.A., Grothaus, L.C., Sandhu, N. *et al.* (1999) Chronic care clinics: a randomized controlled trial of a model of primary care for frail older adults. *J. Am. Geriatr. Soc.*, **47**, 775–783.

Dodge, Y. (2003) *The Oxford Dictionary of Statistical Terms*, Oxford University Press.

Donner, A. and Klar, N. (2000) *Design and Analysis of Cluster Randomised Trials in Health Research*, Arnold, London.

Donner, A., Birkett, N. and Buck, C. (1981) Randomization by cluster. Sample size requirements and analysis. *Am. J. Epidemiol.*, **114**, 906–914.

Eldridge, S.M., Cryer, C., Feder, G.S. *et al.* (2001) Sample size calculations for intervention trials in primary care randomizing by primary care group: an empirical illustration from one proposed intervention trial. *Stat. Med.*, **20** (3), 367–376.

Eldridge, S., Ashby, D., Feder, G. *et al.* (2004) Lessons for cluster randomised trials in the twenty-first century: a systematic review of trials in primary care. *Clin. Trials*, **1**, 80–90.

Eldridge, S., Spencer, A., Cryer, C. *et al.* (2005) Why modelling a complex intervention is an important precursor to trial design: lessons from studying an intervention to reduce falls-related injuries in older people. *J. Health Serv. Res. Policy*, **10** (3), 133–142.

Eldridge, S.M., Ashby, D. and Kerry, S. (2006) Sample size calculations for cluster randomized trials: effect of coefficient of variation of cluster size and analysis method. *Int. J. Epidemiol.*, **35** (5), 1292–1300.

Feder, G., Griffiths, C., Highton, C. *et al.* (1995) Do clinical guidelines introduced with practice-based education improve care of asthmatic and diabetic patients? A randomised controlled trial in general practice in East London. *BMJ*, **311**, 1473–1478.

Gail, M.H., Byar, D.P., Pechacek, T.F. *et al.* (1992) Aspects of statistical design for the Community Intervention Trial for Smoking Cessation (COMMIT). *Control. Clin. Trials*, **13**, 6–21.

Giraudeau, B., Ravaud, P. and Donner, A. (2008) Sample size calculation for cluster randomized cross-over trials. *Stat. Med.*, **27**, 5578–5585.

Griffiths, C., Foster, G., Barnes, N. *et al.* (2004) Specialist nurse intervention to reduce unscheduled asthma care in a deprived multiethnic area: the east London randomised controlled trial for high risk asthma (ELECTRA). *BMJ*, **328**, 144.

Guittet, L., Ravaud, P. and Girandeau, B. (2006) Planning a cluster randomised trial with unequal cluster sizes: practical issues involving continuous outcomes. *BMC Med. Res. Methodol.*, **6**, 17.

Gulliford, M.C., Adams, G., Ukoumunne, O.C. *et al.* (2005) Intraclass correlation coefficient and outcome prevalence are associated in clustered binary data. *J. Clin. Epidemiol.*, **58**, 246–251.

Hannan, P.J., Murray, D.M., Jacobs, D.R. Jr. *et al.* (1994) Parameters to aid in the design and analysis of community trials: intraclass correlations from the Minnesota Heart Health Program. *Epidemiology*, **5**, 88–95.

Hayes, J.H. and Moulton, L.H. (2009) *Cluster Randomised Trials*, Chapman & Hall, Boca Raton.

Hayes, R.J. and Bennet, S. (1999) Simple sample size calculation for cluster-randomized trials. *Int. J. Epidemiol*, **28**, 319–326.

Kelder, S.H., Jacobs, D.R. Jr., Jeffery, R.W. *et al.* (1993) The worksite component of variance: design effects and the Healthy Worker Project. *Health Educ. Res.*, **8**, 555–566.

Kendrick, D., Illingworth, R., Woods, A. *et al.* (2005) Promoting child safety in primary care: a cluster randomised controlled trial to reduce baby walker use. *Br. J. Gen. Pract.*, **55**, 582–588.

Kendrick, T., Burns, T. and Freeling, P. (1995) Randomised controlled trial of teaching general practitioners to carry out structured assessments of their long term mentally ill patients. *BMJ*, **311**, 93–98.

Kerry, S.M. and Bland, J.M. (1998) Statistics notes. Sample size in cluster randomisation. *BMJ*, **316**, 549.

Kerry, S.M. and Bland, J.M. (2001) Unequal cluster sizes for trials in English and Welsh general practice: implications for sample size calculations. *Stat. Med.*, **20** (3), 377–390.

Kinmonth, A.L., Woodcock, A., Griffin, S. *et al.* (1998) Randomised controlled trial of patient centred care of diabetes in general practice: impact on current wellbeing and future disease risk. *BMJ*, **317**, 1202–1208.

Klar, N. and Donner, A. (1997) The merits of matching in community intervention trials: a cautionary tale. *Stat. Med.*, **16**, 1753–1764.

Machin, D., Campbell, M.J., Tan, S.B. *et al.* (2009) *Sample Size Tables for Clinical Studies*, 3rd edn, John Wiley & Sons, Ltd, Chichester.

Murray, D.M. and Short, B. (1995) Intraclass correlation among measures related to alcohol use by young adults: estimates, correlates and applications in intervention studies. *J. Stud. Alcohol.*, **56**, 681–694.

Murray, D.M., Catellier, D.J., Hannan, P.J. *et al.* (2004) School-level intraclass correlation for physical activity in adolescent girls. *Med. Sci. Sports Exerc.*, **36**, 876–882.

NHS Executive (1997) *General Medical Services Statistics, England and Wales 1997*, Department of Health, Leeds.

Oakeshott, P. and Kerry, S. (1999) Development of clinical guidelines. *Lancet*, **353**, 412.

Oakeshott, P., Kerry, S.M. and Williams, J.E. (1994) Randomised controlled trial of the effect of the Royal College of Radiologists' guidelines on general practitioners referrals for radiographic examination. *Br. J. Gen. Pract.*, **44**, 197–200.

Petrie, A. and Sabin, C. (2009) *Medical Statistics at A Glance*, 3rd edn, John Wiley & Sons, Ltd, Chichester.

Reading, R., Harvey, I. and Mclean, M. (2000) Cluster randomised trials in maternal and child health: implications for power and sample size. *Arch. Dis. Child.*, **82**, 79–83.

Richards, S.H., Bankhead, C., Peters, T.J. *et al.* (2001) Cluster randomised controlled trial comparing the effectiveness and cost-effectiveness of two primary care interventions aimed at improving attendance for breast screening. *J. Med. Screen.*, **8** (2), 91–98.

Rose, G. (1985) Sick individuals and sick populations. *Int. J. Epidemiol.*, **14**, 32–38.

Smeeth, L. and Ng, E.S. (2002) Intraclass correlation coefficients for cluster randomized trials in primary care: data from the MRC Trial of the Assessment and Management of Older People in the Community. *Control. Clin. Trials*, **23**, 409–421.

Snedecor, G.W. and Cochran, W.G. (1980) *Statistical Methods*, Iowa State University Press, Ames, IA.

Thomson, A., Hayes, R. and Cousens, S. (2009) Measures of between-cluster variability in cluster randomised trials with binary outcomes. *Stat. Med.*, **28**, 1739–1751.

Tripathy, P., Nair, N., Barnett, S. *et al.* (2010) Effect of a participatory intervention with women's groups on birth outcomes and maternal depression in Jharkhand and Orissa, India: a cluster-randomised controlled trial. *Lancet*, **375**, 1182–1192.

Ukoumunne, O.C., Gulliford, M.C., Chinn, S. *et al.* (1999) Methods for evaluating area-wide and organisation-based interventions in health and health care: a systematic review. *Health Technol. Assess. (Winchester, England)*, **3** (5).

Verma, V. and Le, T. (1996) An analysis of sampling errors for the Demographic Health Surveys. *Int. Stat. Rev.*, **64**, 265–294.

Villar, J., Bakketeig, L., Donner, A. *et al.* (1998) The WHO antenatal care randomised controlled trial: rationale and study design. *Paediatr. Perinat. Epidemiol.*, **12** (Suppl. 2), 27–58.

Watson, L., Small, R., Brown, S. *et al.* (2004) Mounting a community-randomized trial: sample size, matching, selection, and randomization issues in PRISM. *Control. Clin. Trials*, **25**, 235–250.

Yudkin, P.L. and Moher, M. (2001) Putting theory into practice: a cluster randomized trial with a small number of clusters. *Stat. Med.*, **20**, 341–349.

8

The intra-cluster correlation coefficient

The intra-cluster correlation coefficient (ICC) is a measure of the extent of between-cluster variability (Section 1.4) in a cluster randomised trial. In Chapter 7 we outlined the importance of the ICC in calculating sample sizes required for cluster randomised trials; the most popular method of estimating the sample size needed for such a trial requires an estimate of the ICC for the primary outcome. In Section 8.1 we describe the ICC in more detail, articulating different interpretations of this quantity, including the interpretation commonly used in relation to cluster randomised trials.

Estimates of ICC can be found in trial reports, and in publications that provide lists of ICCs for different outcomes in various settings to facilitate future sample size calculations. Patterns in ICCs have also been investigated to better understand likely ICC values for different outcomes in future trials. In Section 8.2 we describe sources of, and patterns in, ICCs. An issue that many researchers in this field have to face is that ICC estimates often lack precision, particularly if they are calculated using data from small trials or pilot studies. To combat this, it is sometimes useful to collect ICC estimates from a number of sources – this reduces the likelihood of using an untypical estimate of an ICC in a sample size calculation. Other researchers have advocated carrying out interim sample size calculations. In Section 8.3 we describe various ways of choosing ICCs from different sources to estimate the ICC for the primary outcome in a putative trial.

A Practical Guide to Cluster Randomised Trials in Health Services Research, First Edition.
Sandra Eldridge and Sally Kerry.
© 2012 John Wiley & Sons, Ltd. Published 2012 by John Wiley & Sons, Ltd.

In addition to estimating ICC values in advance of a trial in order to calculate sample size requirements, it is now considered good practice (and recommended in the extended CONSORT statement for cluster randomised trials – see Chapter 10) to report ICC values in a trial report. The rationale given for this is that it is helpful to future trial investigators, but it is also useful in interpreting trial results. For example, if the ICC for the primary outcome of a trial is considerably larger than expected, then the trial will be underpowered to detect the desired minimally clinically important outcome. ICCs can be estimated in a number of different ways, including directly from some trial analyses. In Section 8.4 we describe methods for estimating ICCs, including a discussion of how to interpret negative ICCs. Finally, in Section 8.5, we discuss uncertainty in ICC estimates including discussion of the construction of confidence intervals for ICCs.

Other measures of between-cluster variation exist, but the ICC is the measure most often used for calculating sample size for cluster randomised trials in health services research, and the measure most frequently referred to and best understood by researchers in this field. In trials in which the outcomes are rates, the between-cluster coefficient of variation of an outcome can also be used as a measure of between-cluster variation. We showed in the previous chapter, however, that the ICC is likely to be a more appropriate measure of between-cluster variation to use in cluster randomised trials except when rates (or proportions) are extreme. Other methods for measuring between-cluster association have been suggested for binary outcomes, such as odds ratios (Ridout, Demetrio and Firth, 1999; Katz *et al.*, 1993). We do not cover these measures in detail in this book.

8.1   What is the ICC?

The ICC is a measure of between-cluster variation; although, as its name suggests it can be thought of as a measure of the homogeneity of individual measures within a cluster. Assuming total variability within a population remains constant, substantial between-cluster variation necessarily implies substantial within-cluster homogeneity; thus within-cluster homogeneity and between-cluster variation are two sides of the same coin. This gives rise to two common interpretations of the ICC as either the proportion of variance due to between-cluster variation or the correlation between members of the same cluster. There are small differences between these interpretations, as we articulate in the following sections, but essentially they are measuring the same quantity (Eldridge, Ukoumunne and Carlin, 2009). A third interpretation of the ICC as a kappa statistic applies only to binary outcomes.

8.1.1   Proportion of variance interpretation

The interpretation of the ICC most familiar to those working in the field of cluster randomised trials is that it is the proportion of variance due to between-cluster variation (Kerry and Bland, 1998; Killip, Mahfoud and Pearce, 2004). For a continuous outcome we assume that within-cluster variance, σ_w^2, is the same in all clusters and, using the same notation as in the previous chapter, the ICC can then be expressed as

$$\rho = \frac{\sigma_b^2}{\sigma_b^2 + \sigma_w^2} \tag{8.1}$$

where σ_b^2 is the between-cluster variance.

The proportion of variance interpretation of the ICC may be expressed slightly differently for binary outcomes. Suppose the prevalence in the population is π. The overall variance of this outcome depends on the prevalence and is $\pi(1 - \pi)$. Consider now a population of clusters. Let the prevalence of the outcome in cluster i be represented by π_i. If clustering is present, π_i will vary between clusters, and then the within-cluster variance $\pi_i(1 - \pi_i)$ will also vary between clusters. Thus the assumption of constant within-cluster variance implicit in Equation 8.1 will not hold. Instead the ICC for a binary outcome is usually expressed as

$$\rho = \frac{\sigma_b^2}{\pi(1 - \pi)} \tag{8.2}$$

8.1.2   Pair-wise correlation interpretation

There is, however, an older interpretation of the ICC as the pair-wise correlation between any two members of the same cluster. More generally this is referred to as the intra-*class* correlation coefficient. It occurs in other fields such as studies of reliability and genetics, and dates back to the early twentieth century (Eldridge, Ukoumunne and Carlin, 2009). Using this interpretation, the ICC can be calculated as a Pearson product-moment correlation (see Section 8.4.2).

8.1.3   Relationship between proportion of variance and pair-wise correlation interpretations

If cluster sizes are finite, the pair-wise correlation between any two members of the same cluster can be negative; whereas because both between-cluster and within-cluster variances must be non-negative, the proportion of variance interpretation allows only non-negative values of the ICC. It is generally believed that in the context of cluster sampling and cluster randomised trials true ICCs are unlikely to be negative (Donner and Klar, 1994; Ferrinho *et al.*, 1992). The interpretations imply the same ICC when the ICC is non-negative.

8.1.4   Kappa interpretation

Starting from an expression for the pair-wise correlation, the ICC for binary outcomes can be rewritten (Mak, 1988) as

$$\rho = \frac{p_s - p_o}{1 - p_o} \tag{8.3}$$

where p_s is the probability that any two subjects from the same cluster have the same outcome, and p_o is the probability that any two subjects from different clusters have the same outcome. The right-hand side of Equation 8.3 indicates the difference between the probability of agreement between outcomes in the same cluster and the probability of agreement between outcomes from different clusters, divided by the maximum possible such difference. This is equal to the kappa index, a measure widely used to quantify chance-corrected agreement between two dichotomous classifications for the same individual (Fleiss, 1981).

8.1.5   Interpretation in cluster randomised trials

In relation to cluster randomised trials, the proportion of variance interpretation of the ICC is used far more than the pair-wise correlation interpretation. Both interpretations originate in the field of cluster sampling, not of trials. Therefore much of the methodological literature in this area assumes that researchers are dealing with a *single* population of clusters with a single overall mean value of the outcome. In cluster randomised trials, however, effective interventions lead to different overall means in different trial arms, and these different arms then essentially represent different populations. This must be taken into account in any attempt to estimate an ICC value for an outcome from the trial, as we explain in Section 8.4. Before considering the estimation of ICCs, however, we describe the various sources of ICC estimates available in the literature, and ways of obtaining ICC estimates for use in sample size calculations.

8.2   Sources of ICC estimates

8.2.1   ICC estimates from trial reports

One source of ICC estimates is published trial reports. It is now fairly common for ICC estimates to be reported alongside effect estimates in such publications. These ICCs can often be estimated directly from the analyses conducted in the trial (see Section 8.4). For analyses conducted at the cluster level, however, an ICC does not naturally arise from the analysis. In a recent review of cluster randomised trials in oral health, 44% (8/18) of authors who conducted an individual-level analysis reported an ICC (Froud *et al.*, 2011). This is a considerable increase on the proportion of trials that reported ICCs in the review by Eldridge *et al.* (2004): 7% (11/152). In that review no distinction was made between trials in which different types of analysis had been used.

   One relatively early example of comprehensive reporting of ICCs was the POST trial (Table 8.1), in which ICCs were reported for 14 outcomes relating to the

Table 8.1 POST: patient and practitioner postal prompts post-myocardial infarction.

Aim: To determine whether postal prompts to patients who have survived an acute coronary event, and to their general practitioners, improve secondary prevention of coronary heart disease

Location and type of cluster: UK general practices

Number of clusters and individual participants: 59 clusters recruited, and 52 randomised and analysed; 328 participants analysed

Interventions: (i) Control: usual care (ii) Intervention: leaflets to patients and letters to practitioners with summary of appropriate treatment based on locally derived guidelines

Primary outcomes: Proportion of patients in whom serum cholesterol concentrations were measured; proportion of patients prescribed β blockers (six months after discharge); and proportion of patients prescribed cholesterol lowering drugs (one year after discharge)

ICCs for primary outcomes:

Whether or not serum cholesterol concentrations were measured = 0.013

Whether or not β blockers were prescribed (six months after discharge) = 0.060

Whether or not cholesterol lowering drugs were prescribed (one year after discharge) = −0.047

Source: Feder *et al.* (1999).

treatment of individuals following discharge from hospital after a myocardial infarction. A more recent example is a trial of guideline-based computerised decision support (Table 8.2). In this trial the clusters were cardiac rehabilitation centres, and ICCs were presented for four outcomes indicating patient concordance.

What neither of these trials does, however, is to report the precision of the ICC estimates, and it is not common to do so in spite of the fact that it is well known that ICCs often have extremely wide confidence intervals. Thus, investigators using such estimates in the sample size calculations for their trials usually have very little idea of the extent of uncertainty attached to them. We return to this issue in Section 8.5. First we consider other sources of ICC estimates.

8.2.2   ICC estimates from lists

An alternative to obtaining an ICC estimate from a previous trial is to look for an estimate amongst the numerous publications that list ICC values for large numbers of outcomes. We listed a selection of such publications in Section 7.1.1. Those publications include ICCs calculated for communities, schools, worksites, hospitals, general practices and other healthcare organisations. Other papers reporting lists of

Table 8.2 Guideline-based computerised decision support in cardiac rehabilitation.

Aim: To determine the extent to which computerised decision support can
   improve concordance of multidisciplinary teams with therapeutic decisions
   recommended by guidelines
Location and type of cluster: Dutch cardiac rehabilitation centres
Number of clusters and individual participants: 21 clusters and 2787 participants
   analysed
Interventions: (i) Control: electronic patient record system providing information
   only (ii) Intervention: electronic patient record system providing information
   and recommendations according to patient's need assessment and guidelines
Primary outcomes: Concordance of multidisciplinary team's therapeutic decision
   about patient with recommendations based on guidelines
ICCs:
Concordance with guideline recommendations over exercise = 0.086
Concordance with guideline recommendations over education = 0.187
Concordance with guideline recommendations over relaxation = 0.479
Concordance with guideline recommendations over lifestyle = 0.110

Source: Goud *et al.* (2009).

ICCs are described in Donner and Klar (2000) and in Murray, Varnell and Blitstein (2004). The papers listed in Donner and Klar include ICCs from studies in which the clusters were communities, neighbourhoods, schools, worksites and families. Those in Murray *et al.* cover communities, schools, worksites and clinics. Such lists may also be available on websites. For example, at the time of writing, a list of ICCs from a number of different studies is currently downloadable from the Health Services Research Unit in Aberdeen (http://www.abdn.ac.uk/hsru/research/research-tools/study-design/). In many of these studies the clusters were doctors or UK general practices.

   The stated rationale for the majority of publications that list ICCs is that the estimates that they provide can be used in future sample size calculations. However, many of the estimates in these papers are taken from epidemiological, population-based surveys and are not directly relevant for cluster randomised trials in health services research, because they do not provide estimates for appropriate clusters such as general practices or hospitals, or for appropriate outcomes. In addition, the population sampled in these surveys may be different from individuals included in cluster randomised trials, and hence the extent of between-cluster variation may differ in the two types of study even if estimates are available for appropriate clusters. Furthermore, as for estimates from individual trials, the estimates in these publications are not usually presented with any indication of precision; although Janjua, Khan and Clemens (2006) is an exception. Thus, identifying an ICC estimate that will reflect the extent of intra-cluster correlation in a putative trial is not without difficulties, and as a result several researchers have not only produced databases of ICCs and listed these in publications, but also investigated patterns in ICC values in order to provide guidance for investigators needing ICC estimates for sample size calculations.

8.2.3   Patterns in ICCs

Considering patterns in ICCs can help investigators planning trials to understand the general level of ICCs in a certain area. This may be particularly useful if no prior ICC for an outcome exists or if there is considerable uncertainty in existing estimates. Several authors have explored patterns in ICCs (Campbell, Fayers and Grimshaw, 2005; Adams *et al.*, 2004; Gulliford *et al.*, 2005; Taljaard *et al.*, 2008; Pagel *et al.*, 2011).

Campbell, Fayers and Grimshaw (2005) investigated the effect of type of outcome (whether this measured a process undertaken by a professional or a clinical or other outcome on participants), type of cluster (primary or secondary care), prevalence of binary outcomes, whether outcome data were collected through self-report or from records, and natural cluster size (Section 1.3.2) on ICC values for a selection of 220 ICCs from 21 largely UK-based studies. They found that process outcomes generally had higher ICC values (median 0.063) than clinical and other outcomes measured on individual participants (median 0.03); a finding confirmed in other studies exploring patterns in ICCs in the field of maternal and perinatal health in a variety of different countries (Taljaard *et al.*, 2008; Pagel *et al.*, 2011). Campbell *et al.* also found that ICCs were generally higher for secondary care settings (median 0.061) than for primary care settings (median 0.045). There was less support for the effect of the other three factors investigated, although there was some suggestion that ICCs for binary outcomes were lower when prevalences were further from 50%. Several other studies have shown a relationship between ICC and natural cluster size, including Donner (1982) and Gulliford, Ukoumunne and Chinn (1999). The natural clusters investigated in these studies were considerably more variable in size than those in Campbell *et al.*'s study, which may account for the discrepant findings.

Adams *et al.* (2004) investigated patterns in ICCs for 1039 ICCs from 31 studies. They found widely differing values of ICCs for the same outcomes, and suggested that ICC values were highly dependent on trial setting, concluding that the precise value of an ICC for a given outcome 'can rarely be estimated in advance' and that 'Studies should be designed with reference to the overall distribution of ICCs and with attention to features that increase efficiency.'

In a separate paper based on the same dataset, Gulliford *et al.* (2005) showed that ICC values were related to the prevalence of a binary outcome with ICC values being lower for extreme prevalences. This finding was confirmed in the study by Taljaard *et al.* (2008). The stronger findings in these studies compared to the Campbell, Fayers and Grimshaw (2005) study may be because of greater numbers of ICCs in the Gulliford *et al.* study, giving the study greater power to detect a trend. ICCs were also measured on larger numbers of individuals in the Taljaard *et al.* study,

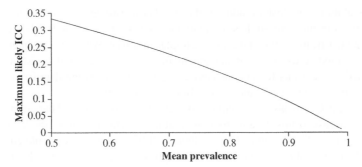

Figure 8.1   Maximum possible ICC by mean prevalence if cluster prevalences follow a unimodal beta distribution.

making these ICCs less susceptible to sampling error. However, it may also be that the relationship is not quite as straightforward as simply a linear decrease in ICC value as prevalences become more extreme; there are sound theoretical reasons for assuming that there is an upper limit to ICC values for a given overall prevalence, which we now illustrate.

Consider the prevalence values of a binary outcome from each cluster in a study. If these prevalences are represented by proportions, then all of the proportions must lie between 0 and 1, and their distribution can then be represented by a beta distribution; a statistical distribution bounded by 0 and 1. The most likely shape of this distribution is unimodal (having one peak) rather than U-shaped with peaks at 0 and 1, or J-shaped with a peak at either 1 or 0. Assuming a unimodal beta distribution, it is possible through algebraic manipulation of formulae representing the shape of the distribution to calculate the maximum possible ICC for different overall prevalences (Figure 8.1). Figure 8.1 suggests that ICCs over 0.35 are unlikely for binary outcomes, and for extreme prevalences ICCs may be even smaller. Nevertheless, high values of the ICC may be observed in some trials as a result of sampling error, and in rare cases when the distribution of ICCs may not be unimodal.

Overall, the work on patterns in ICC values tends to suggest that estimating an ICC value to use in a sample size calculation of a cluster randomised trial may not be as straightforward as picking a single estimate out of a previous trial, particularly for binary outcomes. A possibly more robust strategy is to review a number of ICC estimates for the same or similar outcomes before alighting on a single estimate to use in a sample size calculation. We cover this in the next section.

8.3   Choosing the ICC for use in sample size calculations

One way to estimate an ICC is to guess a value. Over the past 20 years, however, it has become common for investigators to use specific estimates of ICCs in sample size calculations for cluster randomised trials. These estimates can be obtained from publications of previous studies or databanks of ICCs (Section 8.2). They can also be calculated from routine data. For example, in a trial evaluating an intervention aiming to modify dyspepsia management in primary care, an ICC estimate was calculated for referrals for open access endoscopy from routine data from general practices in the same geographic area (Banait *et al.*, 2003).

Finally, ICCs can also be calculated directly from previous trial data if investigators have access to this. In a methodological paper which we describe later in this section (Turner, Thompson and Spiegelhalter, 2005), the authors calculated an ICC for total cholesterol from data from the SHIP trial (Jolly *et al.*, 1999); this ICC was not reported in the main trial publication. However, the lack of precision of ICC estimates and the fact that this precision is rarely calculated or reported means that a single estimate of an ICC value is not particularly robust. In the rest of this section we focus on estimating the ICC for total cholesterol for a putative trial randomising UK general practices, describing the use of single ICC estimates and methods of combining several ICC estimates and/or information about patterns in ICCs. We use the example of total cholesterol and randomisation by UK general practices because this example is used in the methodological paper by Turner, Thompson and Spiegelhalter (2005) which focuses on a method of combining ICCs from various sources that we describe in Section 8.3.4.

8.3.1   Single ICC estimate from an existing source

As an example of a single ICC estimate for total cholesterol from an existing source, we use an estimate of 0.025 calculated from data from the SHIP trial by Turner, Thompson and Spiegelhalter (2005). It has been suggested that in a sample size calculation the upper limit of the confidence interval could be used as a conservative estimate of the ICC. However, confidence intervals for ICCs are usually wide (see Section 8.5); for example in Turner *et al.* the upper limit of the confidence interval for total cholesterol ICC from SHIP is estimated at about 0.08. Thus, using this strategy could result in a substantially larger trial than is necessary. We know of no examples where this upper-limit method has been used. This is perhaps not surprising given the size and logistics of many cluster randomised trials, where even small increases in size can be seen as a considerable extra resource burden.

8.3.2   Single ICC estimate from pilot study

An alternative to using a single ICC estimate from a previous study is to conduct a pilot study and estimate the ICC from the pilot data. If the pilot study is in the same setting as the planned trial and relatively close in time, this might be expected to result in an ICC similar to that likely to occur in the main trial. There are, however, two major disadvantages of calculating ICCs from pilot studies. One is that clusters involved in pilot studies are unlikely to be a random sample from the population of clusters from which the sample for the full trial will be drawn. This makes it difficult to extrapolate from ICCs found in pilot studies to those that might occur in a full trial, using methods of statistical inference which rely on random sampling. The other disadvantage is that even if statistical inference is appropriate, the precision of ICC estimates from pilot studies is likely to be even lower than that from previous trials or larger surveys, because pilot studies will be relatively small.

One simple method of calculating the precision of an ICC is due to Swiger *et al.* (1964), who provided an approximate formula for the variance of an ICC that can be used in the case of binary and continuous outcomes. We present this formula in Section 8.5, where we discuss its use and the precision of ICC estimates in more detail. Based on this formula, Figure 8.2 shows the width of the confidence intervals for ICCs estimated from different sized studies for a fixed ICC value of 0.05, a fairly typical value for outcomes and clusters in health services research. The width of the confidence interval is heavily dependent on the number of individuals in the trial. When the total number of individuals in a study is fewer than 200, the imprecision in any ICC estimate makes its usefulness as a reliable input into a future trial questionable. Pilot studies rarely include more than 200 individuals. This, and the fact that they rarely represent a random sample of any recognisable population, makes them relatively unreliable sources of ICC estimates. The figure also shows

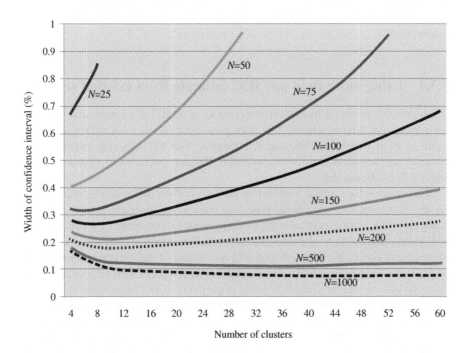

Figure 8.2   Width of ICC confidence interval by number of clusters for selected total sample sizes (N).

that, when the number of individuals in a study is below 200 and fixed, imprecision generally *increases* as the number of clusters increases and there is an optimum number of clusters that will give the most precise estimate of the ICC. This optimum is around 4 or 5 clusters when fewer than 75 individuals are involved in a study, and rises as the number of individuals increases. For ICCs up to about 0.10, the pattern is the same, but for larger ICCs the curves become gradually more U-shaped and begin to slope downwards from left to right for ICCs over 0.5.

8.3.3   Single ICC estimate based on patterns in ICCs

Alternatively, because total cholesterol is a clinical outcome and the mean value of the ICC for a clinical or other participant outcome in Campbell's study of patterns in ICCs was 0.03 (Campbell, Fayers and Grimshaw, 2005), investigators could use this estimate. This strategy for obtaining ICC values is particularly useful when no ICC for a particular outcome can be found from previous studies, and also has the advantage of being extremely quick, since the estimate can be extracted from a single methodological paper and requires no searching of empirical trial and survey literature for specific ICCs. Because it is based on the analysis of a large number of ICCs, this assumed value is likely to be more precise than that in single estimates from previous studies. Its use is limited, however, by the fact that patterns of ICCs have only been studied comprehensively for trials in which general practices are randomised.

8.3.4   Using more than one ICC estimate from existing sources

If it is possible to obtain more than one estimate of an ICC for a particular outcome for a particular type of cluster, this may give more robust information about the value of an ICC for this outcome in a putative trial than a single estimate. The growing number of ICC estimates available through publications (Sections 8.2.2 and 8.2.3) facilitates this.

The question then arises, however, of how to combine different estimates of ICC for the same outcome and cluster type, and there is no generally accepted way of doing this. One option is to take the median, mean or maximum of a collection of ICC values pertaining to the relevant outcome. These options have the advantage of speed and simplicity, although they take no account of the differing nature of different studies which may make some estimates more precise (for larger studies) or more likely to be similar to the ICC found in the putative trial (dependent on setting). Turner, Thompson and Spiegelhalter (2005) present five intra-practice correlation coefficient estimates for total cholesterol, each calculated from the data from a different study: 0.025, 0.016, 0.00003, 0.017 and 0.06. The mean ICC value is 0.0236, the median is 0.017 and the maximum is 0.06. The studies were very different sizes, and the mean ICC weighted simply by number of individuals in each study is 0.01748: very close to the unweighted median. More sophisticated weighting schemes could also be used, possibly taking into account the setting and using the variance of the estimates rather than just the number of individuals in the study.

Turner, Thompson and Spieglehalter (2005) describe a method of combining ICC values using modelling. They use the five ICC estimates from different studies given in the previous paragraph, but also combine these with a number of other ICC estimates for similar outcomes. The estimates for similar outcomes are given a lower weight in the modelling than the estimates for total cholesterol; the reason for their inclusion is that the authors expected the addition of further estimates to increase the precision of the final estimate. They use a number of slightly different modelling methods to produce distributions which reflect the likelihood of the ICC taking a range of values. These distributions are referred to as posterior distributions. Turner *et al.* illustrate how, from a Bayesian perspective, the full information contained in the distribution can be utilized in a sample size calculation as a prior distribution for the ICC. Alternatively the distribution can be summarised using the median and interval between which the central 95% of the distribution lies. For a model incorporating only the five ICC estimates for total cholesterol, the median of the posterior distribution is 0.014 and the central 95% lies between 0 and 0.21. For a more sophisticated model which also incorporates ICC estimates for other outcomes that the authors deemed similar to total cholesterol, the median is 0.015, with the central 95% of the distribution lying between 0.003 and 0.06. This method of modelling has not been widely used by those designing empirical trials, however, possibly because of its relative complexity; many of those estimating sample sizes may not have the technical and/or statistical knowledge required to fit the models, and sample sizes often need to be calculated within a tight time frame, making it impossible to use nonstandard methods that take a considerable amount of time.

8.3.5   Baseline or interim sample size calculations

The reason for wanting a reasonably reliable estimate of the ICC for the primary outcome for a putative trial is to ensure that the sample size has adequate power. A further option for optimising the sample size is to recalculate this based either on baseline data or on a portion of the outcome data part way through the full trial. Either option may give better estimates of sample size required than that based on ICC estimates obtained prior to the start of the trial; although there are difficulties with both approaches. An ICC obtained from baseline data may not reflect that of outcome data partly because an intervention may alter variation in an outcome as well as the general outcome level. If recruitment to the trial is over a long period of time, the trial may be well under way before all baseline data are available, and a late adjustment to the sample size may be difficult. If a portion of outcome data is used (or a portion of baseline data), it is unclear what proportion will result in a reliable ICC estimate. Moreover, depending on time scales, interim calculations based on outcome data may not be feasible.

8.3.6   Comparing different methods

The methods of estimating ICCs described in the previous sections can be classified into three categories: those that require the acquisition of single estimates (single-estimate methods), those that require the acquisition of estimates from more than one study (multiple-estimate methods), and those that require investigators to acquire several estimates and fit fairly sophisticated statistical models (modelling methods). Because of time and technical constraints, the methods requiring the acquisition of a single estimate are likely to remain the methods of choice for those designing cluster randomised trials in the future. Single estimates may be from previous or pilot studies or based on patterns in ICC values. Not many trials have yet used an estimate of ICC based on patterns, but on the grounds of simplicity and likely accuracy this may well be a good choice. Further research on patterns in ICCs would facilitate this.

Table 8.3 shows estimates of ICC for total cholesterol for inputting into the sample size calculation of a putative trial, based on the various methods we have

Table 8.3   ICC estimates, their sources and resulting number of clusters needed for a putative trial with total cholesterol as the primary outcome.

Method	ICC estimate	Number of clusters
Single-estimate methods		
Single estimate from previous study	0.025	25
Estimate based on patterns in ICCs	0.03	26
Multiple-estimate methods		
Mean from collection of estimates from previous studies	0.0236	25
Median from collection of estimates from previous studies	0.017	24
Maximum from collection of estimates from previous studies	0.06	31
Weighted mean from collection of estimates from previous studies	0.0175	24
Modelling methods		
Turner model: median of only total cholesterol outcomes	0.017	24
Turner model: median of total cholesterol and other outcomes	0.015	23
Turner model: 97.5% percentile for only total cholesterol outcomes	0.21	58
Turner model: 97.5% percentile for total cholesterol and other outcomes	0.06	31

presented earlier and divided into the three categories described above. The table also shows the resulting estimated number of clusters required for a cluster randomised trial with fixed cluster size of 10 if the numbers of individuals required in an individually randomised trial was 200. The single-estimate methods give very similar numbers of clusters required in this case, although there is no guarantee that this would be the case more generally. The multiple-estimate methods give results not dissimilar from the single-estimate methods, although using the maximum value found in previous studies requires about five more clusters and is likely to be conservative. Finally, the modelling methods give similar results to the other two methods when the median value from the models is used, but those based on the values below which 97.5% of the posterior distribution lies are again larger and probably conservative. Estimates from these models may be more secure than those based on single studies and general patterns, but they will depend on the single estimates entered into the model, and a reasonably large number of estimates may be needed to avoid the results of the model being unduly affected by unusual values.

8.3.7   Sensitivity analyses

Probably the single most useful piece of advice to those trying to estimate sample size required for a cluster randomised trial is to carry out several calculations inputting different likely values of the ICC to ascertain the sensitivity of the sample size required to these various values. The different ICC values used in the calculations might come from different individual studies or be based on some of the different methods illustrated in the previous section.

8.4   Calculating ICC values

In Sections 8.2 and 8.3, we did not describe how any of the ICC values presented had been calculated. There are, in fact, several methods of calculating ICCs. Different methods are appropriate for different types of outcome. Donner (1986) provides an overview of estimators for continuous outcomes, and Ridout, Demetrio and Firth (1999) for binary outcomes. Three estimation methods are most commonly used by cluster randomised trial investigators: analysis of variance, mixed effects models and generalised estimating equations. Mixed effects models and generalised estimating equations were described in Chapter 6 as methods of analysing cluster randomised trials, but ICC estimates may also be obtained from these models. Estimation of the ICC via analysis of variance and mixed effects models is based on the proportion of variance interpretation of the ICC presented in Section 8.1; while estimation via generalised estimating equations is based on the pair-wise correlation interpretation. As suggested in Section 8.1, there is another method of estimation based on the pair-wise correlation interpretation: the Pearson product-moment correlation coefficient computed over all pairs of individuals within clusters. For completeness we include a section on this method of estimation here, although it is rarely used to calculate the ICC in cluster randomised trials. We begin with estimation using analysis of variance.

8.4.1   Analysis of variance

A simple one-way analysis of variance can be used to calculate ICC values (Donner, 1986). This method can be used for any outcome, but the resulting value must be interpreted with care if the assumptions of analysis of variance are violated. Most standard statistical textbooks provide an introduction to analysis of variance (e.g. Altman, 1991; Kirkwood and Sterne, 2003), and the analysis can be undertaken using standard statistical software.

Analysis of variance provides estimates of the mean squares within and between clusters, MSW and MSB respectively. MSW is an estimate of σ_w^2, the within-cluster variance. MSB varies because of between-cluster and within-cluster variation, and gives an estimate of $m\sigma_b^2 + \sigma_w^2$, where m is the (constant) number of individuals per cluster. Manipulation of these two expressions shows that the proportion of variance interpretation of the ICC expressed in Equation 8.1 can be estimated as

$$\rho = \frac{MSB - MSW}{MSB + (m-1)MSW} \tag{8.4}$$

Note that an ICC estimate calculated from Equation 8.4 may be negative due to chance, even if it is considered impossible for the true value of the ICC to be negative. Some statistical software contains specific commands to calculate ICC values and may truncate ICC values at zero. This can sometimes be helpful, but if, for example, an investigator wishes to collect a number of ICC values together to look at patterns (Section 8.2.3) or to combine the ICCs in some way to form a more robust estimate (Section 8.3.4), this truncation is not helpful as it introduces an upward bias in the overall levels of the ICC values being explored.

When cluster sizes are unequal, m is replaced by m_0 in Equation 8.4 (Donner and Koval, 1980), where

$$m_0 = \bar{m} - \frac{\sum (m_i - \bar{m})^2}{(k-1)N_s} \tag{8.5}$$

$\bar{m}$ is the mean cluster size, m_i is the size of cluster i, k is the number of clusters and N_s is the total number of individuals in the study. This usual analysis of variance calculation of MSB and MSW is appropriate if the ICC is being estimated from a single population: a survey, audit, or pre-intervention or control-group-only data. If researchers wish to estimate the ICC from post-intervention data from a trial, any calculation must take into account differences in outcomes between intervention arms. ICCs can be estimated separately for different trial arms and pooled to provide an overall estimate. MSB and MSW can then be expressed as

$$MSB = \sum_{l=1}^{L} \sum_{i=1}^{k_l} \frac{(Y_{lij} - Y_l)^2}{k - L} \tag{8.6}$$

$$MSW = \sum_{l=1}^{L} \sum_{i=1}^{k_l} \sum_{j=1}^{m_{li}} \frac{(Y_{lji} - Y_{li})^2}{N_c - k}$$

and m_0 becomes

$$m_0 = \frac{N_c - \sum_{l=1}^{L} \sum_{i=1}^{k_l} \frac{m_{li}^2}{N_l}}{k - L}$$

where k denotes the total number of clusters (rather than the number of clusters in each arm; there may be a different number of clusters in each arm). L the total number of intervention arms, N_c the total number of individuals, and the subscript l an individual intervention arm. Y_{ijl} denotes the outcome for the jth individual in the ith cluster in the lth intervention arm, Y_{li} the mean outcome in cluster i in intervention arm l, and Y_l the mean in intervention arm l. In practice the overall ICC can be obtained by combining mean square estimates from separate analyses of variance for the two arms.

Analysis of variance is commonly used to estimate large numbers of ICCs (e.g. Hade $et\ al.$, 2010; Janjua, Khan and Clemens, 2006).

8.4.2   Pearson product-moment correlation coefficient

It is more usual to meet the Pearson product-moment correlation coefficient in relation to considering the association between two measurements taken on the same units than in relation to measuring homogeneity in clusters. In the more usual situation, the correlation lies between 1 and -1 and will be near to one of these values if the two measurements are strongly associated with each other, and near 0 if they are not.

In extending this formulation to intra-cluster correlation, each of our clusters can be viewed as a unit, and each individual within the cluster provides a separate measurement. If there are only two measurements in each cluster this is similar to the usual two-measurement situation described above. To use the Pearson product-moment correlation coefficient in the usual way, one of the measurements in each cluster has to represent a particular variable, say x, and the other measurement has to represent a different variable, say y. The two measurements are said to be perfectly correlated if y can be obtained from x by multiplying by (and/or adding) a constant. If we now consider the pair-wise correlation definition of the ICC in the two-measurement case, the two measurements do not represent two separate variables and the ICC is calculated by calculating the Pearson correlation coefficient between all pairs of measurements in a cluster. This measure can be obtained by writing the paired observations as two columns of figures, and then writing the same columns of figures again underneath, but with the columns switched, and then working out the Pearson correlation of the two columns of figures thus obtained. As a result, perfect intra-cluster correlation occurs only if all measurements within a cluster are *exactly the same*. Usually there are more than two individuals per cluster. Thus the formulation needs some further extension and can be written as

$$\rho = \frac{1}{\sigma^2 k} \sum_i^k \frac{2}{m(m-1)} \sum_{j<n}^m (Y_{ij} - Y)(Y_{in} - Y) \tag{8.7}$$

where Y_{ij} is value of outcome for jth individual in ith cluster, σ^2 is the total variance, and

$$Y = \text{the mean value of the outcome} = \frac{\sum_{i,j} Y_{ij}}{N_s}$$

where N_s is the total number of individuals in the study, assuming as in Equation 8.5 that this is a single population in which the ICC is to be estimated.

Dunn (2004) provides a good introduction to intra-cluster correlation for interested readers, although this is not in the context of cluster randomised trials.

Negative ICC estimates are possible using Equation 8.7. This is not simply a feature of the sampling and estimation processes as it is in analysis of variance. If natural cluster sizes are finite and the ICC is defined as a pair-wise correlation (the basis of Equation 8.7), this can give rise to truly negative ICCs (see Section 8.1.2). When the outcome is continuous, the ICC cannot take a value below $-1/(m_{max} - 1)$, where m_{max} is the largest cluster size (Eldridge, Ukoumunne and Carlin, 2009; Harville, 1997). If, as is not infrequently the case, we conceptualise cluster members as coming from an infinite pool of potential participants in a cluster, then the lower bound for the true ICC in this population is zero. The lower bound is further from zero the smaller the largest natural cluster size in the population, but never goes below -1, the value that occurs when the largest cluster has only two members. This is, in fact, the lower bound for the Pearson correlation coefficient when used in the usual two-measurement situation introduced at the start of this section.

When the outcome is binary, the lower bound value for ρ depends on the overall prevalence as well as the maximum cluster size and is given by

$$\frac{-1}{(m_{max} - 1)} + \frac{\omega(1 - \omega)}{m_{max}(m_{max} - 1)\pi(1 - \pi)}$$

where $\omega = m_{max}\pi - \text{int}(m_{max}\pi)$, and $\text{int}(x)$ is the integer part of x (Ridout, Demetrio and Firth, 1999). As population cluster size tends to infinity, the lower bound becomes zero, as for continuous outcomes.

As for analysis of variance estimation of the ICC, when estimating the ICC from trial data using the Pearson product-moment correlation coefficient it is necessary to estimate ICCs separately by trial arm and then pool these estimates to produce a single ICC estimate for the trial. Unlike analysis of variance estimates, however, estimation via the Pearson product-moment correlation coefficient is rarely used in practice. Software is less readily available and, in addition, previous research indicates that this is a less reliable method of estimating ICC when cluster sizes vary (Fieller and Smith, 1951; Donner and Koval, 1980).

8.4.3   Mixed effects models

Mixed effects models were described in Chapter 6. We distinguished between models for continuous outcomes and models for binary and other types of outcome. We begin with continuous outcomes, which are the most straightforward. To explain the underlying principle of ICC estimation from these models we begin with a simpler model which assumes that the ICC is to be estimated for a single population. This is the one-way random effects model (Donner, 1986). It assumes a probability distribution for the cluster means (usually the normal distribution), and a separate probability distribution for individual outcome measurements within clusters that is identical within each cluster (also usually the normal distribution). The model can then be written as

$$Y_{ij} = \alpha + e_{ij} + \mu_i \qquad (8.8)$$

where

Y_{ij} is the observation for the jth individual in the ith cluster,

α is a constant,

μ_i are cluster-level effects: $\mu_i \sim N(0, \sigma_b^2)$

and e_{ij} are individual-level residual effects: $e_{ij} \sim N(0, \sigma_w^2)$.

σ_b^2 and σ_w^2 are estimated from the model using the methods applicable to mixed effects models such as restricted maximum likelihood and substituted into Equation 8.1 to estimate the ICC. Unlike ICC estimates obtained from analysis of variance, negative estimates cannot arise using these methods.

ICCs can be estimated from mixed effects models in a similar way. As outlined in Section 6.3.3.2, the term 'mixed effects' indicates that a model includes both random and fixed effects. In that chapter we described how mixed effects models appropriate to analysing cluster randomised trials can be specified by adding random effects to various generalised linear models that contain only fixed effects. The same models can be seen as extensions of models containing only random effects, extended by adding a fixed effect to represent the effect of intervention, and further fixed effects to represent further covariates as appropriate. Equation 8.8 extends to an additive mixed effects model on the linear scale. The values of σ_b^2 and σ_w^2 are conditional on the fixed effects in the model. When the only fixed effect is the one representing the intervention, then the variances represent variances *within* each arm. They are assumed identical in all arms. In this way estimation of the ICC using mixed effects models accounts for the different populations in the different intervention arms. Estimation of the ICC using this method is popular and has been used for binary as well as for continuous outcomes when the goal is to estimate ICCs rather than conduct an analysis to estimate the effects of an intervention (e.g. Adams *et al.*, 2004).

Often, however, investigators wish to estimate an ICC as a by-product of an analysis of trial data. This is more complicated for binary outcomes because appropriate mixed effects models for estimating effect sizes for binary outcomes are not linear. Here we focus on the logistic-normal model described in detail in Chapter 6, because this is the most popular method of analysing cluster randomised trials with binary outcomes.

Under this model, the random effect for clusters is fitted on the logistic scale (Section 6.3.3.7); thus between-cluster variance, σ_b^2, is expressed on the logistic scale. The total outcome variance, $\pi(1 - \pi)$, is expressed on the linear scale, however. As a result σ_b^2 and $\pi(1 - \pi)$ are not comparable (Goldstein, Browne and Rasbash, 2002), and there is no closed-form relationship between the between-cluster variance component on the logistic scale and that on the linear scale (Turner, Omar and Thompson, 2001). Consequently, while the ICC can still be *defined* as the ratio of between-cluster variance to total outcome variance on the proportions scale, there is no straightforward expression of this quantity in terms of the parameters of the logistic-normal model. Numerical integration (Evans, Feng and Peterson, 2001), simulation (Goldstein, Browne and Rasbash, 2002), or approximation (Turner, Omar and Thompson, 2001) is required to obtain the ICC from the model parameters.

It is possible to define an alternative ICC for binary outcomes, but this is not the same as the ICC expressed in Equation 8.2. This definition assumes that the binary outcome is derived from an underlying continuous variable that represents the *propensity* of an individual cluster member to have a positive outcome value (Snjiders and Bosker, 1999). Individuals for whom the value of this variable is over a certain threshold have a value of 1 for the binary outcome, while other individuals have a value of 0. The underlying continuous variable is assumed to follow a logistic distribution. As the variance of the standard logistic distribution is $(\Pi^2/3)$, where Π is the mathematical quantity (~ 3.14159), the ICC on the logistic (underlying variable) scale (ρ_l) can be defined as the proportion of the total outcome variance that is due to between-cluster variation on this scale:

$$\rho_l = \frac{\sigma_b^2}{\sigma_b^2 + (\Pi^2/3)} \tag{8.9}$$

On this scale, cluster and individual effects are assumed additive, and the within-cluster variance $\Pi^2/3$ does not depend on cluster prevalence. Table 8.4 shows the values of ρ_l that correspond to values of the ICC on the linear scale, ρ, for various values of prevalence (Eldridge, Ukoumunne and Carlin, 2009). The proportional discrepancy between ρ_l and ρ is greater for larger values of ρ and when the prevalence is further from 50%.

An alternative approach for modelling clustered binary data that does not suffer from the problems described for the logistic-normal model is the beta-binomial model (Ridout, Demetrio and Firth, 1999). This model produces a direct estimate of the ICC as expressed in Equation 8.2 but is hardly ever used to analyse cluster randomised trial data because it is difficult to include individual-level covariates.

Table 8.4 Values of ICC on the logistic scale (ρ_l) given the ICC on the linear scale (ρ) and overall prevalence (π).

ICC on linear scale (ρ)	Overall prevalence (π)				
	0.1	0.2	0.3	0.4	0.5
0.01	0.03	0.02	0.01	0.01	0.01
0.05	0.18	0.10	0.08	0.07	0.06
0.1	0.38	0.21	0.16	0.14	0.13
0.15	0.56	0.33	0.25	0.21	0.21
0.3	[a]	0.65	0.53	0.46	0.44

Source: Eldridge, Ukoumunne and Carlin (2009).
[a]Impossible to obtain result via straightforward simulation, because in the Markov chain Monte Carlo simulation, cluster proportions inevitably reach the value 0, giving an undefined value for prevalence.

8.4.4 Generalised estimating equations

An alternative method of analysing cluster randomised trials is using generalised estimating equations. ICCs can be estimated as a by-product of the analysis. Negative ICCs can arise and, as for the Pearson product-moment correlation, these need not always be assumed to be due to chance, although in most cases they are. This was the method used to calculate ICCs presented in the reports of the Diabetes Manual and ELECTRA trials (Sturt *et al.*, 2008; Griffiths *et al.*, 2004). The analysis of these trials is described in Chapter 6 (Sections 6.3.3.3, 6.3.3.9, 6.3.3.12 and 6.3.3.13). ICCs from generalised estimating equations reflect the degree of clustering on the linear scale, regardless of the scale on which the analysis is conducted.

8.4.5 Negative ICCs

Mixed effects models cannot result in negative ICC estimates, but the other methods of calculating ICCs presented here can. Negative ICC estimates can occur because the true ICC is negative or can be due to chance. Usually, investigators assume the latter, and in most situations this will be the most sensible assumption. True negative ICCs are only possible when natural cluster sizes can be thought of as finite. This is the case when, for example, families or households are randomised. Even then, however, negative ICCs may not be plausible because the outcome, such as prevalence of an infectious disease (Crump *et al.*, 2005) suggests only a positive ICC is possible. Negative ICCs may be plausible when a health professional has finite resources to divide between patients, but usually the most likely explanation for a negative ICC is that it is due to chance. When an analysis results in a negative ICC, the analysis should be redone using a generalised linear model that does not take account of clustering (see Section 6.6), and negative ICCs should never be used in a sample size calculation.

8.5   Uncertainty in ICCs

As already illustrated, ICCs calculated from trial data are often very imprecise. This imprecision can be expressed in terms of the standard errors or equivalently the variances of the estimates. There are three ways of calculating the variances: using an analytic formula, using bootstrap methods or using Bayesian methods.

All the analytic formulae used are approximate and assume that the ICC has been estimated using analysis of variance. Donner and Wells (1986) and Ukoumunne (2002) provide a comprehensive coverage of these formulae. These include Swiger's formula which was mentioned in Section 8.3.2 and has been used in a number of methodological papers (e.g Turner, Thompson and Spiegelhalter, 2005) and Fisher's formula (Fisher, 1970), which was used to calculate ICCs in Pagel *et al.* (2011) and Hade *et al.* (2010). Swiger's formula can be expressed as:

$$\sigma_S^2 = \frac{2(N_c - 1)(1 - \rho)^2 (1 + (m_0 - 1)\rho)^2}{m_0^2 (N_c - k)(k - 1)} \tag{8.10}$$

It thus requires knowledge of the total number of individuals on whom an outcome is measured, N_c, the number of clusters, k, the 'true' ICC, ρ, and m_0 (Equation 8.5). If the ICC and its confidence interval are to be obtained from an original dataset, then all of these quantities will be available. If, however, it is desired to calculate a confidence interval around an ICC obtained from a publication or web-based list, then some of these quantities will need to be approximated. In particular, the ICC estimate can be used as an approximation to the true ICC, and m_0 can be replaced by $\bar{m}$.

Fisher's formula, like Swiger's formula, is based on a large-sample approximation to the variance of an ICC, and can be expressed as:

$$\sigma_F^2 = \frac{2(1 - \rho)^2 (1 + (m_0 - 1)\rho)^2}{N_c(N_c - 1)k} \tag{8.11}$$

Smith (1956) derived an alternative formula that has a more complex form. Other formulae are based on the variance ratio statistics obtained from the analysis of variance, and Fisher also used a method which involves transforming the ICC into a different scale. Donner and Wells (1986) and Ukoumunne (2002) compared the performance of these various methods using simulations. Donner and Wells used simulation scenarios appropriate to studies of families; Ukoumunne simulated data more typical of cluster randomised trials, although cluster size variability was probably underestimated via a Poisson distribution. His work highlights the influence of small numbers of clusters, variable cluster size and non-normality of the distribution of cluster means. Methods based on variance ratios (not presented here) appeared to perform better when numbers of clusters were small. However, these methods rely on output from an analysis of variance and so can only be conducted when the analysts have access to relevant data; this may not be the case in some situations in which a confidence interval around an ICC is desired. A major finding from Ukoumunne's study was that, notwithstanding differences in performance, all methods confirmed the large degree of uncertainty in ICC estimates, suggesting that data from larger studies than typical cluster randomised trials are required to estimate the ICC with a reasonable degree of accuracy. Ukoumunne *et al.* (2003) also explored the performance of bootstrap methods, and Turner, Omar and Thompson (2006) considered the use of Bayesian methods. These methods are conceptually and computationally more intense and do not appear to offer substantial advantages in terms of performance over simpler methods.

8.6   Summary

In this chapter we have provided an introduction to the different ways of interpreting the ICC and described ways of sourcing and estimating the ICC, including estimating the degree of uncertainty around ICC estimates. We have also illustrated the large degree of uncertainty in many ICC estimates and suggested that research that describes patterns in these ICC estimates is particularly useful. Investigators wishing to obtain an estimate of an ICC for a planned trial should not rely on single ICC estimates, and if possible consider the existing evidence on patterns in ICCs alongside any estimates obtained.

References

Adams, G., Gulliford, M.C., Ukoumunne, O.C. *et al.* (2004) Patterns of intra-cluster correlation from primary care research to inform study design and analysis. *J. Clin. Epidemiol.*, **57** (8), 785–794.

Altman, D.G. (1991) *Practical Statistics for Medical Research*, Chapman and Hall.

Banait, G., Sibbald, B., Thompson, D. *et al.* (2003) Modifying dyspepsia management in primary care: a cluster randomised controlled trial of educational outreach compared with passive guideline dissemination. *Br J Gen Pract.* 2003 Feb; **53** (487), 94–100.

Campbell, M.K., Fayers, P.M. and Grimshaw, J.M. (2005) Determinants of the intracluster correlation coefficient in cluster randomized trials: the case of implementation research. *Clin. Trials*, **2** (2), 99–107.

Crump, J.A., Otieno, P.O., Slutsker, L. *et al.* (2005) Household treatment of drinking water with flocculant-disinfectant for preventing diarrhoea in areas with turbid source water in rural western Kenya: cluster randomised controlled trial. *BMJ*, **331** (7515), 478–483.

Donner, A. (1982) An empirical study of cluster randomization. *Int. J. Epidemiol.*, **11** (3), 283–286.

Donner, A. (1986) A review of inference procedures for the intraclass correlation-coefficient in the one-way random effects model. *Int. Stat. Rev.*, **54** (1), 67–82.

Donner, A. and Klar, N. (1994) Cluster randomization trials in epidemiology – theory and application. *J. Stat. Plan. Inference*, **42** (1–2), 37–56.

Donner, A. and Klar, N. (2000) *Design and Analysis of Cluster Randomised Trials in Health Research*, Arnold, London.

Donner, A. and Koval, J.J. (1980) Estimation of intra-class correlation in the analysis of family data. *Biometrics*, **36** (1), 19–25.

Donner, A. and Wells, G. (1986) A comparison of confidence-interval methods for the intraclass correlation-coefficient. *Biometrics*, **42** (2), 401–412.

Dunn, G. (2004) *Statistical Evaluation of Measurement Errors: Design and Analysis of Reliability Studies*, Arnold, London.

Eldridge, S.M., Ashby, D., Feder, G.S. *et al.* (2004) Lessons for cluster randomised trials in the twenty-first century: a systematic review of trials in primary care. *Clin. Trials*, **1**, 80–90.

Eldridge, S.M., Ukoumunne, O.C. and Carlin, J.B. (2009) The intra-cluster correlation coefficient in cluster randomized trials: a review of definitions. *Int. Stat. Rev.*, **77** (3), 378–394.

Evans, B.A., Feng, Z. and Peterson, A.V. (2001) A comparison of generalized linear mixed model procedures with estimating equations for variance and covariance parameter estimation in longitudinal studies and group randomized trials. *Stat. Med.*, **20** (22), 3353–3373.

Feder, G., Griffiths, C., Eldridge, S. *et al.* (1999) Effect of postal prompts to patients and general practitioners on the quality of primary care after a coronary event (POST): randomised controlled trial. *BMJ*, **318** (7197), 1522–1526.

Ferrinho, P., Valli, A., Groeneveld, T. *et al.* (1992) The effects of cluster sampling in an African urban setting. *J. Med.*, **38**, 324–330.

Fieller, E.C. and Smith, C.A.B. (1951) Note on the analysis of variance and intraclass correlation. *Ann. Eugen.*, **16**, 97–104.

Fisher, R.A. (1970) *Statistical Methods for Research Workers*, Hafner, New York.

Fleiss, J.L. (1981) *Statistical Methods for Rates and Proportions*, 2nd edn, John Wiley & Sons, Inc., New York.

Froud, R., Eldridge, S., Diaz Ordaz, K. *et al.* (2011) Quality of cluster randomised controlled trials in oral health: a systematic review of reports published between 2005 and 2009. *Community Dent. Oral Epidemiol.*, in press.

Goldstein, H., Browne, W. and Rasbash, J. (2002) Partitioning variation in multilevel models. *Underst. Stat.*, **1**, 223–232.

Goud, R., de Keizer, N.F., ter Riet, G. *et al.* (2009) Effect of guideline based computerised decisions support on decision making of multidisciplinary teams: cluster randomised trial in cardiac rehabilitation. *BMJ*, **338**, b1440. doi: 10.1136/bmj.b1440

Griffiths, C., Foster, G., Barnes, N. *et al.* (2004) Specialist nurse intervention to reduce unscheduled asthma care in a deprived multiethnic area: the east London randomised controlled trial for high risk asthma (ELECTRA). *BMJ*, **328** (7432), 144.

Gulliford, M.C., Ukoumunne, O.C. and Chinn, S. (1999) Components of variance and intraclass correlations for the design of community-based surveys and intervention studies: data from the Health Survey for England 1994. *Am. J. Epidemiol.*, **149** (9), 876–883.

Gulliford, M.C., Adams, G., Ukoumunne, O.C. *et al.* (2005) Intraclass correlation coefficient and outcome prevalence are associated in clustered binary data. *J. Clin. Epidemiol.*, **58** (3), 246–251.

Hade, E.M., Murray, D.M., Pennell, M.L. *et al.* (2010) Intraclass correlation estimates for cancer screening outcomes: estimates and applications in the design of group-randomized cancer screening studies. *J. Natl. Cancer Inst. Monogr.*, **2010** (40), 97–103.

Harville, D.A. (1997) *Matrix Algebra from A Statistician's Perspective*, Springer, New York, p. 203.

Janjua, N.Z., Khan, M.I. and Clemens, J.D. (2006) Estimates of intraclass correlation coefficient and design effect for surveys and cluster randomized trials on injection use in Pakistan and developing countries. *Trop. Med. Int. Health*, **11** (12), 1832–1840.

Jolly, K., Bradley, F., Sharp, S. *et al.* (1999) Randomised controlled trial of follow up care in general practice of patients with myocardial infarction and angina: final results of the Southampton heart integrated care project (SHIP). The SHIP Collaborative Group. *BMJ*, **318** (7185), 706–711.

Katz, J., Carey, V.J., Zeger, S.L. *et al.* (1993) Estimation of design effects and diarrhea clustering within households and villages. *Am. J. Epidemiol.*, **138** (11), 994–1006.

Kerry, S.M. and Bland, J.M. (1998) The intracluster correlation coefficient in cluster randomisation. *BMJ*, **316** (7142), 1455.

Killip, S., Mahfoud, Z. and Pearce, K. (2004) What is an intracluster correlation coefficient? Crucial concepts for primary care researchers. *Ann. Fam. Med.*, **2** (3), 204–208.

Kirkwood, B.R. and Sterne, J.A.C. (2003) *Essential Medical Statistics*, 2nd edn, Blackwell Science, Oxford.

Mak, T.K. (1988) Analyzing intraclass correlation for dichotomous-variables. *Appl. Stat. – J. R. Stat. Soc. Ser. C*, **37** (3), 344–352.

Murray, D.M., Varnell, S.P. and Blitstein, J.L. (2004) Design and analysis of group-randomized trials: a review of recent methodological developments. *Am. J. Public Health*, **94** (3), 423–432. Review.

Pagel, C., Prost, A., Lewycka, S. *et al.* (2011) Intracluster correlation coefficients and coefficients of variation for perinatal outcomes from five cluster-randomised controlled trials in low and middle-income countries: results and methodological implications. *Trials*, **12**, 151.

Ridout, M.S., Demetrio, C.G.B. and Firth, D. (1999) Estimating intraclass correlation for binary data. *Biometrics*, **55** (1), 137–148.

Smith, C.A.B. (1956) On the estimation of intraclass correlation. *Ann. Hum. Genet.*, **21**, 363–373.

Snjiders, T. and Bosker, R. (1999) *Multilevel Analysis; An Introduction to Basic and Advanced Multilevel Modeling*, Sage, London, p. 223.

Sturt, J.A., Whitlock, S., Fox, C. *et al.* (2008) Effects of the Diabetes Manual 1 : 1 structured education in primary care. *Diabet. Med.*, **25** (6), 722–731.

Swiger, L.A., Harvey, L.R., Everson, D.O. *et al.* (1964) The variance of intraclass correlation involving groups with one observation. *Biometrics*, **20**, 818–826.

Taljaard, M., Donner, A., Villar, J. *et al.* (2008). Intracluster correlation coefficients from the 2005 WHO Global Survey on Maternal and Perinatal Health: implications for implementation research. *Paediatr. Perinat. Epidemiol.*, **22** (2), 117–125.

Turner, R.M., Omar, R.Z. and Thompson, S.G. (2001) Bayesian methods of analysis for cluster randomized trials with binary outcome data. *Stat. Med.*, **20** (3), 453–472.

Turner, R.M., Thompson, S.G. and Spiegelhalter, D.J. (2005) Prior distributions for the intracluster correlation coefficient, based on multiple previous estimates, and their application in cluster randomized trials. *Clin. Trials*, **2** (2), 108–118.

Turner, R.M., Omar, R.Z. and Thompson, S.G. (2006) Constructing intervals for the intracluster correlation coefficient using Bayesian modelling, and application in cluster randomized trials. *Stat. Med.*, **25** (9), 1443–1456.

Ukoumunne, O.C. (2002) A comparison of confidence interval methods for the intraclass correlation coefficient in cluster randomized trials. *Stat. Med.*, **21** (24), 3757–3774.

Ukoumunne, O.C., Davison, A.C., Gulliford, M.C. and Chinn, S. (2003) Non-parametric bootstrap confidence intervals for the intraclass correlation coefficient. *Stat. Med.*, **22** (24), 3805–3821.

9

Other topics

In this chapter we consider the treatment of cluster randomised trials within systematic reviews, cost effectiveness analyses of these trials, process evaluation and data safety and monitoring. These are not issues that directly affect all cluster randomised trials; hence the reason for putting them together in a separate chapter.

The aim of systematic reviews is usually to synthesise evidence in a particular area, drawing on the available literature. In considering systematic reviews in this chapter we cover reviews which include both individually randomised and cluster randomised trials, and reviews which include only cluster randomised trials. The section on systematic reviews (Section 9.1) begins with a discussion of inclusion criteria, then covers quality assessment of cluster randomised trials and assessing heterogeneity in reviews in which cluster randomised trials are present. Three further subsections discuss how to include a trial in a meta-analysis, and the section ends with some remarks about reporting these systematic reviews.

Decision makers appraising the results of trials often require information about cost effectiveness as well as effectiveness. Cost effectiveness analyses are more complicated in cluster randomised trials than in individually randomised trials. In Section 9.2 we describe the additional issues that arise in cluster randomised trials and methods appropriate for undertaking cost effectiveness analyses in these trials, and present the current state of knowledge in this area. This is a rapidly developing field in which there is currently considerable interest.

As discussed in Chapter 3, most cluster randomised trials evaluate complex interventions, and it is often useful in trials of such interventions to conduct a process evaluation to run alongside the quantitative evaluation of outcomes to

A Practical Guide to Cluster Randomised Trials in Health Services Research, First Edition.
Sandra Eldridge and Sally Kerry.
© 2012 John Wiley & Sons, Ltd. Published 2012 by John Wiley & Sons, Ltd.

consider the implementation of the intervention and aid the interpretation of results. We discuss process evaluations in Section 9.3. Finally in Section 9.4 we cover monitoring, both trial monitoring and data monitoring.

9.1   Systematic reviews

A systematic literature review seeks to identify, appraise, select and synthesize high quality research evidence relevant to a particular research question. Many systematic reviews include only trials. In this section we focus on the inclusion of cluster randomised trials in systematic reviews, covering issues related to whether or not to include a trial in a review, how to judge trial quality, potential sources of heterogeneity between trials, including cluster randomised trials in a meta-analysis and how to report reviews including cluster randomised trials. Throughout the section we refer to the Cochrane Handbook (Higgins and Green, 2011), which is available on line and contains helpful guidance for conducting a systematic review including cluster randomised trials. The Cochrane collaboration is an international network that conducts and publishes large numbers of systematic reviews, and also provides resources for those conducting reviews.

9.1.1   Inclusion criteria

Systematic reviewers often use the PICO (population, intervention, comparison, outcome) principle in drawing up criteria for including trials in a systematic review (Sackett *et al.*, 2000). In a review that includes cluster randomised trials, investigators thinking about inclusion criteria need to consider the population of clusters as well as the population of individual participants. For example, the inclusion of the OPERA trial (Table 9.1) in a review of the effect of physical activity on depression might depend not only on the characteristics of the population to be included, but also on whether reviewers include nursing homes as a setting. Interventions may often be complex (see Chapter 3), and investigators must then consider the intervention components, their mode of delivery, the form, content and intensity of interventions to be included. As described in Chapter 3, the intervention for the OPERA trial included exercise classes as a major, but not the only, component. In a review of the effect of exercise on depression, inclusion criteria based on the precise research question should make clear whether reviewers wish to include trials that involve multiple intervention components alongside exercise. In practice, inclusion of this specific trial would also depend on reviewers' judgements about the nature of the intervention from published literature. Comparisons may be made between an intervention and usual care, but more often the control arm receives an active intervention, albeit of lesser intensity or slightly different in nature. Control clusters in the OPERA trial received depression awareness training, whereas in the intervention arm they received a whole-home activity intervention and exercise classes in addition to the depression awareness training. Such a comparison may be

Table 9.1   OPERA: physical activity in residential homes to prevent depression.

Aim: To evaluate the impact on depression of a whole-home intervention to increase physical activity among older people

Location and type of cluster: UK residential and nursing homes for older people

Interventions: (i) Control: depression awareness programme delivered by research nurses (ii) Intervention: depression awareness programme delivered by physiotherapists, plus whole-home package to increase activity among older people, including physiotherapy assessments of individuals, and activity sessions for residents

Primary outcomes: Prevalence of depression (Geriatric Depression Scale) at 12 months (outcome at one time point only; cross-sectional design), change in depression score at 12 months in all those present at baseline (repeated measures on same participants; cohort design), and change in depression score at 6 months in those depressed at baseline (repeated measures on same participants; cohort design)

Source: Underwood *et al.* (2011).

rare amongst trials of the effect of exercise on depression. Thus reviewers should take extra care in defining the settings, interventions and comparisons for reviews likely to involve cluster randomised trials.

For reviews that may include cluster randomised trials, the unit of randomisation is an additional potential inclusion criterion. Investigators must decide whether to include both individually randomised and cluster randomised trials and, if cluster randomised trials are to be included, whether to restrict inclusion to trials with certain types of cluster. This will largely be determined by the aims of the review. Commonly, reviews include all types of trial, but the research question sometimes dictates otherwise. For example, in a review of interventions to reduce maternal mortality (Kidney *et al.*, 2009), the reviewers specified that they wanted to include interventions that were 'community-level'. Cohort studies and trials were included. All the included trials were cluster randomised; an individually randomised trial of a community-level intervention would be very unusual.

9.1.2   Quality

All systematic reviews should consider the quality of identified trials. This aids interpretation of review results. Reviewers may also want to omit poor quality trials from a meta-analysis. Different methods can be used to assess quality. Cochrane currently recommends a domain-based assessment of quality, in which a description is produced of trial procedures in each domain, and a judgement is then made about whether the conduct of the trial within each domain is high quality, medium quality or low quality. The domains are

- Sequence generation

- Allocation concealment

- Blinding of participants, personnel and outcome assessors

- Incomplete outcome data (attrition and exclusions from analysis)

- Selective outcome reporting

- Other sources of bias.

In Chapter 10 we discuss recommendations for reporting these and other quality criteria based on the extended CONSORT statement for cluster randomised trials (Campbell *et al.*, 2004). The CONSORT statement provides a more comprehensive list of quality criteria than the domains listed here. In this chapter we are primarily concerned with those criteria that will affect the interpretation of systematic review results, particularly bias. We briefly outline the main issues to consider when judging the quality of a cluster randomised trial to be included in a systematic review.

Sequence generation and allocation concealment tend not to be contentious in cluster randomised trials. In the OPERA trial (Table 9.1), for example, researchers e-mailed a central randomisation service once a residential home had been recruited. The allocation was made by a statistician independent of the trial using a computer program to minimise the home, and was relayed by e-mail to the researcher, who then communicated the allocation to the home. Because of the passing of information between individuals at the different stages of the process and the use of a computer program for the minimisation, at no point was there an opportunity for either the researcher or the statistician to subvert the allocation. This type of allocation process is not uncommon in cluster randomised trials in health services research. We also describe sequence generation and allocation concealment in Sections 10.4.8–9.

Blinding of participants, personnel and outcome assessors is, however, much less straightforward in cluster randomised trials. The Cochrane Handbook maintains that participants, personnel and outcome assessors should be blind, or investigators should have asserted that the lack of blinding is not going to affect results. In our experience it is rare for authors of cluster randomised trials to assert that lack of blinding will not affect the results, but very common for trial participants and personnel not to be blinded. In fact, it has been argued that in pragmatic trials (which includes most cluster randomised trials – see Section 1.2), lack of blinding is actually a legitimate part of the intervention and that it is acceptable for the knowledge of allocation status to affect outcome because in routine practice individual participants would know that they were receiving the intervention (Roland and Torgerson, 1998). Conversely, others have argued that any lack of blinding automatically results in a lower quality trial. We suggest that the key issue to be addressed here is the likely bias resulting from any unblinding, and that this should be carefully considered by reviewers assessing trial quality. In some cases, reviewers have omitted a consideration of blinding from the quality assessment. For example, Kidney *et al.* (2009) state that they did not use blinding as a quality assessment because blinding of participants or caregivers to intervention types was not possible. They do not, however, mention blinding of outcome assessors, which would usually be considered more important than blinding of participants and caregivers in guarding against bias. We discuss blinding more fully in Section 10.4.11.

In cluster randomised trials it is necessary to take account of both individual participants and clusters when considering attrition from a trial and exclusions from analysis. It is not always possible to assess the loss of clusters to follow-up from a publication. Five out of thirty-four trials in a recent review did not provide enough information for the authors to do this (Eldridge *et al.*, 2008; online Table A: http:// www.bmj.com/content/336/7649/876/suppl/DC1 (last accessed 3 October 2011)). Five trials included in this review lost more than 10% of clusters. When clusters are lost to follow-up this is most likely to be because no participants were recruited into the trial from the cluster, or because of logistic difficulties in taking part in the trial such as lack of time or difficulties with organisation. An example of this is a trial reported by Kulkarni *et al.* (1998), which lost 62% of clusters to follow-up. The proportion of clusters lost to follow-up was similar in both arms and the authors report characteristics of those who provided outcome data and those who did not. These data could be used to judge potential bias caused by the loss of so many clusters.

There is one further important source of bias in cluster randomised trials: identification and recruitment bias, which we discussed extensively in Chapter 2 (Section 2.3). This should always be judged when assessing the quality of a cluster randomised trial included in a systematic review.

A further quality criterion which reviewers should assess is whether the analysis of the trial accounted for clustering. Not accounting for clustering in trial analysis may not necessarily cause bias, but it does result in estimates of standard error that are too small, and this has implications for the inclusion of the trial in a meta-analysis, which we discuss further in Section 9.1.4. If a trial in which investigators failed to account for clustering in the analysis is included in a meta-analysis on the basis of information presented in the trial report, this is likely to give too much weight to the trial results *and* result in a final estimate of effect that is too precise. The reported information can be adjusted to enable the trial to be included with the correct or approximately correct weight, but this is not always straightforward (see Section 9.1.4).

Once reviewers have considered whether clustering was accounted for in the analysis of a trial, and assessed its quality via the domains suggested by Cochrane, a decision must be made about whether to include this trial in any planned meta-analyses. Another factor that impacts on the conduct of meta-analyses is heterogeneity.

9.1.3   Heterogeneity

In the context of systematic reviews, heterogeneity occurs when the difference between intervention effects observed in different trials is greater than one would expect due to chance. It is generally considered good practice to try and identify potential sources of heterogeneity a priori. The existence of heterogeneity can be formally tested using a chi-squared test commonly referred to as a Q-test, although some have argued that this is unnecessary since heterogeneity is almost always present in reviews, and reviews often contain too few studies for the chi-squared test to have adequate power to detect heterogeneity (Higgins and Green, 2011). Instead, the I^2 statistic can be used to assess the likely effect of heterogeneity on meta-analysis results (Higgins and Thompson, 2002; Higgins et al., 2003; Higgins and Green, 2011). This statistic measures the extent of the variation in effect estimates due to heterogeneity rather than chance.

The Cochrane Handbook distinguishes two reasons for heterogeneity: clinical diversity due to variability in participants, interventions and outcomes; and methodological diversity due to study design and potential bias.

A key source of clinical diversity in reviews that contain cluster randomised trials is differences between interventions. We described some of the complexity involved in some interventions evaluated in cluster randomised trials in Chapter 3 and in Section 9.1.1. This complexity often makes it difficult to identify the similarities and differences between different interventions and to understand which might be the most likely sources of heterogeneity in effect. For example, educational interventions may be different in terms of the underlying theory on which the intervention is based, the delivery, the content, the form and the intensity. Any of these could be reasons for heterogeneity of effect within a review. Unfortunately, such interventions are often not described in enough detail in trial reports to enable a reviewer to identify the key differences which might be sources of heterogeneity. Nevertheless in some reviews some differences between interventions are clearer. For example, in a review of community-level interventions to reduce maternal mortality (Kidney et al., 2009), reviewers identified two very distinct types of intervention: one type focusing on education of birth attendants, and the other on reduced frequency but goal-orientated antenatal care. Separate meta-analyses were conducted for each type of intervention.

In addition to aspects of methodological diversity that may result in heterogeneity between individually randomised trials, three further aspects of methodological diversity may result in heterogeneity in reviews in which cluster randomised trials are included: the unit of randomisation, whether or not clustering has been accounted for in the trial, and the design of the trial. This is not intended to be an exhaustive list of relevant aspects but to highlight some specific issues.

We consider the unit of randomisation first. Even when interventions appear similar across trials their introduction via individually randomised or cluster randomised designs may result in heterogeneity. Donner and Klar (2002) suggest that such heterogeneity may exist in a review including cluster randomised trials when there is 'an interaction between the effect of the intervention and the type of unit randomized'. One example of this occurs in a methodological paper based on systematic review data by Hahn et al. (2005). The authors reviewed the effectiveness of hip protectors in individually randomised trials and trials randomising nursing homes. The observed effects of the interventions were greater in cluster randomised trials. Hahn et al. detail a number of potential reasons for this. One plausible view is that when an intervention is delivered to a whole nursing home there is improved compliance, and attitudes towards avoiding falls within a home and general staff behaviour are altered because of staff awareness and interaction. Differences in the way an intervention acts in individually randomised and cluster randomised trials are more likely to occur when the intervention is aimed at changing the behaviour of professionals or individuals within a cluster or the organisation of the cluster: such interventions are likely to act differently on different types of cluster, often because of interaction between professionals and between participants. For other types of intervention, such as those that introduce external elements into a cluster (external-cluster – see Section 2.2.2), or interventions directed primarily at individuals but delivered by health professionals where cluster randomisation is used largely for logistic reasons (individual-cluster – see Section 2.2.2), there may be less scope for interactions that are likely to affect the action of the intervention. For example, in a review of collaborative care for depression in which case managers were introduced to work alongside existing primary care professionals, Gilbody *et al.* (2008) found similar intervention effects in individually randomised and cluster randomised trials; as did Fawzi *et al.* (1993) in a review of the effect of vitamin A supplementation on childhood mortality.

Often the cluster randomised trials included in a review have different units of randomisation (Donner and Klar, 2002; Laopaiboon, 2003), and the action of an intervention may then differ between trials involving different units. It may also differ between trials involving small and large clusters, even when the same types of clusters are randomised. In addition to considering the likelihood of heterogeneity between individually randomised and cluster randomised trials, reviewers should consider the likelihood of heterogeneity between trials with different units of randomisation and with different sized clusters, based on their knowledge of the type of intervention. The classification presented in Chapter 2 (Section 2.2.2) which divides interventions into cluster-cluster, external-cluster, professional-cluster and individual-cluster may be a useful starting point for doing this, although, as discussed in that chapter, interventions are often multifaceted, so that there may be more than one type of intervention within each trial.

If cluster randomised trials do not account for clustering, the variances of effect estimates from these trials will be underestimated and thus appear more precise than they should be. The extent of variability in the data not due to chance, and thus the heterogeneity, will then be overestimated. Gilbody *et al.* (2008) demonstrated this empirically.

The use of a repeated cross-sectional design (Section 5.2) for data collection may also affect heterogeneity. Effects estimated using this design (which is not possible in an individually randomised trial) may differ from those that might be seen in a clustered cohort design (Section 5.2) or an individually randomised design. For example, in OPERA (Table 9.1), using a repeated cross-sectional design, data on prevalence of depression at 12 months were collected from all residents who were present in the residential homes 1 year from the time the home was allocated. Not all of these individuals would have been resident in the home at the time of allocation, and some might only have been resident in the home for 3 months. We might therefore expect some dilution of effect compared to an individually randomised trial in which 12-month data would be collected only on those who had been in the trial and exposed to the intervention for 12 months.

Once sources of heterogeneity have been identified, reviewers must then decide whether to (i) meta-analyse ignoring any heterogeneity (fixed effects meta-analysis), (ii) meta-analyse allowing for heterogeneity (random effects meta-analysis), (iii) meta-analyse only in subgroups within which heterogeneity is reduced, or (iv) allow for and attempt to explain reasons for heterogeneity in a meta-regression. To some extent this decision depends on the nature of research question being addressed by the review, although given the assumption that heterogeneity will be present in most reviews and that there are good reasons for expecting more sources of heterogeneity in a review including cluster randomised trials, a fixed effects meta-analysis is unlikely to be adequate in most reviews. In the review by Hahn *et al.*, (2005) separate meta-analyses of individually randomised and cluster randomised trials appears sensible given the differences in effect size between these two groups of trials; while in the review by Gilbody *et al.* (2008) this would not be necessary. Likewise in the review by Kidney *et al.*, (2009) separate meta-analyses of two very different types of intervention aid interpretation.

9.1.4 Meta-analyses – incorporating cluster randomised trials using the design effect

If a decision has been made to include a cluster randomised trial in a meta-analysis, it is necessary to use a method which allows for clustering. However, many published reviews have not done so (Laopaiboon, 2003). This results in an underestimate of the standard error of the effect estimate from the relevant trials. Consequently too much weight is placed on the results from these trials in a meta-analysis, and the precision of the final effect estimate is also overestimated.

If the analysis in a trial report has allowed for clustering and provides an estimate of the measure of effect (and its confidence interval) that the reviewers wish to summarise in their meta-analysis, it is relatively straightforward to incorporate the trial results directly into the meta-analysis: this trial will have the correct weight in the analysis. However, as we have described in previous chapters, many trial reports contain results of analyses that do not allow for clustering. The results of such trials need to be adjusted before they can be entered into a meta-analysis. There are two methods of doing this; both are suitable for continuous and binary outcomes and are similar in that they involve the calculation of design effects (Section 7.2). Using the first method the incorrect standard error presented in the original trial analysis is corrected by multiplying it by the square root of the design effect. Using the second method, the effective sample size is calculated by dividing the number of participants analysed in the trial by the design effect, and this effective sample size is entered into the meta-analysis. We present the effective sample size method for illustration here.

The effective sample size of a cluster randomised trial is the size of an individually randomised trial designed to answer the same question in the same setting that would produce an effect estimate with the same precision as the cluster randomised trial. The approach is based on the work of Rao and Scott (1992).

From Section 7.2, the usual expression of design effect is

$$Deff = 1 + \rho(m - 1) \tag{9.1}$$

where ρ denotes the ICC, and m is the size of each cluster. This expression is commonly used to estimate sample size required for a cluster randomised trial (see Chapter 7) and also to estimate effective sample size. However, it assumes that all cluster sizes in a trial are the same size, and this is almost never the case. In Section 7.6 we presented an alternative expression for the design effect which allows for variation in cluster size

$$Deff = 1 + \left(\left(cv_c^2 + 1 \right) \bar{m} - 1 \right) \rho \tag{9.2}$$

where $cv_c = \dfrac{s_c}{\bar{m}}$, s_c is the standard deviation of cluster sizes and $\bar{m}$ is the average cluster size. This design effect is beginning to be used for sample size calculations and could be used instead of that presented in Equation 9.1 to calculate effective sample size. In addition to estimates of $\bar{m}$ and ρ, Equation 9.2 requires an estimate of cv_c either from the trial or from other sources.

To use the effective sample size method, the design effect is calculated separately for each arm of the trial and the number of participants in each arm is then divided by the relevant design effect. In addition, for binary data the number of events in each arm must also be reduced by dividing by the relevant design effect, leaving the outcome proportion in each arm unchanged by the adjustment. The adjusted values are then entered into the meta-analysis.

We use data from the POST trial (Table 9.2) as an example. In this trial, 60/157 individuals in the intervention arm and 38/142 in the control arm were prescribed β blockers. Note that this is less than the total number of participants involved in the analysis because some participants did not provide data for this outcome although they did provide data for other outcomes. The intra-cluster correlation coefficient (ICC) for this was 0.06, and 52 clusters were involved: 25 in the intervention arm and 27 in the control arm. Thus the mean cluster size in the intervention arm was 6.3, and in the control arm 5.3. Table 9.3 shows estimates of effective sample size and effective numbers prescribed β blockers that could be included in a meta-analysis, using Equations 9.1 and 9.2. Based on the known variation in cluster size in trials in UK general practice (Eldridge, Ashby and Kerry, 2006), a cv_c of 0.65 was used in Equation 9.2.

A major problem with the effective sample size method is that information required to estimate the design effect is often not available in trial reports. When an estimate of the ICC is not available, external estimates of ICC can be used. It is useful to perform a sensitivity analysis entering different possible values of the ICC if this has not been obtained directly from the trial. There are also techniques for estimating the information needed from the included studies that do provide sufficient data. Donner and Klar (2002) cite two reviews in which this was done

Table 9.2   POST: patient and practitioner postal prompts post myocardial infarction.

Aim: To determine whether postal prompts to patients who have survived an acute coronary event, and to their general practitioners, improve secondary prevention of coronary heart disease

Location and type of cluster: UK general practices

Number of clusters and individual participants: 59 clusters recruited, and 52 randomised and analysed; 328 participants analysed

Interventions: (i) Control: usual care (ii) Intervention: leaflets to patients and letters to practitioners with summary of appropriate treatment based on locally derived guidelines

Primary outcomes: Proportion of patients in whom serum cholesterol concentrations were measured; proportion of patients prescribed β blockers (six months after discharge); and proportion of patients prescribed cholesterol lowering drugs (one year after discharge)

Source: Feder *et al.* (1999).

Table 9.3   Observed and effective sample sizes and number of prescriptions for β blockers in the POST trial.

	Intervention		Control	
	Sample size	Number of prescriptions	Sample size	Number of prescriptions
Observed	157	60	142	38
Effective (Equation 9.1)	119	46	113	30
Effective (Equation 9.2)	106	41	102	27

using regression techniques. Fawzi *et al.* (1993) used a simpler approach of adjusting for clustering by increasing the variance of the effect estimates by 30% for all trials that had not accounted for clustering in the analysis. The figure of 30% was based on the design effects calculated for cluster randomised trials that provided sufficient information to be able to calculate them. However, Laopaiboon (2003) points out that the cluster randomised trials included did not all have the same units of randomisation, and so the same adjustment for all trials may not have been appropriate. If mean cluster size is not available in the trial report it may be possible to obtain this directly from authors. A drawback of the method presented here is that the effective sample size (and numbers of individuals experiencing an event if the outcome is binary) must be rounded before entering into a meta-analysis, and this loses some precision and can be a particular disadvantage for small studies.

Adjusting the standard error by the square root of the design effect (general inverse variance method) does not suffer from this drawback.

Because one of the difficulties of including cluster randomised trials in a meta-analysis is obtaining the relevant data from the trials, some have argued (e.g. Donner and Klar, 2002) that meta-analysis based on individual patient data is even more useful in cluster randomised trials than it is in individually randomised trials.

9.1.5   Other methods of incorporating cluster randomised trials in meta-analyses

A number of other methods have been suggested for incorporating binary outcome data from cluster randomised trials into meta-analyses. The methods that have been suggested focus largely, although not exclusively, on using the numbers of individuals with and without the binary event in each arm provided in trial reports. They include Mantel–Haenszel-based methods which were used by two of the three reviews in Laopaiboon (2003) that allowed for clustering in the meta-analysis. The performance of some of the methods has been compared using data from specific reviews (Donner, Piaggio and Villar, 2001; Darlington and Donner, 2007) and in simulations (Darlington and Donner, 2007). White and Thomas (2005) describe various methods for incorporating standardised mean differences from cluster randomised trials into meta-analyses.

9.1.6   Incorporating stratified and matched trials into a meta-analysis

As discussed in Chapter 5, stratified and matched designs are much more common in cluster randomised than individually randomised trials. The idea behind these designs is that they increase the power of the trial and results are more plausible if trial arms are balanced with respect to prognostic factors. One way of incorporating cluster randomised trials with these designs into a meta-analysis is to use the effective sample size method described in Section 9.1.4 and ignore the trial design. If matching or stratification has been effective, this is likely to lead to a conservative estimate of effect precision with larger standard errors than would occur if the stratification or matching was taken into account (Donner and Klar, 2002). Donner and Klar also describe alternative solutions for stratified and matched designs. The solutions are different for each design. The fundamental problem in incorporating matched designs using methods that rely on calculation of the design effect is estimating the ICC directly from matched pairs. Ignoring the matching enables reviewers to calculate an ICC using the data from the clusters as for a completely randomised design. The alternative approach is to meta-analyse the matched and non-matched trials separately. A different method of meta-analysis must be used for the matched trials based on standard techniques for analysing matched cluster randomised trials (Donner, 1987). For stratified designs, an alternative to ignoring the stratification is to include each stratum in the trial as if it were a separate trial (Donner and Klar, 2002).

9.1.7   Reporting systematic reviews

When reporting reviews that include cluster randomised trials, authors should clearly identify those trials that were cluster randomised. The Cochrane Handbook (Higgins and Green, 2011) recommends that authors do this in their 'table of included studies'. In addition, it is useful to identify the unit of randomisation since this is not always the same in all trials in a review. Reviewers should also report their quality assessment including an assessment of identification and recruitment bias and whether or not clustering was accounted for in the analysis of the trial. Whether or not reviewers conduct a meta-analysis it is useful to report the extent of heterogeneity via, for example, the I^2 parameter. And if a trial is included in a meta-analysis reviewers should report the method used to do this, including, if appropriate, how the ICC was calculated.

9.2   Cost effectiveness analyses (*by Richard Grieve*)

Health decision makers worldwide require evidence not just on effectiveness, but also cost effectiveness, to help decide which interventions to provide (CADTH, 2006; PBAC, 2008; IQWIG, 2009; NICE, 2009). A cost effectiveness analysis compares the relative costs and outcomes of two or more interventions. To help decision makers compare the relative value of a wide range of interventions, such analyses are ideally reported with a generic measure such as quality-adjusted life years (QALY) (Gold *et al.*, 1996). Cost effectiveness analyses are required to include all relevant comparators and to project lifetime costs and health outcomes (NICE, 2009). Hence, they rarely rely on data from a single study, and commonly synthesise evidence from many sources within a decision model (Sculpher *et al.*, 2006). Trials which randomise individual patients provide the best evidence on the short-term effectiveness and costs of the intervention. Here, statistical methods are relatively well developed (Willan and Briggs, 2006; Glick *et al.*, 2007). While early work reported results as incremental costs per QALY gained, it is now recognised that alternative metrics such as incremental net benefits are more amenable to reporting parameter uncertainty. To report incremental net benefits requires a value to be placed against any gain (or loss) in health outcome from the intervention; for example, the National Institute for Health and Clinical Excellence (NICE) recommends that a QALY gain is valued at £20 000 (NICE, 2009). Another recommended metric is to report the probability that the intervention is cost effective, given the data, at alternative levels of willingness to pay for a QALY gained (NICE, 2009).

   Methods guidance for cost effectiveness analyses that use trials where individuals are randomised emphasise the importance of recognising the correlation between costs and outcomes (Willan and Briggs, 2006). For cost effectiveness studies alongside multicentre trials, multilevel models have been proposed that recognise correlation but also allow for the hierarchical nature of the data (Nixon and Thompson, 2005; Manca *et al.*, 2005). In some circumstances, for example when evaluating an area-level intervention, the best available data for the cost effectiveness analysis may come from a cluster randomised trial, which raises additional challenges for the analysis.

9.2.1   Cost effectiveness analyses and cluster randomised trials

Cluster randomised trials provide important information for cost effectiveness analyses evaluating alternative health service and public health interventions, and can also inform the development of clinical guidelines. For these studies to provide a sound basis for decision making, appropriate statistical methods have to be applied, whether these cost effectiveness studies are alongside a single cluster randomised trial, or use information from the trial in a decision model. As Willan (2006) highlights, cost effectiveness analyses of cluster randomised trials raise specific requirements for the analytical method, but have received limited attention.

Firstly, in cost effectiveness analyses of cluster randomised trials, the statistical method has to recognise correlation between costs and outcomes at the level of the individual or the cluster (Gomes *et al.*, 2011a). Secondly, the statistical approach is required to recognise the specific form of clustering (Gomes *et al.*, 2011a). While in cost effectiveness studies alongside multicentre trials data may be hierarchical, individuals within each centre are randomised to alternative treatments. By contrast, in a cluster randomised trial all individuals within a cluster receive the same treatment. This specific form of clustering needs to be recognised by the statistical method; that is, methods developed for multicentre studies are not directly applicable. Furthermore, resource use, unit costs, and hence total costs per patient, may vary widely across clusters, leading to higher ICCs than for health outcomes; for example in the PONDER study (Morrell *et al.*, 2009), the ICC was 0.18 for costs versus 0.05 for outcomes. Thirdly, methods are required that simultaneously allow for both clustering and correlation using bivariate approaches; allowing for clustering in separate univariate analyses of incremental costs and effectiveness is insufficient (Gomes *et al.*, 2011a).

A recent systematic review of cost effectiveness analyses of cluster randomised trials assessed the methodological quality of published studies and examined whether they used methods that recognised clustering and correlation (Gomes *et al.*, 2011a). The review identified 62 papers reporting cost effectiveness analyses that used cluster trials. The results showed that more than 40% of studies adopted statistical methods that completely ignored clustering, and 75% disregarded any correlation between costs and outcomes. Only four studies employed appropriate statistical methods that allowed for both correlation and clustering (Grieve, Nixon and Thompson, 2010; Bachmann *et al.*, 2007; McKenna *et al.*, 2009; Fairall *et al.*, 2010).

The results of cost effectiveness analyses based on a cluster randomised trial can differ according to these methodological choices. Gomes *et al.* (2011a) reanalysed data from a cluster randomised trial (PONDER) to consider the impact of alternative approaches. The trial was of an intervention for preventing postnatal depression (Morrell *et al.*, 2009). Clusters (general practices) were randomised to a routine practice, or screening and behavioural therapy by health visitors. The reanalysis considered the following alternatives. First, the investigators undertook separate ordinary least squares regression analyses for each endpoint, ignoring both the correlation between costs and outcomes and any clustering. The results suggest that, compared to usual care, the intervention had reduced costs, similar QALYs, a positive incremental net benefit (£110), and a relatively high probability (0.8) of being cost effective (Table 9.4). Second, a bivariate regression analysis allowed for correlation between costs and outcomes, but ignored clustering. Here the correlation between the endpoints was low (correlation of 0.05), and the results similar to the previous analysis (Table 9.4). Third, separate multilevel models were fitted for each endpoint; this recognised clustering but assumed the endpoints were uncorrelated. Once clustering was recognised, the uncertainty surrounding the estimated incremental cost was much increased, which reflected the high ICC for costs (0.18). For outcomes, the ICC was smaller (0.05), and the standard error relatively similar to previous analyses. In this example, the point estimate for the incremental cost also changed after recognising clustering; the net effect was that the probability that the intervention was cost effective was reduced to 0.51. Finally, a bivariate multilevel model was considered which simultaneously allowed for clustering and correlation when reporting incremental cost effectiveness. Here estimates were similar to using separate multilevel models for each endpoint.

Table 9.4 Results from the PONDER cost effectiveness analysis according to whether the statistical method accounted for clustering and correlation.

	Neither	Correlation	Clustering	Both
Incremental cost (£)	−72.0	−72.2	−21.4	−22.3
(standard error)	(12.7)	(12.6)	(28.8)	(29.9)
Incremental QALY	0.0019	0.0019	0.0020	0.0018
(standard error)	(0.0015)	(0.0015)	(0.0018)	(0.0017)
Incremental cost per QALY (£)	−37510	−38175	−10715	−12605
Incremental net benefit[a]	110.3	110.0	61.5	57.6
(standard error)	(31.9)	(32.4)	(44.5)	(45.8)
Probability cost effective	0.80	0.79	0.51	0.52

[a]Incremental QALYs valued at £20000 per QALY – a threshold recommended by NICE (2009).

More generally, it is unclear a priori whether the choice of method matters, and hence studies are required to consider analytical methods that can accommodate both clustering and correlation.

9.2.2   Appropriate methods for cost effectiveness analyses of cluster randomised trials

Methods have been proposed for cost effectiveness analyses that allow for the joint estimation of costs and outcomes and accommodate the specific form of clustering present in these studies.

9.2.2.1   Bivariate multilevel models

Multilevel models can recognise the specific form of clustering present in cluster randomised trials, by including parameters that allow for the cluster-specific random effects. They can also allow for the correlation of costs with outcomes. These models can be estimated and interpreted from a frequentist perspective, generally by maximum likelihood, or from a Bayesian perspective implemented with Markov chain Monte Carlo methods, which affords more flexibility. For example, Grieve, Nixon and Thompson (2010) use Markov chain Monte Carlo methods to fit multilevel models that make alternative assumptions about the distribution of costs (normal versus gamma) and allow for individual-level variances to differ across clusters. When fitting such models it is important to use vague priors, and check whether the findings are sensitive to the choice of prior distribution (Lambert *et al.*, 2005).

9.2.2.2   Two-stage bootstrap

In cost effectiveness studies, there may be circumstances, for example when costs have highly skewed distributions, where it may be preferable to avoid assuming particular parametric distributions. For cost effectiveness analyses of cluster randomised trials, Flynn and Peters (2005) suggest a bootstrap algorithm originally proposed by Davison and Hinkley (1997). To recognise the hierarchical nature of the data, the resampling is in two stages: firstly clusters, and then individuals within clusters are resampled at random, with replacement. The bootstrap procedure maintains the individual-level correlation between costs and outcomes by bivariate resampling, and the resampling can also stratify by treatment arm. This is repeated many times with the statistics of interest, for example incremental costs, health outcomes, and the incremental net benefit, reported across the replicates. The probability that the intervention is cost effective given the data is taken as the proportion of bootstrap replicates for which the incremental net benefit is positive. This approach was taken by Fairall *et al.* (2010), who applied the two-stage bootstrap in the PALSA study evaluating educational outreach to increase detection of tuberculosis (Table 10.13). The study found that the probability that the intervention was cost effective exceeded 0.80 at reasonable levels of willingness to pay for a QALY gained. A concern with the bootstrap approach is that it was originally proposed only for studies like PALSA with equal numbers of patients per cluster.

9.2.2.3   Robust variance methods

A simple approach to allowing for both correlation and clustering is to combine approaches such as seeming unrelated regression or generalised estimating equations with a robust variance estimator (Gomes *et al.*, 2011b). Seemingly unrelated regression consists of a system of regression equations that allow residuals to be correlated (Greene, 2003; Wooldridge, 2010). In the context of cost effectiveness analysis, this regression tends to assume that the residuals for costs and health outcomes are drawn from a bivariate normal distribution (Willan and Briggs, 2006). Alternatively, generalised estimating equations can be used, which ensure asymptotically consistent regression parameter estimates, even if the working correlation matrix is misspecified (Hardin and Hilbe, 2003). This holds as long as the model, that is the relationship between the marginal mean and the linear predictor, is correct (Hardin and Hilbe, 2003).

For either system of equations, estimates of incremental costs and outcomes can be obtained by maximum likelihood, assuming that the errors have normal distributions (Gomes *et al.*, 2011b). For either approach, robust standard errors can be reported that allow for the correlation between the endpoints, but also the clustering (Williams, 2000). A concern with such robust variance estimators is that the underlying asymptotic assumptions may not be satisfied in studies with relatively few clusters (Feng, McLerran and Grizzle, 1996). The systematic review of published cost effectiveness analyses using cluster randomised trials (Gomes *et al.*, 2011a) found several studies that used robust variance estimators for univariate analyses (Colvin *et al.*, 2006; Ginnelly *et al.*, 2005), but did not find any studies that took this approach in bivariate analyses.

9.2.3   Current state of knowledge and areas for future research

The methods described are appealing for cost effectiveness analyses of cluster randomised trials because they acknowledge both clustering and correlation. Recent work has compared robust variance estimators (seemingly unrelated regression and generalised estimating equations) with multilevel models and the two-stage bootstrap (Gomes *et al.*, 2011b). This bootstrap procedure extended that proposed by Davison and Hinkley (1997) to more general settings where there are unequal numbers per cluster. The study considered a range of settings faced in practice, including unequal numbers per cluster, few clusters and highly skewed costs. The results showed that the multilevel model and two-stage bootstrap performed well across each of the settings considered. While the robust variance methods also reported unbiased estimates throughout, they gave poor confidence interval coverage in settings with few clusters.

While this study is useful in comparing the alternative methods, further work is required to consider more challenging settings. For example, if data are missing or censored, it is unclear how best to extend approaches such as multilevel models to handle these circumstances. The analytical methods proposed will need modification and testing across the full range of settings faced by cost effectiveness studies that use cluster randomised trials.

9.3   Process evaluation

Process evaluations are carried out concurrently with the running of a trial, and explore the implementation, delivery and receipt of an intervention and how this might have been affected by the trial setting. The primary aim is usually to aid the interpretation of outcomes, and as such these evaluations complement the main function of trials, which is to assess intervention effectiveness. A description of the intervention implementation provided by such evaluations is also useful for those who may want to implement the intervention in other settings.

Process evaluations are relevant for community-based and complex interventions. This makes them particularly appropriate for cluster randomised trials, which are often used to evaluate such interventions (Section 3.2). Brunk and Goeppinger (1990) point out the importance of evaluating the process of implementing a community-based intervention alongside an assessment of impact, suggesting that when such interventions are implemented there is potential for the intervention to be changed or reinvented by those in the field and that it is important for investigators to know about this. They describe this reinvention in the case of a rural community-based intervention implementing self-care for arthritis. More recently, Oakley *et al.* (2006) argue that, for trials evaluating complex interventions, the science of these trials would be improved if process evaluations were conducted as part of the trial evaluation.

Process evaluations often involve both qualitative and quantitative research. They may be relatively small studies or more substantial undertakings. One example of a process evaluation involving substantial research time and resources occurred in the OPERA trial (Ellard *et al.*, 2011). The trial involved the implementation in nursing homes of a whole-home physical activity intervention and a depression awareness programme with the aim of reducing depression. The control arm received the depression awareness programme only (Table 9.1). In the process evaluation, investigators collected quantitative data on recruitment rates for homes and individuals and conducted an in-depth study in six intervention and two control homes purposely chosen to represent the range of types of home included in the trial. The process evaluation was underpinned by a specific theory, the Theory of Change, and structured to evaluate seven key components proposed by Steckler and Linnan (2002). Quantitative data collection from all homes was seen as primary, with qualitative data collection in the small number of homes as complementary. Background data were collected on all homes. Quantitative data collected on staff included attendance at training sessions and satisfaction levels. Quantitative data collected on residents included numbers approached and recruited and whether they attended exercise classes provided in the homes as part of the intervention. Qualitative data were collected in the eight selected homes via observation and interviews with staff and residents. Observation included observing training sessions for staff, exercise classes for residents, general environment in the home, activity of residents, and the consent process.

One of the issues with any evaluation of processes within trials is that such evaluation can itself potentially change behaviour. When the behaviour change induced could affect outcomes, the process evaluation could therefore be seen as part of the intervention. One implication of this is that investigators should carefully consider the extent to which a process evaluation might affect outcomes, and ways of minimising risk of bias that might arise if the intervention and control arms were treated differently within the process evaluation. As outlined in Chapter 3 (Section 3.7), if the aim of evaluating a process is to monitor intervention fidelity, and feedback to clusters to enhance fidelity, then this should be seen as part of the intervention rather than part of a separate process evaluation. A further issue is the bias that can arise if the team responsible for the process evaluation is not kept separate from the main trial research team. It is sometimes difficult to avoid this, however (Ellard et al., 2011), although in such cases investigators should make every effort to minimise bias.

Although Brunk and Goeppinger (1990) made their observations about the importance of process evaluations over 20 years ago, it is only relatively recently that such evaluations have become a common feature of trial evaluation. Nevertheless some of the early cluster randomised trials described in this book did include process evaluations. The COMMIT trial described in Sections 3.1 and 5.1.9 (Corbett et al., 1990) is one example. The Child and Adolescent Trial for Cardiovascular Health (CATCH) is another. For this trial, a series of papers was published in Health Education Quarterly in 1994 describing the process evaluation, including a paper describing the process evaluation protocol (McGraw et al., 1994). This is, however, unusual. Ellard et al. (2011) make a plea for the publication of both protocols and results of process evaluations to advance the science in this area, although they also acknowledge that funding for such evaluations is often minimal. Nevertheless, this looks like an area of research which is set to increase in the near future.

9.4   Monitoring

While process evaluations are designed to be conducted in parallel with trials but not to affect the trial's conduct, other types of monitoring are designed to be implemented during the trial period and if necessary to have an impact on trial conduct. The overall purpose of such monitoring is to ensure good clinical practice in all areas of a trial, particularly in relation to patient rights, safety, confidentiality, balance of harm and benefit, and credibility of data and its interpretation. This usually involves two quite separate processes: monitoring day-to-day procedures at the sites where the trial is taking place, and more arms-length monitoring of data by a data monitoring committee (sometimes also called data safety and monitoring committee or data monitoring and ethics committee).

Not all cluster randomised trials involve monitoring of trial procedures, and not all have data monitoring committees. Whether or not either of these processes occurs in a trial should be dictated by a risk assessment considering the risks to patient safety, confidentiality, rights and data integrity. Generally the risks in cluster randomised trials are lower than in individually randomised trials, while most of the guidance surrounding monitoring processes is designed with higher-risk trials in mind, particularly trials of drugs and other therapeutic products that have yet to be licensed. Nevertheless, both types of monitoring may be useful, and in some countries investigators are coming under increasing pressure to conduct monitoring in all trials. At any rate, an informal risk assessment is good practice; although there is very little guidance on how such assessments should be conducted for trials evaluating the types of interventions that are common in cluster randomised trials.

We have already discussed in Sections 3.7 and 9.3 the benefits of monitoring trial conduct and intervention implementation to explore and enhance intervention fidelity. The precise nature of any monitoring of trial conduct will depend on the sites, organisations and processes involved in the trial, and a risk assessment is recommended to identify specific areas, if any, that would benefit from monitoring. If the trial is multi-site, monitoring should involve, and be similar in, all sites. If laboratories are involved in analysing samples then these could be monitored. Usually, however, the resources for such monitoring are sparse in trials that are not concerned with the development of drugs and other therapeutic products.

Data monitoring via a data monitoring committee is less resource intensive. These committees comprise members independent of the trial team who monitor patient safety and trial efficacy during the trial. Even if the risk to participants in a trial is considered minimal, it is good practice to have some measure of independent oversight to verify probity of trial processes, and if necessary to give advice regarding difficult decisions that may need to be made during the course of the trial (Craig et al., 2008). This independent oversight can be provided by the data monitoring committee. In addition, such a committee can offer advice on the rigour of data collection and how to deal with any difficulties that arise with recruitment and retention in a trial. The committee will usually comprise individuals with expertise in the clinical area on which the trial is focusing, a statistician, and sometimes a lay member. Exactly what the committee does will depend on the features of the trial and the risks involved. It has been recommended that a charter describing how the committee will operate be drawn up at the start of the trial (Sydes et al., 2004; DAMOCLES Study Group and NHS Health Technology Assessment Programme, 2005). Hayes and Moulton discuss data monitoring in cluster randomised trials in more detail (Hayes and Moulton, 2009).

9.5 Summary

In this chapter we have discussed the incorporation of cluster randomised trials in systematic reviews, and cost effectiveness analyses, process evaluation and monitoring for these trials. The results of systematic reviews including cluster randomised trials are potentially important for policy makers, as are the results of cost effectiveness analyses for these trials. While the importance of accounting for clustering in analyses of intervention effectiveness is now widely recognised, appropriate methods are not always being used in systematic reviews or cost effectiveness analyses. In fact, for cost effectiveness analyses, some of the methods are in their infancy. Dissemination of guidance such as the Cochrane Handbook, and attempts to make methods more accessible by publishing detail about methods and appropriate computer code, will encourage the use of appropriate analyses. Process evaluation can be important for understanding the action of complex interventions, and trial and data monitoring can be important for ensuring quality. In the next chapter we consider the quality of cluster randomised trials particularly in relation to reporting.

References

Bachmann, M.O., Fairall, L., Clark, A. *et al.* (2007) Methods for analyzing cost effectiveness data from cluster randomized trials. *Cost Eff. Resour. Alloc.*, **5**, 12.

Brunk, S.E. and Goeppinger, J. (1990) Process evaluation. Assessing re-invention of community-based interventions. *J. Eval. Health Prof.*, **13** (2), 186–203.

CADTH (Canadian Agency for Drugs and Technology in Health) (2006) *Guidelines for the Economic Evaluation of Health Technologies: Canada*, 3rd edn, Canadian Agency for Drugs and Technologies in Health, Ottawa, Canada.

Campbell, M.K., Elbourne, D.R., Altman, D.G. (2004) CONSORT statement: extension to cluster randomised trials. *BMJ*, **328** (7441), 702–708.

Colvin, M., Bachmann, M.O., Homan, R.K. *et al.* (2006) Effectiveness and cost-effectiveness of syndromic sexually transmitted infection packages in South African primary care: a cluster randomised trial. *Sex. Transm. Infect.*, **82**, 290–294.

Corbett, K., Thompson, B., White, N. *et al.* (1990) Process evaluation in the Community Intervention Trial for Smoking Cessation (COMMIT). *Int. Q. Community Health Educ.*, **11** (3), 291–309.

Craig, P., Dieppe, P., Macintyre, S. *et al.* (2008) Developing and evaluating complex interventions: the new Medical Research Council guidance. *BMJ*, **337**, a1655. doi: 10.1136/bmj.a1655

DAMOCLES Study Group and NHS Health Technology Assessment Programme (2005) A proposed charter for clinical trial data monitoring committees: helping them to do their job well. *Lancet*, **365** (9460), 711–722.

Darlington, G.A. and Donner, A. (2007) Meta-analysis of community-based cluster randomization trials with binary outcomes. *Clin. Trials*, **4** (5), 491–498.

Davison, A.C. and Hinkley, D.V. (1997) *Bootstrap Methods and Their Applications*, Cambridge University Press, Cambridge.

Donner, A. (1987) Statistical methodology for paired cluster designs. *Am. J. Epidemiol.*, **126**, 972–979.

Donner, A. and Klar, N. (2002) Issues in the meta-analysis of cluster randomized trials. *Stat. Med.*, **21**, 2971–2980.

Donner, A., Piaggio, G. and Villar, J. (2001) Statistical methods for the meta-analysis of cluster randomized trials. *Stat. Methods Med. Res.*, **10**, 325–338.

Eldridge, S., Ashby, D., Bennett, C. *et al.* (2008) Internal and external validity of cluster randomised trials: systematic review of recent trials. *BMJ*, **336** (7649), 876–880.

Eldridge, S.M., Ashby, D. and Kerry, S. (2006) Sample size calculations for cluster randomized trials: effect of coefficient of variation of cluster size and analysis method. *Int. J. Epidemiol.*, **35** (5), 1292–1300.

Ellard, D.R., Taylor, S.J., Parsons, S. *et al.* (2011) The OPERA trial: a protocol for the process evaluation of a randomised trial of an exercise intervention for older people in residential and nursing accommodation. *Trials*, **12**, 28.

Fairall, L., Bachmann, M.O., Zwarenstein, M. *et al.* (2010) Cost-effectiveness of educational outreach to primary care nurses to increase tuberculosis case detection and improve respiratory care: economic evaluation alongside a randomised trial. *Trop. Med. Int. Health*, **15** (3), 277–286.

Fawzi, W.W., Chalmers, T.C., Herrera, M.G. *et al.* (1993) Vitamin A supplementation and child mortality. *J. Am. Med. Assoc.*, **269**, 898–903.

Feder, G., Griffiths, C., Eldridge, S. *et al.* (1999) Effect of postal prompts to patients and general practitioners on the quality of primary care after a coronary event (POST): randomised controlled trial. *BMJ*, **318**, 1522–1526.

Feng, Z.D., McLerran, D. and Grizzle, J. (1996) A comparison of statistical methods for clustered data analysis with Gaussian error. *Stat. Med.*, **15** (16), 1793–1806.

Flynn, T.F. and Peters, T.J. (2005) Cluster randomised trials: another problem for cost-effectiveness ratios. *Int. J. Technol. Assess. Health Care*, **21** (3), 403–409.

Gilbody, S., Bower, P., Torgerson, D. *et al.* (2008) Cluster randomized trials produced similar results to individually randomized trials in a meta-analysis of enhanced care for depression. *J. Clin. Epidemiol.*, **61** (2), 160–168.

Ginnelly, L., Sculpher, M., Buyke, C. *et al.* (2005) Determining the cost effectiveness of a smoke alarm give-away program using data from a randomized controlled trial. *Eur. J. Public Health*, **15**, 448–453.

Glick, H.A., Doshi, J.A., Sonnad, S.S. *et al.* (2007) *Economic Evaluation in Clinical Trials*, 1st edn, Oxford University Press, Oxford.

Gold, M.R., Siegel, J.E., Russell, L.B. *et al.* (eds) (1996) *Cost-Effectiveness in Health and Medicine*, Oxford University Press, NewYork.

Gomes, M., Grieve, R., Nixon, R. and Edmunds, W.J. (2011a) Statistical methods for cost-effectiveness analyses that use data from cluster randomized trials: a systematic review and checklist for critical appraisal. *Med. Decis. Making.* May 24. [Epub ahead of print]. doi: 10.1177/0272989X11407341

Gomes, M., Ng, E.S., Grieve, R. *et al.* (2011b) Developing appropriate analytical methods for cost-effectiveness analyses that use cluster randomized trials. *Med. Decis. Making*, Med Decis Making. 2011 Oct 19. [Epub ahead of print]

Greene, W.H. (2003) *Econometric Analysis*, Prentice Hall, Upper Saddle River, NJ.

Grieve, R., Nixon, R. and Thompson, S.G. (2010) Bayesian hierarchical models for cost-effectiveness analyses that use data from cluster randomized trials. *Med. Decis. Making*, **30** (2), 163–175.

Hahn, S., Puffer, S., Torgerson, D.J. and Watson, J. (2005) Methodological bias in cluster randomised trials. *BMC Med. Res. Methodol.*, **5**, 10.

Hardin, J.W. and Hilbe, J.M. (2003) *Generalized Estimating Equations*, Chapman & Hall/CRC, Boca Raton.

Hayes, J.H. and Moulton, L.H. (2009) *Cluster Randomised Trials*, Chapman & Hall, Boca Raton.

Higgins, J.P.T. and Green, S. (eds) (2011) Cochrane Handbook for Systematic Reviews of Interventions Version 5.1.0 (Updated March 2011). The Cochrane Collaboration. Available from www.cochrane-handbook.org (last accessed 30 Sep 2011).

Higgins, J.P.T. and Thompson, S.G. (2002) Quantifying heterogeneity in a meta-analysis. *Stat. Med.*, **21**, 1539–1558.

Higgins, J.P.T., Thompson, S.G., Deeks, J.J. *et al.* (2003) Measuring inconsistency in meta-analyses. *BMJ*, **327**, 557–560.

IQWIG (Institute for Quality and Efficiency in Health Care) (2009) *Methods for Assessment of the Relation of Benefits to Costs in the German Statutory Health Care System*, Institute for Quality and Efficiency in Health Care, Cologne, Germany.

Kidney, E., Winter, H.R., Khan, K.S. *et al.* (2009) Systematic review of effect of community-level interventions to reduce maternal mortality. *BMC Pregnancy Childbirth*, **9**, 2.

Kulkarni, K., Castle, G., Gregory, R. *et al.* (1998) Nutrition Practice Guidelines for Type 1 Diabetes Mellitus positively affect dietitian practices and patient outcomes. *J. Am. Diet. Assoc.*, **98**, 62–70.

Lambert, P.C., Sutton, A.J., Burton, P.R. *et al.* (2005) How vague is vague? A simulation study of the impact of the use of vague prior distributions in MCMC using WinBUGS. *Stat. Med.*, **24**, 2401–2428.

Laopaiboon, M. (2003) Meta-analyses involving cluster randomization trials: a review of published literature in health care. *Stat. Methods Med. Res.*, **12** (6), 515–530.

Manca, A., Rice, N., Sculpher, M.J. *et al.* (2005) Assessing generalisability by location in trial-based cost-effectiveness analysis: the use of multilevel models. *Health Econ.*, **14**, 471–485.

McGraw, S.A., Stone, E.J., Osganian, S.K. *et al.* (1994) Design of process evaluation within the Child and Adolescent Trial for Cardiovascular Health (CATCH). *Health Educ. Q.*, **1994** (Suppl. 2), S5–S26.

McKenna, C., Bojke, L., Manca, A. *et al.* (2009) Shoulder acute pain in primary health care: is retraining GPs effective? The SAPPHIRE randomized trial: a cost-effectiveness analysis. *Rheumatology*, **48** (5), 558–563.

Morrell, C.J., Slade, P., Warner, R. *et al.* (2009) Clinical effectiveness of health visitor training in psychologically informed approaches for depression in postnatal women: pragmatic cluster randomised trial in primary care. *BMJ*, **338**, a3045.

NICE (National Institute for Health and Clinical Excellence) (2009) *Methods for the Development of NICE Public Health Guidance*, National Institute for Health and Clinical Excellence, London, UK.

Nixon, R.M. and Thompson, S.G. (2005) Incorporating covariate adjustment, subgroup analysis and between-centre differences into cost-effectiveness evaluations. *Health Econ.*, **14**, 1217–1229.

Oakley, A., Strange, V., Bonell, C. *et al.* (2006) Process evaluation in randomised controlled trials of complex interventions. *BMJ*, **332** (7538), 413–416.

PBAC (Pharmaceutical Benefits Advisory Committee) (2008) *Guidelines for Preparing Submissions to the Pharmaceutical Benefits Advisory Committee.* Department of Health and Ageing, Australian Government, Canberra, Australia.

Rao, J.N.K. and Scott, A.J. (1992) A simple method for the analysis of clustered binary data. *Biometrics*, **48**, 577–585.

Roland, M. and Torgerson, D.J. (1998) What are pragmatic trials? *BMJ*, **316**, 285.

Sackett, D.L., Straus, S.E., Richardson, W.S. *et al.* (2000) *Evidence-Based Medicine: How to Practice and Teach*, Churchill Livingstone, London.

Sculpher, M., Claxton, K., Drummond, M. *et al.* (2006) Whither trial-based economic evaluation for trial-based decision-making? *Health Econ.*, **15**, 677–688.

Steckler, A. and Linnan, L. (eds) (2002) *Process Evaluation for Public Health Interventions and Research*, Jossey-Bass, San Francisco.

Sydes, M.R., Spiegelhalter, D.J., Altman, D.G. *et al.* (2004) Systematic qualitative review of the literature on data monitoring committees for randomized controlled trials. *Clin. Trials*, **1** (1), 60–79.

Underwood, M., Eldridge, S., Lamb, S. *et al.* (2011) The OPERA trial: protocol for a randomised trial of an exercise intervention for older people in residential and nursing accommodation. *Trials*, **12**, 27.

White, I.R. and Thomas, J. (2005) Standardized mean differences in individually-randomized and cluster-randomized trials, with applications to meta-analysis. *Clin. Trials*, **2**, 141–151.

Willan, A. and Briggs, A. (2006) *Statistical Analysis of Cost-Effectiveness Data*, John Wiley & Sons, Ltd, Chichester.

Willan, A.R. (2006) Statistical analysis of cost-effectiveness data from randomized clinical trials. *Expert Rev. Pharmacoecon. Outcomes Res.*, **6**, 337–346.

Williams, R.L. (2000) A note on robust variance for cluster-correlated data. *Biometrics*, **56**, 645–646.

Wooldridge, J.M. (2010) *Econometric Analysis of Cross Section and Panel Data*, MIT Press, Cambridge, MA.

10

Trial reporting

We introduced the concepts of internal and external validity of a trial in Chapter 1 and described steps which could be taken to enhance both internal and external validity when selecting and recruiting clusters and individual cluster members in Chapter 2. Internal validity is also enhanced by having sufficient numbers of clusters and participants (Chapter 7) and appropriate analyses (Chapter 6). The final stage in conducting a trial is the main trial report, where the results of the trial are presented. Good quality reporting is essential to ensure results are interpreted and applied correctly and any limitations of the trial are understood by the reader. The main part of this chapter (Section 10.4) is structured around the CONSORT (Consolidated Standards of Reporting Trials) statement (Moher *et al.*, 2010). This statement gives guidelines for reporting randomised trials in general, in the form of a checklist, with an extension to cover cluster randomised trials. There are, however, two steps which can be taken earlier in the process which will make the trial findings more robust. These are the registration of the trial, and publication of the trial protocol (Section 10.2). First we will consider what is meant by trial quality and its relationship with trial reporting (Section 10.1), including some background to the CONSORT statement.

10.1 Trial quality and reporting quality

In the context of trials, quality has been defined as 'the confidence that the trial design, conduct, analysis, and presentation have minimized or avoided biased

A Practical Guide to Cluster Randomised Trials in Health Services Research, First Edition.
Sandra Eldridge and Sally Kerry.
© 2012 John Wiley & Sons, Ltd. Published 2012 by John Wiley & Sons, Ltd.

comparisons of the interventions under evaluation' (Moher and Schulz, 1998; Moher, Jadad and Tugwell, 1996). A well designed and analysed trial may be compromised through poor reporting. On the other hand, where logistical, financial or ethical issues have compromised the trial's internal validity, good transparent reporting allows the reader to assess the effect of the trial's shortcomings on the results. Sometimes these compromises are intrinsic to the particular research question. Cluster randomised trials in particular often attempt to answer questions where high internal and external validity is hard to achieve. Evidence from such trials, transparently reported, can still make a useful contribution to the evidence base to answer a particular research question.

Assessing quality from trial reports does have disadvantages. The relevant information may not always be included in a report, because some aspects of trial quality are not usually reported, or because space restrictions in journals prevent authors from reporting all aspects, or because authors are unaware of the importance of reporting certain aspects. Information on trial quality could be collected directly from trial investigators. This information would be more time consuming to collect, however, and less readily accessible than information from a trial report; and may suffer from different sorts of response bias. Various checklists have been proposed in order to assess the quality of the evidence from randomised trials. Some, such as the CASP checklist (www.casp-uk.net/ (last accessed 20 June 2011)), are more useful for critical appraisal of an individual trial; while other scoring systems, for example the Jadad score (Jadad *et al.*, 1996), are more commonly used in systematic reviews of randomised trials. The evidence on the relationship between quality judged by reports and quality judged in other ways is mixed (Liberati, Himel and Chalmers, 1986; Soares *et al.*, 2004). Uncertainty about the information obtained as a result of assessing quality from trial reports does not, however, invalidate the use of a checklist as a basis for describing what constitutes a high-quality trial.

10.1.1   Checklists for assessing the quality of cluster randomised trials

There have been a number of reviews of cluster randomised trials which have attempted to assess their quality via a checklist. The first, Donner, Brown and Brasher (1990), included 16 trials. It assessed whether the trial authors (i) provided a justification for cluster randomisation, (ii) had accounted for clustering in the sample size calculation, (iii) had accounted for clustering in the analysis (iv) provided a baseline comparison of possible confounders by treatment arm, (v) used covariates in the analysis, and (vi) described loss to follow-up. Since this early quality assessment, there have been a number of others (e.g. Puffer, Torgerson and Watson, 2003; Isaakidis and Ioannidis, 2003; Eldridge *et al.*, 2004, 2008). Many have assessed whether or not clustering has been accounted for in the sample size calculation and analysis, but the other items in the checklist have not been consistent. Most reviews have included a limited range of journals and/or been conducted in a specific area.

These reviews articulate the general quality of cluster randomised trials over the past 30 years and, where relevant, we refer to the results of these reviews in this chapter.

Two major quality issues which apply to cluster randomised trials in a different way from other randomised trials are appropriate sample size calculations and analysis. If analyses do not account for clustering correctly then effect size estimates will be unbiased, but there is a risk of a false statistically significant result, and thus the interpretation of the trial can be affected. If sample size calculations do not account for clustering the interpretation may in incorrect in the opposite direction.

There is very little research which provides an empirical basis for the strength of the association between attributes of cluster randomised trials and bias in trial results. Criteria for assessing quality are usually based on theoretical arguments, or on an assumption that criteria that apply to individually randomised trials will also apply to cluster randomised trials.

Ukoumunne *et al.* (1999) were the first to provide a list of recommendations specific to the conduct of cluster randomised trials. Box 10.1 lists a subset of the recommendations in their publication; the recommendations that we have omitted relate to studies in which clustering is present but which are not necessarily trials. Some of their recommendations are difficult to assess from a publication. For example, the recommendation to 'consider different approaches to repeated measures in prospective evaluations' relates to making a decision at the design stage about whether to take repeat measures on the same individuals or on separate samples of individuals over time. This recommendation could not be assessed from a publication: although the authors might have carried it out, they would almost certainly not report it. Some recommendations, for example to consider using stratification or matching, may not apply in every circumstance, and for others the precise

---

> Justify use of cluster as the unit of allocation or observation
>
> Allow for clustering in sample size calculation
>
> Consider using matching or stratification when appropriate
>
> Include a sufficient number of clusters
>
> Consider different approaches to repeated measures
>
> Allow for clustering in analysis
>
> Allow for confounding in analysis
>
> Include estimates of intra-cluster correlation (ICC) or components of variance in trial publications.
>
> Source: Ukoumunne *et al.* (1999).

Box 10.1   Recommendations for the design and analysis of cluster randomised trials

details will vary from trial to trial; for example the assessment of a sufficient number of clusters. In addition, it will not always be necessary to allow for confounding in the analysis, and so this recommendation will not always be appropriate. Thus, while these recommendations are useful pointers for those designing trials, some are not very easy to use for those assessing trial quality from a publication. Nevertheless, some of the recommendations, such as justifying the use of a clustered design, are incorporated into an extended CONSORT statement (Campbell, Elbourne and Altman, 2004), as we describe later in this section.

Donner and Klar (2000) list strategies for successful cluster randomised trials. These are not the same as quality criteria, however, and again several would be difficult to assess from published reports; for example whether investigators had estimated their minimal clinically important effect realistically, or considered stratification or matching. Some of these criteria also appear in the CONSORT statement specifically extended for cluster randomised trials (Campbell, Elbourne and Altman, 2004).

10.1.2 CONSORT statement for reporting trials

Several pieces of research have shown that the reporting of certain attributes of individually randomised trials is associated with bias (Schulz *et al.*, 1995; Khan *et al.*, 1996). Such research contributed towards the publication of the CONSORT statement in 1996 (Begg *et al.*, 1996). This statement is the best known guide for reporting randomised controlled trials. Devised jointly by the Standards of Reporting Trials Group (1994) and the Working Group on Recommendations for Reporting of Clinical Trials in the Biomedical Literature (1994), this statement was designed to be based, as far as possible, on evidence about trial attributes that appear to have a marked influence on the size of estimates of effect. Earlier attempts to provide guidance about assessing trial quality did not have this aim.

The CONSORT statement contains a checklist of items (Section 10.4; Table 10.1) plus a detailed rationale for the inclusion of each of them. Some items have a stronger empirical or theoretical justification than others, and some are more strongly linked to quality. The statement has been updated several times in line with new evidence about trial attributes that affect quality, most recently in 2010 (Moher *et al.*, 2010). It is used by many journal editors as a basis for assessing the suitability of trial reports for inclusion in their journal; although the purpose of the CONSORT statement is to improve reporting and transparency, not to assess the trial quality (Moher *et al.*, 2010).

The criteria listed in the CONSORT statement for randomised controlled trials apply equally to cluster randomised trials. For example, item 2b in the CONSORT statement requires that specific objectives and hypotheses should be given. This is so that readers can assess outcomes against the stated objectives and hypotheses. This requirement is exactly the same in cluster randomised trials as in any other randomised trial. Nevertheless there are particular issues related to the quality of cluster randomised trials that mean some of the CONSORT criteria need to be expanded or adapted.

Table 10.1 CONSORT 2010 checklist of information to include when reporting a randomised trial, with extensions to cluster, pragmatic and non-pharmacological trials.

Section/Topic	Item No	Checklist item for main CONSORT checklist with cluster extension in italics	Additional items for pragmatic and non pharmacological trials	Reported on page No.
	1a	Identification as a *cluster*^a randomised trial in the title		
	1b	Structured summary of trial design, methods, results, and conclusions (for specific guidance see CONSORT for abstracts)	*Non pharmacological:* In the abstract, description of the experimental treatment, comparator, care providers, centres, and blinding status	
Background and objectives	2a	Scientific background and explanation of rationale *(including the rationale for using a cluster design)*	*Pragmatic:* Describe the health or health service problem that the intervention is intended to address and other interventions that may commonly be aimed at this problem	
	2b	Specific objectives and hypotheses, *and whether they pertain to the individual level, the cluster level or both*		
Trial design	3a	Description of trial design (such as parallel, factorial) including allocation ratio		
	3b	Important changes to methods after trial commencement (such as eligibility criteria), with reasons		
Participants	4a	Eligibility criteria for participants *and clusters*	*Pragmatic trials:* Eligibility criteria should be explicitly framed to show the degree to which they include typical participants and/or, where applicable, typical providers (e.g., nurses), institutions (e.g., hospitals), communities (or localities e.g., towns) and settings of care (e.g., different healthcare financing systems) *Non pharmacological:* When applicable, eligibility criteria for centres and those performing the interventions	
	4b	Settings and locations where the data were collected		

(Continued)

Interventions	5	The interventions for each group with sufficient details to allow replication, including how and when they were actually administered, *and whether they pertain to the individual level, the cluster level or both*
		Pragmatic trials: Describe extra resources added to (or resources removed from) usual settings in order to implement intervention. Indicate if efforts were made to standardise the intervention or if the intervention and its delivery were allowed to vary between participants, practitioners, or study sites
		Pragmatic trials: Describe the comparator in similar detail to the intervention
		Non pharmacological: When applicable, eligibility criteria for centres and those performing the interventions
		Non pharmacological: Description of the different components of the interventions and, when applicable, descriptions of the procedure for tailoring the interventions to individual participants
		Non pharmacological: Details of how the interventions were standardized
		Non pharmacological: Details of how adherence of care providers with the protocol was assessed or enhanced
Outcomes	6a	Completely defined pre specified primary and secondary outcome measures, including how and when they were assessed, and *whether they pertain to the individual level, the cluster level or both*
		Pragmatic trials: Explain why the chosen outcomes and, when relevant, the length of follow up are considered important to those who will use the results of the trial
	6b	Any changes to trial outcomes after the trial commenced, with reasons

Table 10.1 (*Continued*)

Section/Topic	Item No	Checklist item for main CONSORT checklist with cluster extension in italics	Additional items for pragmatic and non pharmacological trials	Reported on page No.
Sample size	7a	How total sample size was determined (including method of calculation, number of clusters, cluster size, a coefficient of intra cluster correlation (ICC or k), and an indication of its uncertainty)	Pragmatic trials: If calculated using the smallest difference considered important by the target decision maker audience (the minimally important difference) then report where this difference was obtained Non pharmacological: When applicable, details of whether and how the clustering by care providers or centres was addressed	
	7b	When applicable, explanation of any interim analyses and stopping guidelines		
Randomisation Sequence generation	8a	Method used to generate the random allocation sequence	Non pharmacological: When applicable, how care providers were allocated to each trial group	
	8b	Type of randomisation; details of any restriction (such as blocking and block size)		
Allocation Concealment mechanism	9	Mechanism used to implement the random allocation sequence (such as sequentially numbered containers), describing any steps taken to conceal the sequence until interventions were assigned and specifying that allocation was based on clusters rather than individuals		
Implementation	10	Who generated the random allocation sequence, who enrolled participants, and who assigned participants to interventions		
Blinding	11a	If done, who was blinded after assignment to interventions (for example, participants, care providers, those assessing outcomes) and how	Pragmatic trials: If blinding was not done, or was not possible, explain why Non pharmacological: Whether or not those administering co interventions were blinded to group assignment Non pharmacological: If blinded, method of blinding	
	11b	If relevant, description of the similarity of interventions	Non pharmacological: Description of the similarity of interventions	

Statistical methods	12a	Statistical methods used to compare groups for primary and secondary outcomes indicating how clustering was taken into account	Non pharmacological: When applicable, details of whether and how the clustering by care providers or centres was addressed
	12b	Methods for additional analyses, such as subgroup analyses and adjusted analyses	
Participant flow (a diagram is strongly recommended)	13a	For each group, the numbers of clusters and participants who were randomly assigned, received intended treatment, and were analysed for the primary outcome	Pragmatic: The number of participants or units approached to take part in the trial, the number which were eligible, and reasons for non participation should be reported Non pharmacological: The number of care providers or centres performing the intervention in each group and the number of patients treated by each care provider or in each centre
	13b	For each group, losses and exclusions after randomisation, together with reasons	
Implementation of intervention	New item		Non pharmacological: Details of the experimental treatment and comparator as they were implemented
Recruitment	14a	Dates defining the periods of recruitment and follow up	
	14b	Why the trial ended or was stopped	
Baseline data	15	A table showing baseline demographic and clinical characteristics for each group for the individual and cluster levels as applicable	Non pharmacological: When applicable, a description of care providers (case volume, qualification, expertise, etc.) and centres (volume) in each group
Numbers analysed	16	For each group, number of clusters and participants (denominator) included in each analysis and whether the analysis was by original assigned groups	
Outcomes and estimation	17a	For each primary and secondary outcome, results for each group, for the individual or cluster level as applicable, and the estimated effect size and its precision (such as 95% confidence interval) and a coefficient of intra-cluster correlation (ICC or k) for each primary outcome.	
	17b	For binary outcomes, presentation of both absolute and relative effect sizes is recommended	

(Continued)

Table 10.1 (*Continued*)

Section/Topic	Item No	Checklist item for main CONSORT checklist with cluster extension in italics	Additional items for pragmatic and non pharmacological trials	Reported on page No.
Ancillary analyses	18	Results of any other analyses performed, including subgroup analyses and adjusted analyses, distinguishing pre specified from exploratory		
Harms	19	All important harms or unintended effects in each group (for specific guidance see CONSORT for harms)		
Discussion				
Limitations	20	Trial limitations, addressing sources of potential bias, imprecision, and, if relevant, multiplicity of analyses	*Non pharmacological:* In addition, take into account the choice of the comparator, lack of or partial blinding, and unequal expertise of care providers or centres in each group	
Generalisability	21	Generalisability (external validity, applicability) *to individuals and/ or clusters (as relevant)* of the trial findings.	*Pragmatic:* Describe key aspects of the setting which determined the trial results. Discuss possible differences in other settings where clinical traditions, health service organisation, staffing, or resources may vary from those of the trial	
			Non pharmacological: Generalizability (external validity) of the trial findings according to the intervention, comparators, patients, and care providers and centres involved in the trial	
Interpretation	22	Interpretation consistent with results, balancing benefits and harms, and considering other relevant evidence		
Other information				
Registration	23	Registration number and name of trial registry		
Protocol	24	Where the full trial protocol can be accessed, if available		
Funding	25	Sources of funding and other support (such as supply of drugs), role of funders		

aThe addition of 'cluster' is our own; the wording of this item has been changed since the cluster extension was written. Reproduced by permission of CONSORT.

10.1.3   Extension to the CONSORT statement for cluster randomised trials

Elbourne and Campbell (2001) published a discussion paper on extending the CONSORT statement to cluster randomised trials, and an extended statement was published in 2004 (Campbell, Elbourne and Altman, 2004). This statement now plays a similar role in promoting high quality reporting of cluster randomised trials as the original CONSORT statement plays in promoting high quality reporting of randomised controlled trials more generally.

A full explanation of each of the adaptations, and examples of good practice, are given in the extended statement (Campbell, Elbourne and Altman, 2004). Because of space limitations these examples are often extremely brief and do not apply to any particular area in which cluster randomised trials are common. In this chapter we take each of the 25 items in turn, including those where no adaptations have been made, and briefly discuss their application to cluster randomised trials in health services research, and the rationale and meaning of any adaptations, referencing sections in the book where some of the relevant issues are discussed in more detail.

10.1.4   Other extensions to the CONSORT statement

The CONSORT statement is aimed at trials with a two-arm parallel design, although most recommendations apply equally well to other designs, such as inferiority, equivalence, factorial and crossover trials. Extensions to cover some particular situations have been published and all are available on the CONSORT website; more are planned. Box 10.2 lists those currently available.

Since many cluster randomised trials are also pragmatic trials and test non-pharmacological interventions, recommendations from the relevant extended statements have been added to Table 10.1. As with the cluster randomised trials, work is under way to update the various CONSORT extensions to reflect the 2010 checklist (www.consort-statement.org (last accessed 29 June 2011)).

10.2   Steps to improve trial reporting in the early stages of the trial

Two items on the CONSORT checklist require action during the early stages of the trial. Firstly the trial should be registered before the first participant is randomised; and secondly it is useful if the trial protocol is published before the start of the data analysis.

10.2.1   Trial registration

There have been many calls for randomised trials to be registered over the last 25 years (Simes, 1986; Tonks, 1999; De Angelis *et al.*, 2004) and for information about

---

Design extensions

- Cluster trials
- Non-inferiority and equivalence trials
- Pragmatic trials

Intervention extensions

- Herbal medicinal interventions
- Non-pharmacological treatment interventions
- Acupuncture interventions

Data extensions

- Harms
- Abstracts

Source: http://www.consort-statement.org/extensions/ (last accessed 29 June 2011).

Box 10.2   Extensions to the CONSORT statement

the trials to be made publicly available. The main stimulus behind this move has come from drug trials where evidence of drug efficacy can be biased in favour of new drugs, because trials which do not show effectiveness are less likely to be published than those which show more positive results. A review of unpublished and published data on the effectiveness of selective serotonin re-uptake inhibitors for treating depression in children showed harms outweighed benefits when unpublished data were included in a meta-analysis, whereas published data alone showed a more positive result (Whittington *et al.*, 2004). The published data had led to some children being prescribed these drugs and suffering from serious adverse effects as a result.

While very few cluster randomised trials test interventions where misleading evidence is likely to do serious harm to an individual patient, non-publication of cluster randomised trials is nevertheless an important issue. Such trials are often large and expensive, but even so may struggle to recruit sufficient clusters and participants and so risk being underpowered to detect important differences; even small effect sizes at a population level can be important (Section 7.1.4). Yet trialists may have collected information which could be used in systematic reviews and meta-analyses if others were aware of the trial's existence. In addition, cluster randomised trials are often difficult to carry out owing to the complexity of recruitment and delivering the intervention. If the trial needed to be abandoned because of

To mitigate against publication bias – the under reporting of trials with disappointing, negative, or inconclusive results – which misleads researchers conducting systematic reviews and doctors making decisions based on published evidence.

To prevent unnecessary duplication of research effort, while encouraging appropriate replication and confirmation of results.

To alert researchers to gaps in the knowledge base.

To foster international collaboration among researchers and stimulate recruitment to clinical trials, enhancing their chances of success.

To provide reliable intelligence about ongoing trials that will help funding bodies target their money where it is most needed.

To aid recruitment to trials by direct appeal to the public.

To enable research into research. Who is doing what, and how?

To improve accessibility and therefore credibility of research performed by the pharmaceutical industry.

To satisfy public demand for unbiased evidence on the effectiveness of treatments, and to promote the public accountability of medical research in general.

Source: Tonks (1999).

Box 10.3   Reasons for registering trials

practical problems, it is important to make this knowledge available to other researchers in order to avoid such problems in the future. A good example of this is the UK BEAM pilot trial, which was redesigned because of biased recruitment (Farrin *et al.*, 2005). Information from this pilot trial has been very useful in developing future good practice (Eldridge *et al.*, 2008).

Tonks (1999) lists several reasons why trials should be registered (Box 10.3). This list was written mainly for individually randomised trials, but most points apply equally well to cluster randomised trials. Assisting recruitment is probably less relevant to cluster randomised trials, as normally individuals are deliberately selected because they belong to a participating cluster; and few cluster randomised trials involve the pharmaceutical industry.

Trial registration in an approved trial registration database will involve providing a minimum set of details about the trial including specifying the primary outcome. Selective reporting of outcome can lead to bias in the reported results (Moher *et al.*, 2010). Pre-specifying the primary outcome at the start of the trial protects against such bias and is a useful aid to robust trial reporting.

Since September 2004, it has been the policy of the International Committee of Medical Journal Editors (ICMJE) only to consider for publication those trials which have been registered before the enrolment of the first participant (De Angelis *et al.*, 2004). The ICMJE website gives guidance on acceptable registries (http://www. icmje.org/faq_clinical.html (last accessed 2 June 2011)).

10.2.2 Publication of trial protocol

Registration requires some details of the trial to be made publicly available, but this will be only a small part of the information contained in the trial protocol. It is a good idea to publish the protocol before the data are analysed; the protocol can then be referenced in the main trial report. Two examples of protocols come from the OPERA and PRISM trials (Underwood *et al.*, 2011; Lumley *et al.*, 2003).

Prior publication of the protocol restricts the likelihood of undeclared *post hoc* changes to the trial methods and selective outcome reporting (Moher *et al.*, 2010). Alternatively the protocol may be published on the website of the journal publishing the trial's primary results, or on the website of the author's employer. The SPIRIT (Standard Protocol Items For Randomized Trials) initiative has yet to report but aims to give a checklist of items to be included in a trial protocol (Equator network 2011).

10.3 Reporting randomised trials in journal and conference abstracts

Although journal abstracts are covered in the main CONSORT checklist (item 1b, Table 10.1), they have also been the subject of a separate CONSORT extension (Hopewell *et al.*, 2008) which covers conference abstracts as well; so we present abstracts here as a separate section. Conference abstracts are usually the only written record of an oral presentation, and only half of randomised controlled trials reported in conference proceedings are subsequently published in full (Scherer, Langenberg and von Elm, 2007). Journal abstracts are usually available free to all readers on the internet, while journals may charge a fee for the full text for non-subscribers; although some readers will use abstracts to decide whether to seek more information about a trial, many will simply base their assessment of the trial on the information in the abstract. It is therefore important that abstracts of randomised trials are clear, transparent and contain key details. The checklist is given in Table 10.2. Although the trial design item includes 'cluster' as an option, there has been no formally agreed extension of the abstract checklist for cluster trials; the additions in italics are our own, but we have not changed any other wording.

A full discussion of the role of abstracts and the checklist items is given in Hopewell *et al.* (2008). Most of the items in this checklist are also included in the main CONSORT checklist discussed in Section 10.4, although they must be reported more succinctly in an abstract. There are two items which are included in the abstract checklist only.

Table 10.2 Items to include when reporting a randomized trial in a journal or conference abstract (Hopewell *et al.*, 2008); extensions for cluster trials given in italics are our own.

Item	Description	Reported on line number
Title	Identification of the study as *cluster* randomized	
Authors[a]	Contact details for the corresponding author	
Trial design	Description of the trial design (e.g. parallel, cluster, non-inferiority)	
Methods		
Participants	Eligibility criteria for participants *and clusters* and the settings where the data were collected	
Interventions	Interventions intended for each group	
Objective	Specific objective or hypothesis	
Outcome	Clearly defined primary outcome for this report	
Randomization	How *clusters* and participants were allocated to interventions *and whether participants and those taking consent were blind to allocation status*	
Blinding (masking)	Whether or not participants, care givers, and those assessing the outcomes were blinded to group assignment	
Results		
Numbers randomized	Number of *clusters and* participants randomized to each group	
Recruitment	Trial status	
Numbers analysed	Number of *clusters and* participants analysed in each group	
Outcome	For the primary outcome, a result for each group and the estimated effect size and its precision	
Harms	Important adverse events or side effects	
Conclusions	General interpretation of the results	
Trial registration	Registration number and name of trial register	
Funding	Source of funding	

[a]This item is specific to conference abstracts. Reproduced by permission of CONSORT.

Recruitment item; trial status: authors should report whether the trial is still ongoing, closed to recruitment, or closed to follow-up. If the trial has stopped earlier than planned, or if an interim analysis is being carried out, it is important to explain why.

Authors: for a conference presentation, contact details should be given to enable readers to contact the author for more information about the trial and the final results if the trial is ongoing.

Box 10.4 gives an example of an abstract from a cluster randomised trial report. The title describes the study as cluster randomised, the setting is described, the clusters are specified as dwellings, and the numbers of clusters and participants are given, both at randomisation and follow-up. The trial follow-up is ongoing, but it is unclear from the abstract that the interim analysis was pre-planned, although this is stated in the full text. The trial registration number and the name of the register are given as well as funding details. The authors' details are given elsewhere in the document.

10.4   Application of CONSORT statement to cluster randomised trials

The extension of the CONSORT statement to cluster randomised trials (Campbell, Elbourne and Altman, 2004) was published in 2004; the main CONSORT checklist was subsequently updated in 2010 (Moher *et al.*, 2010). Table 10.1 reproduces the 2010 checklist together with the 2004 extended checklist for cluster randomised trials. Except for item 1, title and abstract, the statements which were amended to allow for clustering have remained unchanged between 2004 and 2010, although there has been some reordering of the first six items. The CONSORT statement refers to treatment or intervention *groups* rather than *arms*. We have not changed this wording in any tables or quotes but in the chapter text we use the term *arms* to be consistent with terminology used in the rest of the book.

10.4.1   Item 1a: Information in title

As for individually randomised trials, those conducting cluster randomised trials should include in the title some wording which indicates that their trial is randomised. The additional recommendation to specify the allocation by cluster in either the title or the abstract (adaptation of item 1) is justified in the extended CONSORT statement because this ensures accurate indexing of trials in Medline. Medline is the National Library of Medicine database of publications. In this database, publications are indexed according to subject matter and methodology by attaching key terms known as Medical Subject Headings (MeSH) to each publication. Randomised controlled trials are indexed with their own headings but, as yet,

Efficacy and safety of a modified killed-whole-cell oral cholera vaccine in India: an interim analysis of a cluster-randomised, double-blind, placebo-controlled trial

Methods

In this double-blind trial, 107 774 non-pregnant residents of Kolkata, India, aged one year or older, were cluster randomised by dwelling to receive two doses of either modified killed-whole-cell cholera vaccine (n = 52 212; 1966 clusters) or heat-killed *Escherichia coli* K12 placebo (n = 55 562; 1967 clusters), both delivered orally. Randomisation was done by computer-generated sequence in blocks of four. The primary endpoint was prevention of episodes of culture-confirmed *Vibrio cholerae* O1 diarrhoea severe enough for the patient to seek treatment in a healthcare facility. We undertook an interim, per-protocol analysis at two years of follow-up that included individuals who received two completely ingested doses of vaccine or placebo. We assessed first episodes of cholera that occurred between 14 days and 730 days after receipt of the second dose. This study is registered with ClinicalTrials.gov, number NCT00289224.

Findings

31 932 participants assigned to vaccine (1721 clusters) and 34 968 assigned to placebo (1757 clusters) received two doses of study treatment. There were 20 episodes of cholera in the vaccine group and 68 episodes in the placebo group (protective efficacy 67%; one-tailed 99% CI, lower bound 35%, $p < 0.0001$). The vaccine protected individuals in age-groups 1.0–4.9 years, 5.0–14.9 years, and 15 years and older, and protective efficacy did not differ significantly between age-groups ($p = 0.28$). We recorded no vaccine-related serious adverse events.

Funding

Bill & Melinda Gates Foundation, Swedish International Development Cooperation Agency, Governments of South Korea, Sweden, and Kuwait

Source: Sur *et al.* (2009).

Box 10.4 Extracts from the abstract of a report of an ongoing cluster randomised trial.

cluster randomised trials are not. The MeSH system is also used in the Cochrane database. Thus, perhaps a better reason for specifying allocation by cluster in either the title or the abstract of a report is that this aids those searching for cluster randomised trials within electronic databases. For example, Eldridge *et al.* (2004) conducted a large review of cluster randomised trials published between 1997 and 2000. They attempted to identify cluster randomised trials in primary care in any journals within this time span. They did not have the capacity to hand search all journals, and so attempted to devise an electronic search strategy to identify cluster randomised trials. This proved impossible because of the lack of consistency amongst authors in the way that they indicated that the trial was cluster randomised. The idea of searching electronically for cluster randomised trials in primary care had to be abandoned. An electronic search for randomised trials in primary care was undertaken instead. Abstracts and/or full texts were then read to establish whether or not each trial was cluster randomised. The simple inclusion of the word 'cluster' in the title or the abstract would have enabled the use of an electronic search. Trials are more likely to be included in future reviews or meta-analyses if they are easily identifiable. Recent experience indicates that 'cluster randomised' in the title is becoming more common (e.g. Sur *et al.*, 2009; Kaczorowski *et al.*, 2011).

The 2010 version of the CONSORT statement clearly recommends 'randomised' in the title; while the 2001 version on which the cluster randomised trial extension is based does not separate title and abstract. Therefore the recommendation to include 'cluster' in the title is ours, but seems consistent with the 2010 checklist.

Item 1b was covered in Section 10.3.

10.4.2   Item 2: Background information

As for individually randomised trials, authors should explain the scientific background and rationale for their cluster randomised trial. Because most of the interventions evaluated in cluster randomised trials are complex (see Chapter 3), it is necessary to explain the rationale for the elements of the complex intervention as well as the scientific rationale for investigating the particular medical condition. This includes, if appropriate, describing the theory on which the intervention is based and the reason why this particular complex intervention has been chosen. The latter may involve a brief description of any development work undertaken prior to the trial. An example of a report in which theory and development work are briefly described is the Diabetes Manual trial, extracts of which are reported in Table 10.3. The development work for this trial was also described in Section 4.1.

The additional recommendation in the extended statement is that authors should include a rationale for the clustered design; the reason being that it is unethical to expose individuals to research unnecessarily and, because of the need to allow for between-cluster variability, more people are included in a cluster randomised trial. In Chapter 1 we described the various reasons that a cluster randomised trial is likely to be undertaken in health services research. Investigators should explain which of these reasons (there may be more than one) apply in their trial. In three reviews of

Table 10.3   Diabetes Manual trial: manual and structured care to improve outcomes.

Aim: To determine the effects of the Diabetes Manual on glycaemic control, diabetes-related distress and confidence to self-care of patients with type 2 diabetes

Location and type of cluster: UK general practices

Number of clusters and individual participants: 48 clusters analysed; 202 individual participants analysed

Interventions: (i) Control: usual care (ii) Intervention: education of nurses, followed by one-to-one structured education of patients via a self-completed manual and nurse support, and audiotapes

Primary outcome: HbA1c level

Description of the intervention:

> The Diabetes Manual was developed using social learning theory to employ self-efficacy enhancing strategies such as positive mastery experiences, vicarious learning, emotional adjustment and verbal persuasion [references]. Using the Medical Research Council complex intervention framework [references], the intervention development work [reference to figure] commenced in 2001 with a needs assessment focus group study followed by a primary care survey of people living with diabetes and simultaneous general practitioner (GP) and practice nurse interviews to identify desirable programme content [references]. In 2003, lay and health professional development panels were established to explore the theoretical approach, develop the curriculum and write the Diabetes Manual workbook, audio tape scripts and nurse training course. Nurse training syllabus development followed [references].

Description of cluster eligibility and the characteristics of eligible clusters:

> General practices in which the nurse had undertaken post registration diabetes care training were invited to participate from June 2004 to November 2005. Practices were drawn from 24 Primary Care Trusts across the West Midlands, UK. This population is characterized by urbanization, ethnic diversity, seasonal population transience and high social deprivation.

Source: Sturt *et al.* (2008).

cluster randomised trials (Donner, Brown and Brasher, 1990; Isaakidis and Ioannidis, 2003; Eldridge *et al.*, 2004), less than a quarter of trial reports include a rationale for conducting a cluster randomised trial: the most common reason reported is that the intervention is aimed at the clusters and it is therefore logistically impossible to randomise at an individual level. Three examples of reporting the reasons for conducting a cluster randomised trial are given in Tables 10.4 to 10.6.

The 2010 CONSORT checklist contains an additional item, 'Trial design' (item 3), under 'Methods', and in the full explanation recommends that researchers who use designs which will lead to larger sample sizes, including cluster randomised

Table 10.4   Shared care development for long term mental illness.

Aim: To determine the effects of Mental Health Link, a facilitation-based quality improvement programme designed to improve communication between community mental health teams and systems of care with a general practice

Location and type of cluster: UK general practices

Number of clusters and individual participants: 23 clusters analysed; 322 participants analysed

Interventions: (i) Control: usual care (ii) Intervention: quality improvement programme facilitated by trained researchers working with small groups of professionals and managers from each practice and its associated community mental health team

Primary outcome: Patients' satisfaction with care and perception of unmet need

Reason for cluster randomisation

> Facilitation programmes, as a subtype of organisational interventions, although ultimately aiming to improve the health of patients, work through changing practitioner beliefs and behaviour to develop systems and improve practice during contact with patients. We therefore used a […] cluster-based randomised controlled trial to evaluate the Mental Health Link intervention by looking at its impact on three levels: practice, practitioner, and patient.

Source: Byng *et al.* (2004).

Table 10.5   ELECTRA: asthma liaison nurses to reduce unscheduled care.

Aim: To determine whether asthma specialist nurses, using a liaison model of care, reduce unscheduled care in a deprived multiethnic setting

Location and type of cluster: UK general practices

Number of clusters and individual participants: 44 clusters analysed; 319 participants analysed

Interventions: (i) Control: a visit promoting standard asthma guidelines; patients were checked for inhaler technique (ii) Intervention: patient review in a nurse-led clinic and liaison with general practitioners and practice nurses comprising educational outreach, promotion of guidelines for high risk asthma, and ongoing clinical support

Primary outcome: Unscheduled care for acute asthma over one year, and time to first unscheduled attendance ,

Reason for cluster randomisation:

> We used a pragmatic cluster randomised controlled design, as an important element of the intervention addressed clinicians in general practice

Qualifications of nurses used to implement the intervention:

> Two specialist nurses were accredited by the National Respiratory Training Centre in Stratford, East London

---

Source: Griffiths *et al.* (2004).

Table 10.6   Early stimulation for undernourished children in Jamaica.

Aim: To assess the feasibility of integrating early psychosocial stimulation into primary care for undernourished children, and to determine the effect on children's development and mothers' knowledge and practices of childrearing

Location and type of cluster: Jamaican clinics

Interventions: (i) Control: usual care (ii) Intervention: specially trained community health aides visited homes weekly for half an hour and demonstrated play activities involving the mother and child

Primary outcome: Griffiths mental development scale

Number of clusters and individual participants: 18 clusters analysed; 129 participants analysed

Reason for cluster randomisation:

We randomised by clinic not by child as it was not feasible for the children to receive different treatments within the same clinic.

Source: Powell *et al.* (2004).

designs, explain their choice. This may be a more appropriate place for authors to justify their design, as we describe in the next section.

The extended statement recommends that it is made clear whether objectives pertain to cluster or individual level, in order to aid statistical interpretation; the assumption being that interpretation should match objectives. In the majority of cluster randomised trials in health services research, objectives pertain to the individual level. For example, in the ELECTRA trial (Table 10.5), the objective was to determine whether asthma liaison nurses could reduce unscheduled care, an objective focused on the patients. On the other hand, Table 10.7 describes an intervention which was aimed at changing the test ordering behaviour of general practices, and therefore the research objectives are at the cluster level. Trial objectives were listed as a separate item, item 5, in previous versions of CONSORT, but are now listed under 'Introduction, background and objectives'. The wording of the item is unchanged.

10.4.3   Item 3: Trial design

Most cluster randomised trials use a two-arm parallel design which sets out to test whether a new intervention is superior to current practice. Other possible designs are multi-arm parallel, crossover and factorial designs, and trials which are designed to assess non-inferiority or equivalence. In addition, matched designs are not uncommon in cluster randomised trials. This item also encompasses describing the unit of randomisation, and recommends that authors explain their choice of design. To some extent this overlaps with the cluster extension recommendations for item 2.

It may also be helpful to provide the allocation ratio. Although most cluster randomised trials use a 1 : 1 ratio, not all do. For example the OPERA trial used a 1 : 1.5 ratio (Table 10.8).

Table 10.7   Improving screening for carriers of haemoglobin disorders.

Aim: To investigate the feasibility of improving screening for carriers of haemoglobin disorders in general practice by using a nurse facilitator to work with primary care teams and the relevant haematology laboratories

Location and type of cluster: UK general practices

Interventions: (i) Control: usual care (ii) Intervention: posters, leaflets, formal education sessions

Primary outcome: Number of requests for screening tests for haemoglobin disorders

Data collection: The number of requests for screening was obtained from the laboratory at baseline and at the end of the intervention period

Source: Modell *et al.* (1998).

Table 10.8   OPERA: physical activity in residential homes to prevent depression.

Aim: To evaluate the impact on depression of a whole-home intervention to increase physical activity among older people

Location and type of cluster: UK residential and nursing homes for older people

Number of clusters randomised and analysed: 78

Number of residents recruited: 1060

Interventions: (i) Control: depression awareness programme delivered by research nurses (ii) Intervention: depression awareness programme delivered by physiotherapists plus whole-home package to increase activity among older people, including physiotherapy assessments of individuals, and activity sessions for residents

Primary outcome: Prevalence of depression (Geriatric Depression Scale) at 12 months and change in depression score

Allocation ratio:

> To reduce NHS [National Heath Service] treatment costs we are using an unbalanced randomisation:- 1 intervention home: 1.5 control homes

Changes to inclusion criteria (reported in protocol paper):

> One pilot home and one home recruited early in the study were dementia specialist homes, but we found that the proportion of residents able to complete the questions for our primary outcome measure (the geriatric depression scale – 15 item version) was small and concluded that recruiting such homes was not the best use of our resources

Source: Underwood *et al.* (2011).

Most trial protocols specify in detail how the trial will be conducted. However, as the trial progresses there may be unforeseen circumstances which lead to changes from the original design. For example, there may be changes to the eligibility criteria, how the interventions are delivered, randomisation allocation ratio or duration of follow-up. The OPERA trial originally planned to include residential homes for people with dementia, but later the inclusion criteria were changed (Table 10.8).

The data monitoring committee may also recommend trial protocol changes as the trial progresses. An explanation of any changes to the original protocol as designed and submitted to the ethics committee, and the role of any independent advisors, should be given.

10.4.4   Item 4: Description of participants

Because there are two levels of inference, cluster and individual, eligibility must be reported for both. This is not usually difficult; although, if cluster eligibility is simply geographical, it may be helpful to readers unfamiliar with the geographical area to describe the characteristics of clusters in this area and how they might differ from clusters in other areas where the intervention might be implemented. The Diabetes Manual trial (Table 10.3) provides an example of a description of cluster eligibility and the characteristics of eligible clusters.

It is also important to describe the setting in which the trial takes place (see also Section 2.1.1). The selection criteria or characteristics of those performing the intervention should also be described. Although in some cluster randomised trials the intervention may be performed by the clusters themselves, some external-cluster interventions use additional staff to implement the intervention or part of it, as in the ELECTRA trial. The qualifications of the nurses in this trial are described in Griffiths *et al.* (2004) and reproduced in Table 10.5.

10.4.5   Item 5: Description of interventions

'The reports of thousands of trials are never acted on because their published reports do not describe the interventions in enough detail' (Boutron *et al.*, 2008). Many cluster randomised trials comprise non-pharmacological interventions. Protocols and funding applications may contain fuller descriptions of interventions than main trial reports; we have illustrated this with three examples in Chapter 3 (Tables 3.3–3.5). However, such documents are often not publicly available, and published protocols tend to be shorter than the protocols to which research teams work.

Describing interventions adequately is often difficult, particularly given space constraints in journals (Nation *et al.*, 2003; Davidson *et al.*, 2003). One way of dealing with this issue in a publication is to describe the intervention briefly in the text, with detail in a box, or on the journal's website. Griffiths *et al.* (2007) used a box to summarise key intervention components (Box 10.5) and also put a copy of the four-page guidelines, 'Tuberculosis screening in primary care', on the journal's website, with a short summary in the text of the article (see Table 10.9).

Panel: **Implementation of screening**

Practice visits

A tuberculosis specialist nurse and a local academic GP (CG) made one educational outreach visit to each intervention practice to promote tuberculosis screening and raise awareness of tuberculosis as a local public health concern, and distributed copies of local tuberculosis screening guidelines with algorithms (webappendix).

Computer prompts

We incorporated prompts into the template for the practice computer system used for registration health check consultations to remind clinicians to ask the screening questions stipulated in the guidelines. These prompts comprised READ* coded items, such that a searchable code was entered in response to a positive answer to a screening question.

Equipment

We provided equipment for tuberculin skin testing: Heaf heads and guns, and tuberculin.

Support

We arranged telephone support by a tuberculosis specialist nurse for advice and to receive referrals.

Financial incentive

A financial incentive of £7 (€10.2; US$12.9) was paid to the practice for every tuberculin skin test.

*READ codes are a coded thesaurus of clinical terms that enable clinicians to make effective use of computer systems. The codes facilitate the access of information within patient records to enable reporting, auditing, research, automation of repetitive tasks, electronic communication and decision support. The READ code is named after James Read who was a GP.
Source: Griffiths *et al.* (2007).

Box 10.5   Screening for tuberculosis in primary care: panel summarising the implementation of screening

Table 10.9   Screening for tuberculosis in primary care.

Aim: To assess a programme to promote screening for tuberculosis in a UK primary healthcare district

Location and type of cluster: UK general practices

Number of clusters randomised: 50

Interventions: (i) Control: usual care (ii) Intervention: an outreach programme that promoted screening for tuberculosis in people registering in primary care

Primary outcome: The proportion of new cases of active tuberculosis identified in primary care

Intervention description in text of journal article:

> The educational visits to practices lasted an hour, were attended by the general practitioners and practice nurses, and used the social influence model of behaviour change. [references] At this visit, the two educators discussed recommendations from local tuberculosis screening guidelines, taught tuberculin skin testing using the Heaf method, and imported screening prompts into the practice computer system, and demonstrated their use. We discussed screening at health checks for newly registering patients and promoted awareness during routine consultations. The tuberculosis specialist nurse telephoned practices a week later to reinforce the education and deal with any difficulties in skin testing. The nurse continued to contact practices throughout the study to provide supplies for tuberculosis testing, and to provide encouragement.

Source: Griffiths *et al.* (2007).

In an effort to improve the clarity of reporting of complex interventions, Perera, Heneghan and Yudkin (2007) developed a graphical method of describing interventions. This has been used in the reports of several cluster randomised trials. Figure 10.1 shows the diagram applied to a trial of a language promotion programme for slow to talk toddlers (Table 10.10). The components are regarded as either objects or activities. Objects are represented by squares (to reflect their fixed nature) and activities by circles (to reflect their flexibility). Different component are given different letters with a key. In Figure 10.1 the screening questionnaire is an object, which will be the same for all patients; whereas the 'You Make The Difference' sessions are activities, the exact content of which may vary from group to group.

The extended CONSORT statement recommends that investigators should report whether the interventions used in the trial 'pertain to the cluster level or the individual level or both'. This recommendation relates to the *administration* of the intervention.

10.4.6   Item 6: Outcomes

In the methods section authors should clearly define pre-specified primary and secondary outcome measures, including how and when they were assessed. A fuller

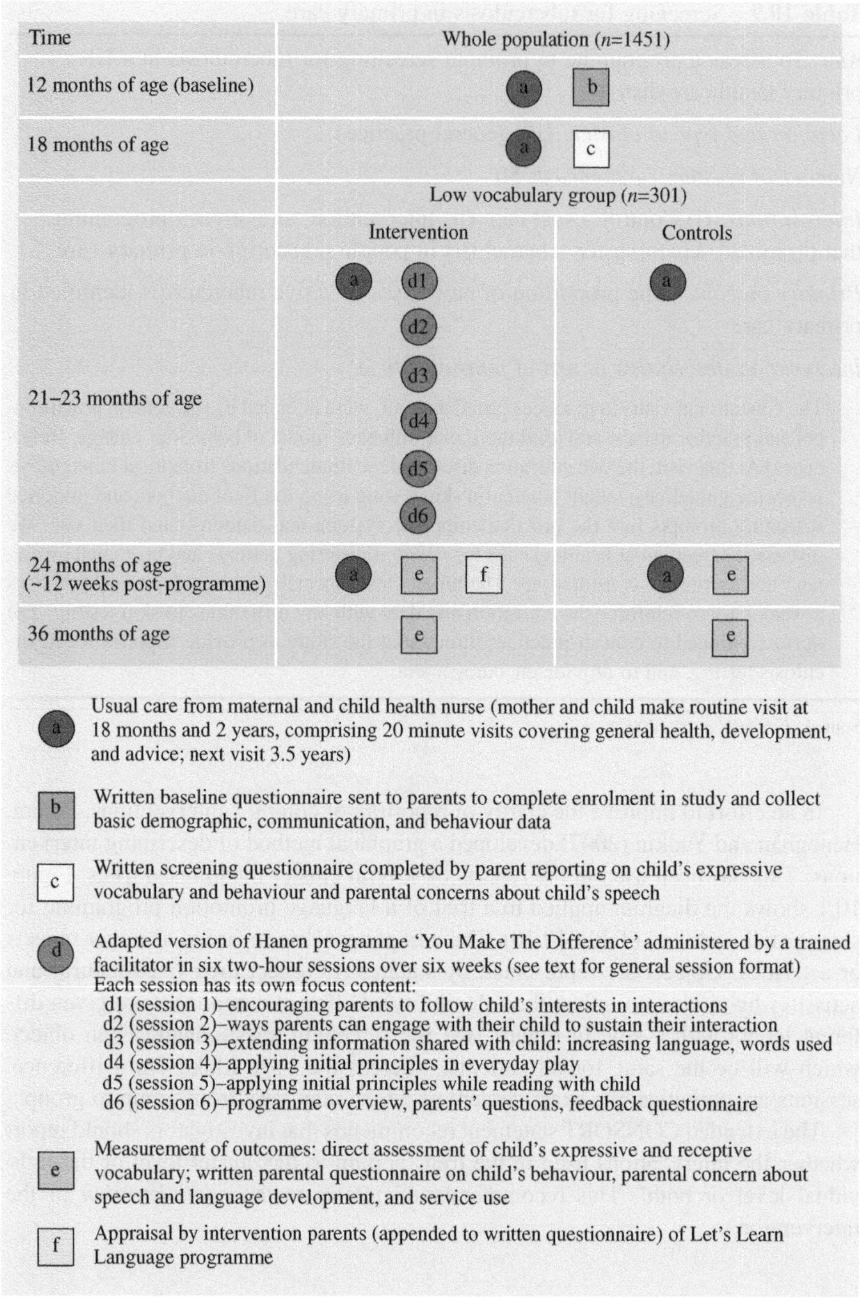

Time	Whole population (n=1451)	
12 months of age (baseline)	ⓐ b	
18 months of age	ⓐ c	
	Low vocabulary group (n=301)	
	Intervention	Controls
21–23 months of age	ⓐ d1 d2 d3 d4 d5 d6	ⓐ
24 months of age (~12 weeks post-programme)	ⓐ e f	ⓐ e
36 months of age	e	e

ⓐ Usual care from maternal and child health nurse (mother and child make routine visit at 18 months and 2 years, comprising 20 minute visits covering general health, development, and advice; next visit 3.5 years)

b Written baseline questionnaire sent to parents to complete enrolment in study and collect basic demographic, communication, and behaviour data

c Written screening questionnaire completed by parent reporting on child's expressive vocabulary and behaviour and parental concerns about child's speech

ⓓ Adapted version of Hanen programme 'You Make The Difference' administered by a trained facilitator in six two-hour sessions over six weeks (see text for general session format) Each session has its own focus content:
d1 (session 1)–encouraging parents to follow child's interests in interactions
d2 (session 2)–ways parents can engage with their child to sustain their interaction
d3 (session 3)–extending information shared with child: increasing language, words used
d4 (session 4)–applying initial principles in everyday play
d5 (session 5)–applying initial principles while reading with child
d6 (session 6)–programme overview, parents' questions, feedback questionnaire

e Measurement of outcomes: direct assessment of child's expressive and receptive vocabulary; written parental questionnaire on child's behaviour, parental concern about speech and language development, and service use

f Appraisal by intervention parents (appended to written questionnaire) of Let's Learn Language programme

Figure 10.1   Graphical display of trial to improve language development in slow to talk toddlers. Reproduced from Outcomes of population based language promotion for slow to talk toddlers at ages 2 and 3 years: Let's learn language cluster randomised controlled trial. © 2011 with permission from BMJ Publishing Group Ltd.

Table 10.10   Let's Learn Language to promote language in slow to talk toddlers.

Aim: To determine the benefits of a low intensity parent–toddler language promotion programme delivered to toddlers identified as slow to talk on screening in universal services

Location and type of cluster: Canadian maternal and child health clinics

Number of clusters analysed: 38

Number of individuals analysed: 274

Interventions: (i) Control: usual care (ii) Modified 'You Make The Difference' programme over six, weekly sessions for parents

Primary outcome: Expressive language as measured by the Preschool Language Scale-4

Source: Wake *et al.* (2011).

discussion of bias introduced by selective reporting is given in Section 10.4.17. Whether outcomes are measured at the individual or cluster level has implications for the appropriate analysis of the outcome data (see Section 6.3), and so should be reported. As with all protocol changes after the trial has commenced, those affecting the outcomes should be reported, with reasons.

10.4.7   Item 7: Sample size and interim analyses

The issue of the appropriate sample size for cluster randomised trials has been highlighted in a number of reviews of cluster randomised trials and in other publications. In six reviews (Donner, Brown and Brasher, 1990; Simpson, Klar and Donner, 1995; Chuang, Hripcsak and Jenders, 2000; Isaakidis and Ioannidis, 2003; Eldridge *et al.*, 2004; Varnell *et al.*, 2004) published before or at about the same time as the extended CONSORT statement, fewer than a quarter of the trial reports indicated that the sample size had been estimated correctly, although more recent reviews indicate that the situation appears to be improving (Puffer, Torgerson and Watson, 2003; Eldridge *et al.*, 2008).

In terms of reporting sample size calculations, the extended CONSORT statement recommends that authors report the number of clusters, cluster size (i.e. the number of subjects sampled per cluster) and the ICC, with some measure of uncertainty on the latter. An example of a simple sample size statement is given in Box 7.1.

'Cluster size' here is slightly ambiguous, since clusters may not always be the same size and the cluster sizes expected may differ from actual cluster sizes. When cluster sizes are expected to vary authors should report, at the very minimum, the expected mean cluster size on which their sample size was based (or should give enough information for readers to be able to calculate this). Sample size requirements actually depend on the variability in cluster size (see Section 7.6), usually measured by either the coefficient of variation of cluster size or expected minimum and maximum cluster size. There are few examples of trial reports where these quantities have been reported. The extract below describes how variability in cluster size has been taken into account in one trial. The authors referenced the relevant methodology paper by Eldridge *et al.* (2006).

> There were 85 state-funded mixed-sex schools in the greater Santiago area with >1 class per year group. We randomly selected four classes for study in those schools with more than four per year group. Therefore schools participating in the study had 2, 3 or 4 classes in the trial, yielding a mean year group size of 125 (SD 40), and a mean cluster size for analysis of 80 (SD 26) assuming 80% consent and retention rates [...] Using Eldridge *et al.*'s formula for inflation of sample size in cluster randomised trials with unequal cluster sizes, we calculated we needed to invite 2634 students from 20.3 schools in order to maintain 90% power for the primary analysis. We therefore aimed to recruit and randomise 22 schools. (Araya *et al.*, 2011)

Item 7b, related to interim analyses, has been added to the 2010 statement. Selective reporting of interim analyses and multiple 'looks' at the data leading to premature trial closure or early reporting can result in bias. It is important to know whether the trial was stopped prematurely and how the decision was taken, and the role of independent committees such as a data monitoring committee in the decision. It is rare for cluster randomised trials to be stopped early, however.

10.4.8   Item 8: Generation of random allocation sequence

A description of the generation of the random allocation sequence reassures readers that random allocation was performed correctly. As for individually randomised trials, authors of cluster randomised trial reports should detail whether the random allocation involved any restrictions. The 2010 version of the CONSORT checklist covers all types of restricted randomisation, including minimisation. These are described in Moher *et al.* (2010) and in Chapter 5 (Section 5.1). The extended CONSORT statement added matching, which is rarely used outside cluster randomised trials owing to the difficulty of matching individual participants. Whatever the method, authors should report details of factors used to balance arms (whether by stratification, minimisation, matching or some other method) and how these factors were categorised. If using stratification, block size and whether or not block size varied randomly should be reported. If minimisation is used this is usually via a computer program and can be with or without a random element. Authors should describe or reference the program used and whether or not a random element was incorporated. In the ELECTRA trial (Table 10.5), the authors report the use of a minimisation program and specify the minimisation factors used. The cut-off points defining the levels are given in an accompanying table. The program used includes a random element, although this is not explicitly mentioned in the paper.

> We randomised practices to intervention and control groups using a minimisation program, [reference to program] stratifying by partnership size, training practice status, hospital admission rate for asthma, employment of practice nurse, and whether the

practice nurse was trained in asthma care [refers to table which gives categories for stratification factors]. (Griffiths *et al.*, 2004)

10.4.9   Item 9: Allocation concealment

By definition, allocation in cluster randomised trials is by cluster, and the extended CONSORT statement recommends specifying that this is the case. Allocation concealment is seen as the cornerstone to avoiding bias in randomised controlled trials. This usually means making sure that the individual who allocates participants to their respective intervention arms either never knows which arm they are in (remains blinded by placebo control); or does not know it until she or he is about to inform the participants (usually at the same time that the participants are recruited). Unlike placebo-controlled trials, it is common for clusters to be recruited at one time point and randomised some time later. Between these two time points the cluster allocation must be made and communicated to the individual who will relay this information to the cluster. The principles behind allocation concealment require that this individual does not have the opportunity to subvert the randomisation schedule. This is usually relatively straightforward to ensure, because the identity of the clusters is established at the point of allocation and cannot be altered by the individual who simply relays that allocation to the clusters. An example of this, from the OPERA trial, is described in Section 9.1.2. In fact, bias is much more likely to occur at the patient enrolment stage as described in Section 2.3. Investigators should report whether or not allocation was concealed, and more detail if it was not.

10.4.10   Item 10: Who generated allocation sequence, enrolled participants and assigned participants to their groups

The general purpose of this item is to ensure that readers of the trial report can assess whether there has been any bias caused by unblinded individuals carrying out these various tasks. Although there is no addition to this item in the extended CONSORT statement, it should be specified whether the tasks are carried out for clusters or individuals. The generation of allocation sequence and assignment clearly apply to clusters and, because there are no ethical and duty of care considerations towards clusters in the same way as there are towards patients, there is more flexibility around who contacts clusters and how; it need not be an individual who a priori knows anything about the cluster, and contact can be by telephone. In these circumstances the potential for subversion of the randomisation schedule (if this has not been ruled out as described in the previous section) is lessened. Additionally, allocation may be less open to subversion because it is less clear what would be achieved by it. Sometimes the potential relationship between clusters and trial outcome may be more obvious. For example, in the OPERA trial in nursing homes, it may have been easier, given the considerable variation in home environment and characteristics of residents, for investigators who had visited homes to assess the extent to which an individual home might promote this relatively intensive intervention and the extent to which residents might benefit from it. In all circumstances clear reporting enables the reader to make a judgement for themselves about the integrity of the allocation process.

Enrolment, in contrast with generation of randomisation sequence and assignment, may refer to enrolment of clusters or enrolment of participants. While those enrolling both clusters and individuals should ideally be blind to allocation status, this is not always the case for cluster randomised trials (Section 2.3). Figure 2.2 in Section 2.3.5 lists four questions which can identify whether or not there is likely to be bias in the enrolment of participants. We suggest that these questions are used to guide reporting, and that any potential bias is recognised in the trial limitations (Section 10.4.20).

In the following statement, from Godwin *et al.* (2010), it is clear how investigators protected against recruitment bias; while in the trial presented in Table 10.11, the authors discuss the potential for bias in the trial limitations.

> Cluster randomization was conducted. After all the physician's eligible consenting patients had baseline data collected, the physician and all his participating patients were randomized as a cluster to either the intervention arm or the control arm of the study. The research assistant (RA) collecting the baseline data contacted the project coordinator

Table 10.11   Promoting child safety by reducing baby walker use.

Aim: To evaluate the effectiveness of an educational package provided by midwives and health visitors to reduce baby walker possession and use

Location and type of cluster: UK groups of general practices sharing a health visitor (between 1 and 4 practices)

Number of clusters and individual participants: 46 clusters analysed; 1008 participants analysed

Interventions: (i) Control: usual care (ii) Intervention: trained midwives and health visitors delivered an educational package to mothers to be, at 10 days postpartum and 3–4 months later, to discourage baby walker use or encourage safe use for those who already had baby walkers

Primary outcome: Possession and use of a baby walker

Recruitment: By midwives and health visitors during pregnancy after randomisation

Discussion of recruitment bias:

> There was some evidence of imbalance between the treatment arms at baseline, which may reflect post-randomisation recruitment bias. This could have arisen either by midwives inadvertently selecting women to participate on the basis of midwives' perceptions about their propensity to use a walker, or by women becoming aware that the trial was aimed at reducing baby walker use prior to giving consent and choosing whether or not to participate based on this knowledge.

Source: Kendrick *et al.* (2005).

to determine random assignment; the project coordinator held the randomization schedule but was not aware of which physician was about to be randomized. This process provided masking of the randomization. (Godwin *et al.*, 2010)

10.4.11 Item 11: Blinding

The previous item deals with blinding during enrolment and allocation, while this item is concerned with what happens after randomisation; that is, reducing bias through ensuring blinding of individual trial participants, those delivering the intervention, and those assessing outcomes. The issue of blinding is often quite different in cluster randomised from individually randomised trials. In cluster randomised trials, 'delivery of the intervention' could mean an intervention component aimed at clusters or at individuals; in many trials there are intervention components at both levels. Those delivering an intervention aimed at clusters, such as a training course, cannot be blind to intervention status; neither can health professionals delivering an educational, advice or similar intervention component within clusters. The IRIS trial contains both these types of components (Table 10.12). The relevant question is whether bias will ensue as a result of this unblinding (see also Section 9.1.2). If those delivering the intervention are seen as an integral part of the intervention, and random allocation has not been subverted, then there is little potential for bias, unless those delivering the intervention in the control arm suffer from 'resentful

Table 10.12   IRIS: training to increase identification and referral of victims of domestic violence.

Aim: To test the effectiveness of a training and support programme for general practice teams targeting identification of women experiencing domestic violence, and referral to specialist domestic violence advocates

Location and type of cluster: UK general practices

Intervention: (i) Control: usual care (ii) Intervention: multidisciplinary training sessions in each practice electronic prompts in the patient record and referral pathway to a named domestic violence advocate as well as feedbackon referrals and reinforcement over the course of a year. Posters were displayed in the practice, and leaflets were available

Primary outcome: Number of referrals of women aged over 16 to advocacy services based in specialist domestic violence agencies recorded in the general practice records

Consent required by clusters: Yes

Consent required by participants: No

Comment: Outcome data were obtained from practice notes by researchers, and no patient-identifiable data taken outside practices. Additional screening for domestic violence in consultations was not expected to affect usual care negatively

Source: Feder *et al.* (2011).

demoralisation'– a tendency not to treat participants as well as they might otherwise do because they are disappointed at not receiving the intervention. It is to be hoped that this does not happen in a clinical setting. Investigators should report whether health professionals involved in the trial, and individual participants, were blind or not. Following the recommendation in the CONSORT extension for pragmatic trials, it may also be useful to explain why certain individuals could not be blind. A discussion of any potential bias should be included in the discussion section of the report.

It has generally been accepted that the blinding of those who assess outcomes is important in order to avoid bias. In many cases it is straightforward to blind outcome assessors; but when, for example, the assessment has to be carried out by researchers going into a cluster setting where the intervention status will become obvious – because of posters on the walls, templates on computers, or things said by the professionals in the clusters – this may prove to be difficult. In the IRIS trial (Table 10.12) this problem was circumvented by validating outcome data collection using researchers who knew nothing about the trial and who were escorted into and out of the cluster (general practices) by a trial researcher who acted as a shield between them and any information that might unblind them. Where unblinding occurs accidentally, for example by an individual cluster member revealing their allocation, this may unblind the whole cluster, not just one individual. Accordingly, a much greater proportion of the data may be affected than in the case of a single unblinding incident occurring in an individually randomised trial.

10.4.12   Item 12: Statistical methods

The requirement for a trial report fully to describe the statistical methods used applies to all trial types. The extended CONSORT statement additionally specifies that for cluster randomised trials investigators should report how clustering was taken into account in the analysis. Reviews have shown that cluster randomised trials are more likely to account for clustering in the analysis than in the sample size. Almost 90% of trials in a recent review in primary care did so (Eldridge et al., 2008). It may be that reporting in the journals selected for the review, in which cluster randomised trial reports are relatively common, is better than in other journals, but nevertheless there is some reason to be optimistic about the extent to which investigators are using appropriate methods of analysis, particularly in health services research. There are usually several ways in which the data can be analysed, and authors should provide sufficient information to be able to replicate the analysis if the data were available, including the model adopted for analysis, software used and method of fitting. In our experience in searching for examples for this book, this is rarely done.

Because many cluster randomised trials are stratified or minimised, it is appropriate to include stratification or minimisation factors in the analysis. Other factors are also often included. Reviews by Donner, Brown and Brasher (1990) Isaakidis and Ioannidis (2003) and Eldridge et al. (2004) found that 83%, 31% and 52%

respectively of trials included covariates in their analysis. If covariates are included in an analysis, these should be clearly specified.

10.4.13   Item 13: Participant flow

CONSORT recommends that the flow of clusters and individuals through the trial is displayed in a flow chart. A clear flow chart is more difficult to produce for a cluster randomised trial because of the necessity of showing the flow of both individuals and clusters. Figure 10.2 shows the layout recommended in the extended CONSORT statement. In this layout, only the flow of clusters through the trial is

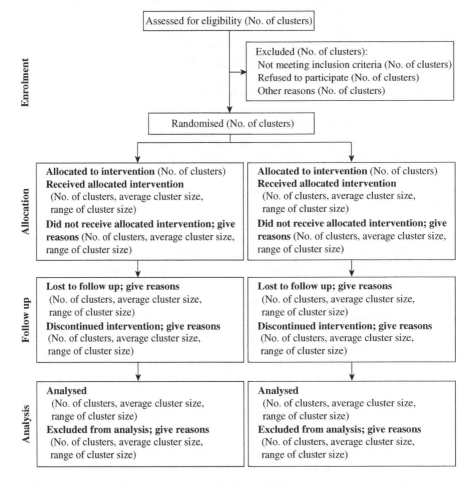

Figure 10.2   Format recommended by CONSORT for flow diagram of the progress of clusters and individuals through the phases of a randomised trial. Reproduced by permission of CONSORT.

shown. Since clusters are the units of randomisation, from a statistical point of view this is the correct layout to use. In a cluster randomised trial, however, it is important that investigators also adequately report the flow of individuals through their trial. This can be achieved by adding information about individuals to the flow chart, albeit in a way which does not makes the flow chart incomprehensible. Alternatively, a second flow chart could be presented, but this takes up valuable space in a publication and readers are likely to want to compare the information for clusters and individuals, so having this information on the same figure is probably preferable. Because of the various different design features of cluster randomised trials (see Chapter 5), here we present several flow charts for recently published trials which illustrate ways of constructing these charts for different situations.

In Figure 10.3 we present a flow chart used in a recent cluster randomised trial (Table 10.13) which we feel adequately captures most of the relevant information required. It is common to begin with randomised clusters but not to describe how these were selected, or any who refused or were ineligible. In this example some attempt has been made to include this information; there are 236 primary care clinics in the state, of which 200 were eligible. The reasons why 36 were excluded are given at the bottom of the figure, but the CONSORT extension recommends an 'excluded' box in the main flow chart. It is not clear how the 40 randomised clinics were chosen from the 200 eligible, although the text of the paper states that these were the 40 largest. Explaining how many clusters were approached and how many were eligible is particularly important for pragmatic trials. The bottom box shows the number of clusters analysed. This information is often absent in flow charts presented in reports of cluster randomised trials, which tend to focus on the flow of individuals through the trial.

Figure 10.4 shows the flow chart for a cluster randomised trial where data on the effectiveness of the intervention were obtained from repeated cross-sectional surveys. Students completed questionnaires about their knowledge and awareness of depression, but different students were included at the two time points, before and after the intervention. This departs from the structure recommended in Figure 10.2 in order to make clear that the samples are different students, making a total of over 5000 students in each arm, approximately 2500 in each arm at each time point. This example illustrates the difficulties of using the same flowchart structure for all cluster randomised trials.

Where possible the number of clusters and participants who received the intervention should be reported, in order to aid interpretation of the results (see Section 10.4.22).

An example of reporting how many clusters received an intervention is provided by Modell et al. (1998):

> The first sessions were completed at the end of 1995, and the intervention year started in January 1996. The second and third sessions were offered at the middle and end of 1996. Ten practices accepted all three sessions, two accepted two, and one accepted one. The haemoglobinopathy counsellors attended seven of the final sessions. Ten of the 13 control practices accepted the offer of a 30–40 minute training session after the intervention year. (Modell et al., 1998)

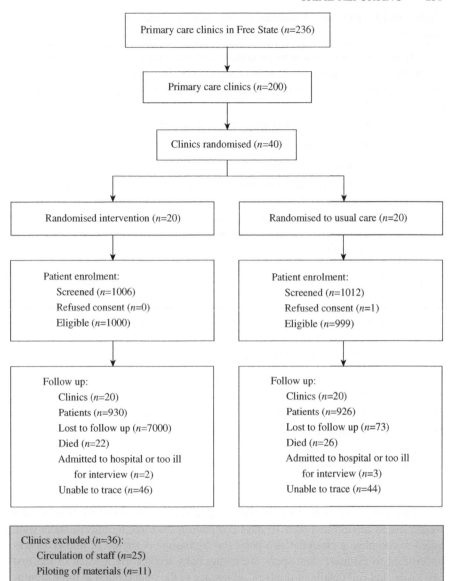

Figure 10.3   Example of flow chart from the PALSA trial of education outreach for tuberculosis (Table 10.13). Reproduced from Effect of educational outreach to nurses on tuberculosis case detection and primary care of respiratory illness: pragmatic cluster randomised controlled trial. L.R. Fairall, M. Zwarenstein, E.D. Bteman et al., 331, 7519, © 2005 with permission from BMJ Publishing Group Ltd.

Table 10.13 PALSA: Educational outreach to increase tuberculosis case detection.

Aim: To develop and implement an educational outreach programme for the integrated case management of priority respiratory diseases, and to evaluate its effects on respiratory care and detection of tuberculosis among adults attending primary care clinics

Location and type of cluster: Primary care clinics in South Africa

Number of clusters analysed: 40

Number of individuals analysed: 1856

Interventions: (i) Control (ii) Intervention: between two and six educational outreach sessions delivered by trainers from the health department

Primary outcome: Detection of tuberculosis

Source: Fairall *et al.* (2005).

Table 10.14 Educational intervention to increase depression awareness among students.

Aim: To assess the effectiveness of an intervention to educate students about depression

Location and type of cluster: UK colleges of one university

Interventions: (i) Control (ii) Intervention: postcards and posters on depression and its treatment

Outcomes: Student awareness that depression can be treated effectively

Data collection: Repeated cross-sectional surveys

Number of clusters randomised: 28

Source: Merritt *et al.* (2007).

In the baby walker trial (Table 10.11), midwives were asked to discuss baby walker use at recruitment then 10 days postpartum. At three months mothers were asked to complete a checklist as a basis for discussion. A survey of midwives was undertaken to estimate time spent discussing baby walker use at each of the first two visits, and full details of mothers' adherence to the intervention at three months was given in the flow chart (Figure 10.5). The number of clusters invited to participate and the number recruiting patients are shown, but it would have been better if the number of clusters followed-up was also given.

10.4.14   Item 14: Recruitment

The recommendation to define the dates of recruitment and follow-up applies equally to individually and cluster randomised trials.

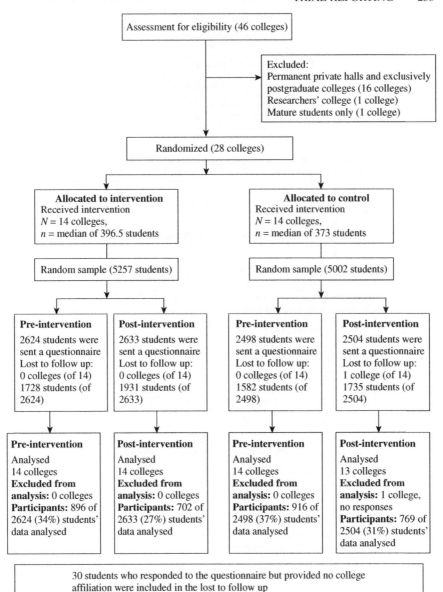

Assessment for eligibility (46 colleges)

Excluded:
Permanent private halls and exclusively
postgraduate colleges (16 colleges)
Researchers' college (1 college)
Mature students only (1 college)

Randomized (28 colleges)

Allocated to intervention
Received intervention
N = 14 colleges,
n = median of 396.5 students

Allocated to control
Received intervention
N = 14 colleges,
n = median of 373 students

Random sample (5257 students)

Random sample (5002 students)

Pre-intervention

2624 students were
sent a questionnaire
Lost to follow up:
0 colleges (of 14)
1728 students (of
2624)

Post-intervention

2633 students were
sent a questionnaire
Lost to follow up:
0 colleges (of 14)
1931 students (of
2633)

Pre-intervention

2498 students were
sent a questionnaire
Lost to follow up:
0 colleges (of 14)
1582 students (of
2498)

Post-intervention

2504 students were
sent a questionnaire
Lost to follow up:
1 college (of 14)
1735 students (of
2504)

Pre-intervention

Analysed
14 colleges
**Excluded from
analysis:** 0 colleges
Participants: 896 of
2624 (34%) students'
data analysed

Post-intervention

Analysed
14 colleges
**Excluded from
analysis:** 0 colleges
Participants: 702 of
2633 (27%) students'
data analysed

Pre-intervention

Analysed
14 colleges
**Excluded from
analysis:** 0 colleges
Participants: 916 of
2498 (37%) students'
data analysed

Post-intervention

Analysed
13 colleges
**Excluded from
analysis:** 1 college,
no responses
Participants: 769 of
2504 (31%) students'
data analysed

30 students who responded to the questionnaire but provided no college
affiliation were included in the lost to follow up

Figure 10.4   Example of flow chart from the depression awareness trial (Table 10.14). R.K. Merritt, J.R. Price, J. Mollison, J.R. Gedison, Psychological Medicine, *37, 363–372, reproduced with permission from Cambridge University Press © 1969.*

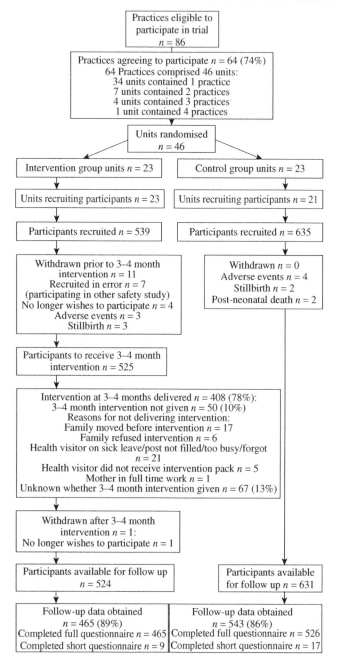

Figure 10.5   Example of flow chart from the baby walker trial (Table 10.11). Kendrick D., Illingworth R., Woods, A., et al., Promoting child safety in primary care: a cluster randomised controlled trial to reduce baby walker use. British Journal of General Practice *2005; (55) 517: 582–588.*

10.4.15   Item 15: Baseline data

Information pertaining to baseline data for individuals in each intervention arm is usually included in reports of individually randomised trials as a prelude to the main analyses, as an indication that correct procedures have been followed and to enable readers to assess the extent of imbalance between the arms. The extended CONSORT statement suggests that this information should be presented for both clusters and individuals. The reason for this is that imbalance can occur at both levels and potentially affect results. In fact, imbalance at both levels may be more likely to occur in cluster randomised trials; at cluster level because there is a small number of clusters, and at individual level because randomisation at cluster level does not guarantee that individual-level characteristics will be balanced. For example, in the POST trial (Table 10.15), although allocation to intervention arms was minimised on factors that might influence the effect of the intervention, there was considerable imbalance in the proportions of individuals on β blockers at baseline (33% in the intervention arm and 23% in the control arm).

Presentation of cluster and individual baseline characteristics by trial arm status can usually be effected via a single table in which the top half shows baseline cluster characteristics in each intervention arm and the bottom half shows baseline individual characteristics, or visa versa. In Figure 10.6 we present an example of good

Table 10.15   POST: Practitioner and patient postal prompts post-myocardial infarction.

Aim: To determine whether postal prompts to patients who have survived an acute coronary event, and to their general practitioners, improve secondary prevention of coronary heart disease

Location and type of cluster: UK general practices

Number of clusters analysed: 52

Number of individuals analysed: 328

Minimisation factors: (i) Patients per principal <1600/1600–2200/>2200 (ii) Practice nurse yes/no (iii) Number of partners 1/2/>3 (iv) Training status yes/no (v) Facilitated education session on guidelines for coronary heart disease yes/no

Interventions: (i) Control: usual care (ii) Intervention: leaflets to patients and letters to general practitioners with summary of appropriate treatment based on locally agreed guidelines

Outcomes: Proportion of patients in whom serum cholesterol concentrations were measured; proportion of patients prescribed β blockers (six months after discharge); and proportion of patients prescribed cholesterol lowering drugs (one year after discharge)

Source: Feder *et al.* (1999).

Characteristic	Outreach group	Control group
Clinics		
No. of clinics	20	20
Median total no. of adult attendances a quarter	12 749	12 935
Median no. of nurses per clinic	9	8.5
Tuberculosis treatment service available	19 (95)	20 (100)
24-hour emergency service available	4 (20)	2 (10)
Median distance (km) from local referral hospital	7.0	5.5
Patients		
No. of patients	1000	999
Women	643 (64.3)	660 (66.1)
Mean age (years)	44.9	44.2
Education:		
Never attended school	169 (17.0)	154 (15.4)
Attended primary school only	464 (46.6)	433 (43.4)
Attended secondary school	363 (36.4)	410 (41.1)
Employment:		
Employed	155 (15.6)	209 (21.0)
Unemployed without welfare	569 (57.2)	557 (56.0)
Receiving welfare	271 (27.2)	230 (23.1)
Smoking history:		
Current	164 (16.5)	193 (19.4)
Past	313 (31.4)	300 (30.1)
Never	519 (52.1)	504 (50.6)
Mean pack year history (smokers only)	8.9	8.3

Figure 10.6   Baseline characteristics of clinics and patients in PALSA trial (Table 10.13). Reproduced from Effect of educational outreach to nurses on tuberculosis case detection and primary care of respiratory illness: pragmatic cluster randomised controlled trial. L.R. Fairall, M. Zwarenstein, E.D. Bteman et al., 331, 7519, © 2005 with permission from BMJ Publishing Group Ltd.

practice taken from the PALSA trial (Table 10.13). In the review by Eldridge *et al.* (2004), 57% of trials reported baseline comparisons of individual characteristics and 48% reported baseline characteristics of clusters.

10.4.16   Item 16: Numbers analysed

The number of participants followed up should be included in the flow chart, but the number analysed may vary between outcomes. In an individually randomised trial it is recommended that participants are analysed in the arms to which they were randomised whether or not they receive the intervention as intended – intention to treat analysis (Section 6.5). True intention to treat analysis includes all individuals in the arm to which they were randomised. The problem is that most trials have missing data. Data may be missing for a variety of reasons: refusal to complete follow-up questionnaires, moved away, death of participants or technical reasons such as equipment failure. Consequently, true intention to treat analysis cannot be carried out without imputation of missing data (Altman, 2009). The terms 'intention to treat' and 'modified intention to treat' are used inconsistently (Abraha and Montedori, 2010); consequently the latest CONSORT checklist (Moher *et al.*, 2010) recommends specifying which cases have been included in each analysis and describing clearly any methods for dealing with missing data. While many cluster randomised trials retain all the randomised clusters, missing data at the participant level is common. It may be sufficient to report the clusters remaining in the trial in the flow chart and the numbers of participants for each outcome alongside the analysis for that outcome. Table 10.16 is reproduced from Feder *et al.* (1999) and shows the numbers included in the analysis of each outcome. The accompanying text explains that data on cholesterol could only be collected on patients recruited in the first half of the study.

10.4.17   Item 17: Outcomes and estimation

In common with individually randomised trials, a summary of results for each arm for each outcome should be given for cluster randomised trials, along with the estimated effect size and a measure of its precision. Additionally for cluster randomised trials an estimate of the ICC or coefficient of variation of the outcome should be given. This enables readers to check the assumptions in the sample size calculations and helps with planning future studies. This is illustrated in Table 10.16. The odds ratio is adjusted for clustering using the method described in Section 6.3.1 for those outcomes for which the observed ICC was negative; it was set to zero to calculate adjusted odds ratios, confidence intervals (CIs), and chi-squared statistics.

Moher *et al.* (2010) recognise that selective reporting is a common problem in randomised trials, and recommend that all planned primary and secondary end points are presented. Table 10.16 is the first few lines of a much larger table from the paper (Feder *et al.*, 1999), which lists all primary and secondary outcomes.

Table 10.16   POST: prescribing outcome variables by intervention. Values are percentages (numbers) unless stated otherwise.

Variable	Intervention group ($n = 172$)	Control group ($n = 156$)	Estimated ICC	Adjusted odds ratio (95% CI)	Adjusted χ^2 statistic	P-value
Cholesterol lowering drugs	28 (23/81)	19 (16/83)	−0.047	1.7 (0.8 to 3.4)	1.9	>0.05
β blocker[a]	38 (60/157)	27 (38/142)	0.060	1.7 (0.9 to 3.0)	0.9	>0.05
Aspirin[a]	90 (141/157)	91 (127/139)	−0.018	0.9 (0.4 to 1.9)	0.0	>0.05

Source: Feder *et al.* (1999).
[a]Patients with contraindications were removed from these analyses.

For binary outcomes CONSORT recommends that effects are presented as both a risk difference and an estimate of relative effect; either an odds ratio or relative risk. If a logistic regression model (see Section 6.3.3 for details of appropriate methods) is used for the main analysis, then the odds ratio and confidence interval that results from this analysis should both be presented. The risk difference can then be presented without a confidence interval to aid interpretation of the results, or a confidence interval for the risk difference that does not allow for clustering can be adjusted to allow for clustering by multiplying the standard errors by the square root of the observed design effect.

10.4.18   Item 18: Ancillary analyses

Multiple analyses of the same data set will give rise to a greater chance of false positive findings (Moher *et al.*, 2010). Whether or not ancillary analyses were pre-planned or exploratory should be stated clearly. Box 10.6 gives a number of different types of analysis that might be undertaken: many of them applicable to all randomised trials. The following statement describes a number of ancillary analyses and makes it clear the subgroup analyses were pre-planned.

> We also undertook a sensitivity analysis and a per protocol analysis to estimate the effect of exposure to the intervention or group attendance on outcomes. Pre-planned analyses were also conducted to examine those participants whose risk factors were above target ranges at baseline—that is, HbA1c >7%, systolic blood pressure >130 mm Hg, and cholesterol concentration >4.8 mmol/L. (Smith *et al.*, 2004)

Relevant to all randomised trials

- Per protocol analyses; restricting the analysis to those who received the intervention as planned

- Different ways of dealing with missing data; complete case analysis where only cases with complete data are included, or available case where all cases are included where possible; imputation methods for missing data

- Process variables

- Subgroup analyses

- Adjusted analyses including additional covariates other than stratification factors.

Relevant to cluster randomised trials only

- When the ICC is negative analyses that do not allow for clustering should be the main analysis, although in an analysis plan it might be considered as ancillary, because if the ICC is non-negative it will not be necessary (Section 6.6)

- Analyses using different weighting of the participants (Section 6.3.1)

- Cluster-level analyses or adapted individual-level analyses if there is some doubt about the validity of individual-level analyses because of the trial design and characteristics (Section 6.6).

Box 10.6   Different ancillary analyses that may be performed

A problem which is more acute for cluster randomised trials than individually randomised trials is the variety of valid methods of analysis available (Chapter 6) which may give rise to different interpretations of the results (Campbell *et al.*, 2000). It is generally seen as good practice to develop an analysis plan (Section 6.6) before looking at the data, so that the analysis is hypothesis driven rather than data driven. Steps which have been taken to protect against data-driven analysis should be specified in the methods.

10.4.19   Item 19: Adverse events

Because of the nature of interventions evaluated in cluster randomised trials, adverse events are extremely rare. Although we expect there are some other examples, the only cluster randomised trials in which we are aware of any adverse events being reported are those conducted in residential and nursing homes for older people, such as OPERA (Underwood *et al.* 2011).

10.4.20   Item 20: Limitations

Researchers should objectively consider the limitations of their trial, in particular any possible sources of bias that would affect its internal validity. For cluster randomised trials this will include any potential identification and recruitment bias (Section 2.3) and how any features of the trial design, such as the need for informed consent, may have biased the intervention effect. The implications of multiple hypothesis testing and difficulties in achieving sufficient power should be discussed, as well as the implication of lack of blinding. Cluster randomised trials often randomise a smaller number of units than individually randomised trials, and there is greater potential for imbalance between the randomised arms.

The following examples illustrate different limitations which commonly occur in cluster randomised trials:

- **Outcomes and power of the trial**

  Our study was limited by having power to measure changes in the proportion of cases identified, rather than changes in identification rate. Measurement of this change would have needed a much larger sample size than was feasible in this study. (Table 10.9; Griffiths *et al.*, 2007)

- **Effect of the intervention on routine care being delivered in the intervention arm**

  A further potential limitation is that the presence of a peer support intervention within a practice could have motivated the entire team to provide better diabetes care. The process evaluation and the data relating to prescribing, however, did not suggest differences in delivery of diabetes care between intervention and control practices. (Smith *et al.*, 2011)

- **Whether the control arm can be considered to represent usual care**

  In our opinion, the control group was not a real control group but was in fact another intervention group. The practice nurses were very experienced and eager to participate in the study and were highly motivated to improve the quality of care. It seems that the nurses in our study were early adopters of innovations in primary care and that the overall performance of the nurses was high, which made it difficult to attain a contrast between the groups with one training course. (Koelewijn-van Loon *et al.*, 2009).

This trial compared cardiovascular risk management in nurse-led clinics, where a multifaceted intervention including risk assessment, risk communication, a decision aid and adapted motivational interviewing was compared with a minimal nurse-led intervention.

The potential for recruitment and/or identification bias should also be discussed if appropriate. This was covered in Section 10.4.10.

10.4.21   Item 21: Generalisability

Generalisability refers to the extent to which study results can be applied to other individuals or settings. Although a single trial cannot be expected to produce results that are directly relevant to all individuals and all settings, results should be reported in such a way that healthcare professionals, managers and community leaders can judge for themselves to whom they might reasonably be applied (Rothwell, 2006). This is perhaps as important as internal validity in judging the quality of trials as a basis for healthcare policy, but has been poorly reported in cluster randomised trials, possibly because, while journals may explicitly ask authors to discuss the strengths and weaknesses of their study, discussion of generalisability is seldom explicitly requested (Eldridge *et al.*, 2008). It is included as a separate item in the CONSORT checklist to emphasise its importance.

The following examples describe different aspects of external validity:

• **Discussion of the cluster and setting characteristics**

  The intervention was carried out in small towns and rural primary care clinics in a poor province with a high rate of tuberculosis and HIV infection. It was delivered by existing staff, and was effective despite the low number of educational contacts, reportedly due to difficulties accommodating visits in clinic schedules [...] The Free State and other provinces are adapting educational outreach for HIV/AIDS and implementing it widely. We suggest that in other lower and middle income countries where non-physicians provide primary care, equipping middle managers as outreach trainers is feasible within existing constraints on staff and could improve quality of care. (Table 10.13; Fairall *et al.*, 2005)

• **Discussion of the generalisability of the intervention and participants**

  Our experience suggested that while physicians review the results of patients monitoring [sic] and take those into consideration, their management decision is likely based on many different objective and subjective pieces of information. In an attempt to duplicate this, we tried not to change usual practice in the intervention group except for the fact that the patients had, and were asked to use, home BP [blood pressure] monitors. Apart from the provision of standard guidelines, we gave no instruction regarding frequency of visits, which medication to use or how and when to adjust medication dosage. We asked only that they attempt to treat to target and that they review the patients monitoring record when they came in for a visit. We did not involve other health care professionals, and we did not ask the patients to adjust their own medications, and the physician was free to use whatever pieces of data they had (office BP; patient's stress level; knowledge of the patient and his/her social, psychological and medical conditions). We did not exclude people with various cardiovascular diseases or diabetes. Hence, this was a very heterogeneous population typical of primary care. (Godwin *et al.*, 2010)

10.4.22   Item 22: Interpretation

Authors should give a general interpretation of the results in the context of current evidence, avoiding selecting only studies that support the results. A recent systematic review may be useful in summarising previous research, but one including cluster randomised trials may not be available; the nature of cluster randomised trials means that trial replication and consequent synthesis is often less likely. For complex interventions, literature may be available regarding the effectiveness of some components. In the report of a trial of a cardiovascular health awareness programme (Kaczorowski *et al.*, 2011), authors cite a previous review of community programmes for the prevention of cardiovascular disease.

> The modest success of previous community-wide cardiovascular prevention initiatives has been attributed to many factors, including the potency, duration, and penetration of the interventions, secular trends in morbidity and mortality from cardiovascular disease, and methodological weaknesses [authors refer to Pennant *et al.* (2010)]. Most have failed to detect changes in cardiovascular risk factors or mortality that could unequivocally be attributed to the interventions. Although the importance of small shifts in the distribution of risk factors on the overall cardiovascular health of the population has been underscored repeatedly in the literature [references], robust evidence supporting community-wide interventions to such shifts remains sparse. (Kaczorowski *et al.*, 2011)

10.4.23   Other information

The final three items on the checklist, trial registration, protocol, and funding source have been discussed earlier in this chapter (Sections 10.2 and 10.3).

10.5   Summary

Several previous reviews of cluster randomised trials have suggested that these are poorly reported (e.g. Eldridge *et al.*, 2004), although more recent reviews indicate some improvement (e.g. Eldridge *et al.*, 2008). Nevertheless, further improvements are needed to maximise the potential benefits to patients, the healthcare system and the general population from the research being undertaken.

The CONSORT statement is the most widely followed guidance for reporting trials and now includes recommendations specific to cluster randomised trials, and other recommendations for pragmatic and non-pharmacological trials which are relevant to cluster randomised trials. In this chapter we have described the application of the CONSORT statement to cluster randomised trials; in particular the importance of reporting how potential biases have been avoided or reduced, clearly describing the intervention and various aspects of a trial in relation to *both* clusters *and* individuals, and transparently reporting how the sample size calculation and analysis account for clustering. Because cluster randomised trials are frequently complex, such high quality reporting may pose a challenge if journals impose word limits on trial reports. Nevertheless, with the advent of online publishing, norms in relation to publishing are becoming more fluid. We strongly recommend that authors of trials follow the CONSORT guidance in reporting all aspects of their trial. This will ensure that high quality evidence from cluster randomised trials has the best chance of making an impact on practice and policy. The Equator network website (Equator network 2011) contains the most up-to-date information on trial reporting, and in due course should contain an updated extension of the CONSORT statement to cluster randomised trials.

References

Abraha, I. and Montedori, A. (2010) Modified intention to treat reporting in randomised controlled trials: systematic review. *BMJ*, **340**, c2697. doi: 10.1136/bmj.c2697

Altman, D.G. (2009) Missing outcomes in randomised trials: addressing the dilemma. *Open Med.*, **3**, e51–e53.

Araya, R., Montgomery, A.A., Fritsch, R. *et al.* (2011) School-based intervention to improve the mental health of low-income, secondary school students in Santiago, Chile (YPSA): study protocol for a randomized controlled trial. *Trials*, **12**, 49.

Begg, C., Cho, M., Eastwood, S. *et al.* (1996) Improving the quality of reporting of randomized controlled trials. The CONSORT statement. *JAMA*, **276** (8), 637–639.

Boutron, I., Moher, D., Altman, D.G. *et al.* (2008) Extending the CONSORT statement to randomized trials of nonpharmacologic treatment: explanation and elaboration. *Ann. Intern. Med.*, **148**, 295–309.

Byng, R., Jones, R., Leese, M. *et al.* (2004) Exploratory cluster randomised controlled trial of shared care development for long-term mental illness. *Br. J. Gen. Pract.*, **54** (501), 259–266.

Campbell, M.K., Mollinson, J., Steen, N. *et al.* (2000) Analysis of cluster randomized trials in primary care: a practical approach. *Fam. Pract.*, **17**, 192–196.

Campbell, M.K., Elbourne, D.R. and Altman, D.G. (2004) CONSORT statement: extension to cluster randomised trials. *BMJ*, **328** (7441), 702–708.

Chuang, J.H., Hripcsak, G. and Jenders, R.A. (2000) Considering clustering: a methodological review of clinical decision support system studies. *Proc. AMIA Symp.*, **2000**, 146–150.

Davidson, K.W., Goldstein, M., Kaplan, R.M. *et al.* (2003) Evidence-based behavioral medicine: what is it and how do we achieve it? *Ann. Behav. Med.*, **26** (3), 161–171.

De Angelis, C., Drazen, J.M., Frizelle, F.A. *et al.* (2004) Clinical trial registration: a statement from the International Committee of Medical Journal Editors. *N. Engl. J. Med.*, **351**, 1250–1251.

Donner, A. and Klar, N. (2000) *Design and Analysis of Cluster Randomised Trials in Health Research*, Arnold, London.

Donner, A., Brown, K.S. and Brasher, P. (1990) A methodological review of non-therapeutic intervention trials employing cluster randomization, 1979–1989. *Int. J. Epidemiol.*, **19** (4), 795–800.

Elbourne, D.R. and Campbell, M.K. (2001) Extending the CONSORT statement to cluster randomized trials: for discussion. *Stat. Med.*, **20** (3), 489–496.

Eldridge, S.M., Ashby, D., Feder, G.S. *et al.* (2004) Lessons for cluster randomised trials in the twenty-first century: a systematic review of trials in primary care. *Clin. Trials*, **1**, 80–90.

Eldridge, S.M., Ashby, D. and Kerry, S. (2006) Sample size calculations for cluster randomized trials: effect of coefficient of variation of cluster size and analysis method. *Int. J. Epidemiol.*, **35** (5), 1292–1300.

Eldridge, S., Ashby, D., Bennett, C. *et al.* (2008) Internal and external validity of cluster randomised trials: systematic review of recent trials. *BMJ*, **336** (7649), 876–880.

Equator Network (2011) Reporting guidelines under development. http://www.equator-network.org/resource-centre/library-of-health-research-reporting/reporting-guidelines-under-development/reporting-guidelines-under-development/ (last accessed 2 June 2011).

Fairall, L.R., Zwarenstein, M., Bateman, E.D. *et al.* (2005) Effect of educational outreach to nurses on tuberculosis case detection and primary care of respiratory illness: pragmatic cluster randomised controlled trial. *BMJ*, **331** (7519), 750–754.

Farrin, A., Russell, I., Torgerson, D. *et al.* (2005) Differential recruitment in a cluster randomized trial in primary care: the experience of the UK back pain, exercise, active management and manipulation (UK BEAM) feasibility study. *Clin. Trials*, **2** (2), 119–124.

Feder, G., Griffiths, C., Eldridge, S. *et al.* (1999) Effect of postal prompts to patients and general practitioners on the quality of primary care after a coronary event (POST): randomised controlled trial. *BMJ*, **318**, 1522–1526.

Feder, G., Agnew Davies, R., Baird, K. *et al.* (2011) Identification and Referral to Improve Safety (IRIS) of women experiencing domestic violence: a cluster randomised controlled trial of a primary care training and support programme. *Lancet*, Oct 12 [epub ahead of print].

Godwin, M., Lam, M., Birtwhistle, R. *et al.* (2010) A primary care pragmatic cluster randomized trial of the use of home blood pressure monitoring on blood pressure levels in hypertensive patients with above target blood pressure. *Fam. Pract.*, **27** (2), 135–142.

Griffiths, C., Foster, G., Barnes, N. *et al.* (2004) Specialist nurse intervention to reduce unscheduled asthma care in a deprived multiethnic area: the east London randomised controlled trial for high risk asthma (ELECTRA). *BMJ*, **328** (7432), 144.

Griffiths, C., Sturdy, P., Brewin, P. *et al.* (2007) Educational outreach to promote screening for tuberculosis in primary care: a cluster randomised controlled trial. *Lancet*, **369** (9572), 1528–1534.

Hopewell, S., Clarke, M., Moher, D. *et al.* (2008) CONSORT for reporting randomized controlled trials in journal and conference abstracts: explanation and elaboration. *PLoS Med.*, **5** (1), e20. doi: 10.1371/journal. pmed.0050020

Ioannidis, J.P., Evans, S.J., Gotzsche, P.C. *et al.* (2004) Better reporting of harms in randomized trials: an extension of the CONSORT statement. *Ann. Intern. Med.*, **141**, 781–788.

Isaakidis, P. and Ioannidis, J.P. (2003) Evaluation of cluster randomized controlled trials in sub-Saharan Africa. *Am. J. Epidemiol.*, **158** (9), 921–926.

Jadad, A.R., Moore, R.A., Carroll, D. *et al.* (1996) Assessing the quality of reports of randomized clinical trials: is blinding necessary? *Control. Clin. Trials*, **17** (1), 1–12.

Kaczorowski, J., Chambers, L.W., Dolovich, L. *et al.* (2011) Improving cardiovascular health at population level: 39 community cluster randomised trial of Cardiovascular Health Awareness Program (CHAP). *BMJ*, **342**, d442.

Kendrick, D., Illingworth, R., Woods, A. *et al.* (2005) Promoting child safety in primary care: a cluster randomised controlled trial to reduce baby walker use. *Br. J. Gen. Pract.*, **55** (517), 582–588.

Khan, K.S., Daya, S., Collins, J.A. *et al.* (1996) Empirical evidence of bias in infertility research: overestimation of treatment effect in crossover trials using pregnancy as the outcome measure. *Fertil. Steril.*, **65** (5), 939–945.

Koelewijn-van Loon, M.S., van der Weijden, T., van Steenkiste, B. *et al.* (2009) Involving patients in cardiovascular risk management with nurse-led clinics: a cluster randomized controlled trial. *CMAJ*, **181**, E267–E274.

Liberati, A., Himel, H.N. and Chalmers, T.C. (1986) A quality assessment of randomized control trials of primary treatment of breast cancer. *J. Clin. Oncol.*, **4** (6), 942–951.

Lumley, J., Small, R., Brown, S. *et al.* (2003) PRISM (Program of Resources, Information and Support for Mothers) Protocol for a community-randomised trial (ISRCTN03464021). *BMC Public Health*, **3**, 36.

Merritt, R.K., Price, J.R., Mollison, J. *et al.* (2007) A cluster randomized controlled trial to assess the effectiveness of an intervention to educate students about depression. *Psychol. Med.*, **37** (3), 363–372.

Modell, M., Wonke, B., Anionwu, E. *et al.* (1998) A multidisciplinary approach for improving services in primary care: randomised controlled trial of screening for haemoglobin disorders. *BMJ*, **317**, 788–791.

Moher, D. and Schulz, K.F. (1998) Randomized controlled trials in cancer: improving the quality of their reports will also facilitate better conduct. *Ann. Oncol.*, **9** (5), 483–487.

Moher, D., Jadad, A.R. and Tugwell, P. (1996) Assessing the quality of randomized controlled trials. Current issues and future directions. *Int. J. Technol. Assess. Health Care*, **12** (2), 195–208.

Moher, D., Hopewell, S., Schulz, K.F. *et al.* (2010) CONSORT 2010 Explanation and Elaboration: updated guidelines for reporting parallel group randomised trials. *BMJ*, **340**, c869.

Nation, M., Crusto, C., Wandersman, A. *et al.* (2003) What works in prevention. Principles of effective prevention programs. *Am. Psychol.*, **58** (6–7), 449–456.

Pennant, M., Davenport, C., Bayliss, S. *et al.* (2010) Community programs for the prevention of cardiovascular disease: a systematic review. *Am. J. Epidemiol.*, **172**, 501–516.

Perera, R., Heneghan, C. and Yudkin, P. (2007) Graphical method for depicting randomised trials of complex interventions. *BMJ*, **334**, 127–129.

Powell, C., Baker-Henningham, H., Walker, S. *et al.* (2004) Feasibility of integrating early stimulation into primary care for undernourished Jamaican children: cluster randomised controlled trial. *BMJ*, **329** (7457), 89.

Puffer, S., Torgerson, D. and Watson, J. (2003) Evidence for risk of bias in cluster randomised trials: review of recent trials published in three general medical journals. *BMJ*, **327** (7418), 785–789.

Rothwell, P.M. (2006) Factors that can affect the external validity of randomised controlled trials. *PLoS Clin. Trials*, **1** (1), e9.

Scherer, R.W., Langenberg, P. and von Elm, E. (2007) Full publication of results initially presented in abstracts. *Cochrane Database Syst. Rev.* 2 (Art. No.: MR000005). doi: 10.1002/14651858.MR000005.pub3

Schulz, K.F., Chalmers, I., Hayes, R.J. *et al.* (1995) Empirical evidence of bias. Dimensions of methodological quality associated with estimates of treatment effects in controlled trials. *JAMA*, **273** (5), 408–412.

Simes, R.J. (1986) Publication bias: the case for an international registry of Clinical Trials. *J. Clin. Oncol.*, **4**, 1529–1541.

Simpson, J.M., Klar, N. and Donner, A. (1995) Accounting for cluster randomization: a review of primary prevention trials, 1990 through 1993. *Am. J. Public Health*, **85** (10), 1378–1383.

Smith, S., Bury, G., O'Leary, M. *et al.* (2004) The North Dublin randomized controlled trial of structured diabetes shared care. *Fam. Pract.*, **21** (1), 39–45.

Smith, S.M., Paul, G., Kelly, A. *et al.* (2011) Peer support for patients with type 2 diabetes: cluster randomized controlled trial. *BMJ*, **342**, d715. doi: 10.1136/bmj.d715

Soares, H.P., Daniels, S., Kumar, A. *et al.* (2004) Bad reporting does not mean bad methods for randomised trials: observational study of randomised controlled trials performed by the Radiation Therapy Oncology Group. *BMJ*, **328** (7430), 22–24.

Sturt, J.A., Whitlock, S., Fox, C. *et al.* (2008) Effects of the Diabetes Manual 1 : 1 structured education in primary care. *Diabet. Med.*, **25** (6), 722–731.

Sur, D., Lopez, A.L., Kanungo, S. *et al.* (2009) Efficacy and safety of a modified killed-whole-cell oral cholera vaccine in India: an interim analysis of a cluster-randomised, double-blind, placebo-controlled trial. *Lancet*, **374** (9702), 1694–1702. doi: 10.1016/S0140-6736(09)61297-6

Standards of Reporting Trials Group (1994) A proposal for structured reporting of randomized controlled trials. *JAMA*, **272**, 1926–1931.

Tonks, A. (1999) Registering clinical trials. *BMJ*, **319**, 1565–1568.

Ukoumunne, O.C., Gulliford, M.C., Chinn, S. *et al.* (1999) Methods for evaluating area-wide and organisation-based interventions in health and health care: a systematic review. *Health Technol. Assess. (Winchester, England)*, **3**, iii–i92.

Underwood, M., Eldridge, S., Lamb, S. *et al.* (2011) The OPERA trial: protocol for a randomised trial of an exercise intervention for older people in residential and nursing accommodation. *Trials*, **12**, 27.

Varnell, S.P., Murray, D.M., Janega, J.B. *et al.* (2004) Design and analysis of group-randomized trials: a review of recent practices. *Am. J. Public Health*, **94** (3), 393–399.

Wake, M., Tobin, S., Girolametto, L. *et al.* (2011). Outcomes of population based language promotion for slow to talk toddlers at ages 2 and 3 years: let's Learn Language cluster randomised controlled trial. *BMJ*, **343**, d4741. doi: 10.1136/bmj.d4741

Whittington, C.J., Kendall, T., Fonagy, P. *et al.* (2004) Selective serotonin reuptake inhibitors in childhood depression: systematic review of published versus unpublished data. *Lancet*, **363**, 1341.

Working Group on Recommendations for Reporting of Clinical Trials in the Biomedical Literature (1994) Call for comments on a proposal to improve reporting of clinical trials in the biomedical literature. *Ann. Intern. Med.*, **121**, 894–895.

Index

A Practical Guide to Cluster Randomised Trials in Health Services Research, First Edition.
Sandra Eldridge and Sally Kerry.
© 2012 John Wiley & Sons, Ltd. Published 2012 by John Wiley & Sons, Ltd.

Printed and bound by CPI Group (UK) Ltd, Croydon, CR0 4YY

27/10/2024

14580140-0003